Grandma Putt's

Old-Time
VINEGAR,
GARLIC,
BAKING SODA,
and 101 More
PROBLEM
SOLVERS

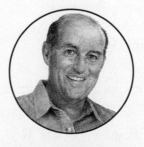

www.jerrybaker.com

Other Jerry Baker Books:

Jerry Baker's Solve It with Vinegar!
Jerry Baker's Speed Cleaning Secrets!
America's Best Practical Problem Solvers
Jerry Baker's Can The Clutter!
Jerry Baker's Homespun Magic
Jerry Baker's Supermarket Super Products!
Jerry Baker's It Pays to Be Cheap!

Healing Fixers Mixers & Elixirs
Grandma Putt's Home Health Remedies
Nature's Best Miracle Medicines
Jerry Baker's Supermarket Super Remedies
Jerry Baker's The New Healing Foods
Jerry Baker's Amazing Antidotes
Jerry Baker's Anti-Pain Plan
Jerry Baker's Oddball Ointments, Powerful Potions, and Fabulous Folk Remedies
Jerry Baker's Giant Book of Kitchen Counter Cures

Jerry Baker's The New Impatient Gardener
Jerry Baker's Supermarket Super Gardens
Jerry Baker's Dear God...Please Help It Grow!
Secrets from the Jerry Baker Test Gardens
Jerry Baker's All-American Lawns
Jerry Baker's Bug Off!
Jerry Baker's Terrific Garden Tonics!
Jerry Baker's Backyard Problem Solver
Jerry Baker's Green Grass Magic
Jerry Baker's Great Green Book of Garden Secrets
Jerry Baker's Old-Time Gardening Wisdom

Jerry Baker's Backyard Birdscaping Bonanza
Jerry Baker's Backyard Bird Feeding Bonanza
Jerry Baker's Year-Round Bloomers
Jerry Baker's Flower Garden Problem Solver
Jerry Baker's Perfect Perennials!

To order any of the above, or for more information on Jerry Baker's amazing home, health, and garden tips, tricks, and tonics, please write to:

Jerry Baker, P.O. Box 1001
Wixom, MI 48393

Or, visit Jerry Baker online at:
www.jerrybaker.com

Grandma Putt's
Old-Time
VINEGAR, GARLIC, BAKING SODA, and 101 More PROBLEM SOLVERS

2,500 Super Solutions for Your Home, Health, and Garden

by Jerry Baker, America's Master Gardener®

Published by American Master Products, Inc.

Executive Editor: Kim Adam Gasior
Managing Editor: Cheryl Winters-Tetreau
Production Editor: Stacy Mulka
Writer: Vicki Webster
Copy Editor: Nanette Bendyna
Interior Design and Layout: Sandy Freeman
Cover Design: Kitty Pierce Mace
Indexer: Nan Badgett

Publisher's Cataloging-in-Publication (Provided by Quality Books, Inc.)

Baker, Jerry.
    Grandma Putt's old-time vinegar, garlic, baking soda, and 101 more problem solvers : 2,500 super solutions for your home, health, and garden / Jerry Baker.
        p. cm.
    Includes index.
    ISBN 978-0-922433-77-3

    1. Home economics. 2. Health.
3. Gardening.   I. Title.

TX158.B294 2006   640
QBI05-600163

Published by American Master Products, Inc. / Jerry Baker

Printed in the United States of America
30 28 26 27 29 hardcover

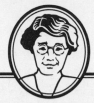

CONTENTS

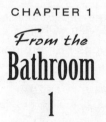
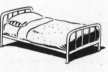
V

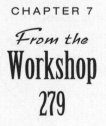
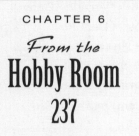

INTRODUCTION

I guess I'm just an old-fashioned kind of guy. I don't see the appeal of all the stuff lining store shelves these days. I mean, how many different kinds of cough medicine do we need, when a simple onion syrup works as well as any of 'em? The same goes for pricey stain removers; none of 'em does the job better than good old-fashioned denture cleaning tablets. And what about these fancy spa treatments? With a little buttermilk or some garden-fresh fruit, you can whip up the most fabulous facial in town—at a fraction of the cost!

One of the things I love to do most is discover amazing ways to put common household items to use—like using alcohol to clean the chrome on my appliances or turning a pillowcase into a laundry bag for my grandson in college. In fact, I've already written a couple of books about my discoveries—and boy, did people love 'em! Now, wherever I go, folks come up to me and say, "Hey, Jer, I know you're a garden guy from way back, but you've become a regular reuse artist! Where'd you ever learn this stuff?"

Well, I'll tell you where: from a remarkable lady named Ethel Grace Puttnam, a.k.a. my Grandma Putt. When I was growing up at her house, money was in pretty short supply—and, with World War II raging overseas, so was just about everything else. But did that stop Grandma from letting the good times roll? No, siree! Using good old Yankee ingenuity, she found ways to do whatever needed to be done by tapping the hidden powers of whatever products she had on hand. And you can, too!

In these pages, I'll take you on a room-by-room tour of Grandma's laboratory—which also happened to be her house and garden. Along the way, you'll learn scads of super-simple, money-saving secrets, such as:

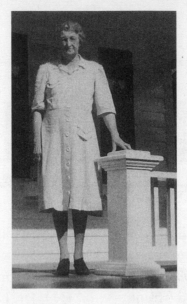

➤ Old-time remedies, routines, tonics, and toddies that'll cure whatever ails you and yours—with no unpleasant side effects.

➤ Grandma's grooming aids and beauty treatments that will keep every member of your family looking great—at a fraction of the cost of newfangled commercial versions.

➤ Tips, tricks, treats, and toys that are guaranteed to delight the day-lights out of your children, grand-children, pets—and you, too!

➤ Simple, nontoxic cleaners and easy-as-pie organizing aids that make it a breeze to keep your whole house as clean as a whistle and neat as a pin.

➤ Potent potions, fabulous formu-las, and just plain great ideas that'll help make your outdoor green scene as much of a showstopper as Grandma's was.

But that's not all! Because Grandma's spirit of adventure lives on, we'll take a look at dozens of products that arrived on the scene after she'd departed her earthly home—but that probably fill your house to burstin'! You'll dis-cover a gazillion great, Grandma-worthy uses for everything from the hair dryer in your bath-room to the coffee filters in your kitchen to the fabric-softener sheets in your laundry room.

Our tour ends, appropriately, in the attic—that three-dimensional scrapbook that holds so many of Grandma's (and our own) tucked-away treasures. But they don't have to stay there, just gathering dust. In Chapter 8, I'll tell you about a passel of well-used and well-loved things I've found in Grandma Putt's attic, and the ways my family and I use them today. With luck, those tips will inspire you to unearth objects from your own past, and put them where you can enjoy them every day—just as Grandma did!

So what are we waiting for? Step inside for our old-time house tour!

CHAPTER ONE

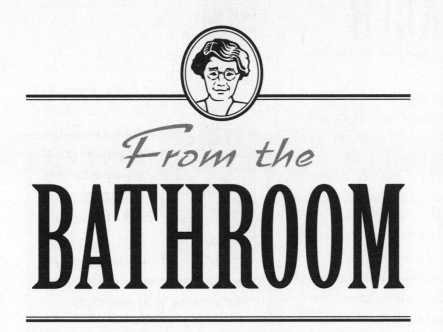

From the

BATHROOM

To your
HEALTH

As a youngster, I sure picked up my share of bumps, bruises, and strained muscles. But the pain never lasted long, because Grandma Putt knew exactly what to do: She'd rush to the freezer and pull out a reusable ice pack that she always kept on hand. Here's how she made it—and you can, too: Mix 1 part isopropyl (rubbing) **ALCOHOL** with 2 parts water, then pour the solution into a hot water bottle (but don't fill it; leave room for expansion). Squeeze out all of the air, insert the plug, and put the bottle in the freezer. Because alcohol doesn't freeze, the contents will be slushy rather than rock hard—and

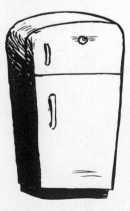

all the more comfortable on your achin' body. (If you'd like to modernize this procedure, you can use a heavy-duty, zip-top plastic freezer bag.)

TIP A run-in with poison ivy is never fun—to put it mildly! But Grandma taught me that if you act fast, you can lessen the effects of the rash, or even head it off entirely. All you need to do is swab the affected skin with rubbing **ALCOHOL,** which will cut

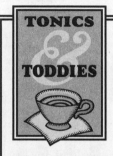

TONICS & TODDIES

HAPPY TIMES BUBBLE BATH

Feeling down in the dumps? Try one of Grandma Putt's no-fail pick-me-uppers—a good soak in an old-fashioned bubble bath. This was her favorite recipe, which makes enough for one bath.

½ cup of Dr. Bronner's Peppermint Soap®*
1 tbsp. of sugar
1 egg white

Mix all of the ingredients together. Turn on the tap to the temperature level of your choice, and pour the mixture under the running water. Then ease into the tub, sit back, and say, "Ahhhh...."

* Or substitute ½ cup of liquid hand soap and a few drops of your favorite scented oil.

through the plant's toxic oil and dilute it. Then, wash the area with soap and water.

TIP You say your new dress shoes are too tight? Here's an old-time solution that will prevent painful blisters: Saturate a cotton ball with rubbing **ALCOHOL,** and rub it on the inside of each shoe at the tight spots. Then go out and dance the night away. For permanent relief, take that footgear to a cobbler for professional stretching.

TIP Even some beneficial insects can deliver nasty bites or stings. Whenever that happened at our place, Grandma would dissolve two **ANTACID TABLETS** in a glass of water. Then she'd moisten a soft cloth with the solution, and hold it on the bite for 20 minutes.

TIP Get rid of corns and calluses by mashing five **ASPIRIN** tablets and adding equal parts of water and lemon juice (just enough to make a thick paste). Apply the mixture to the annoying c-spot. Wrap the area in a warm towel, put a plastic bag over your foot, and leave it on for 10 minutes. Take off the wrappings, and scrub with a pumice stone.

In Grandma's Day

Can you imagine a time when **ASPIRIN** didn't exist? Well, Grandma Putt could. This potent painkiller arrived on the scene when she was a girl—and it almost didn't make it then. A French chemist named Charles Gerhardt invented the substance in 1853, but after a few tests, he lost interest. Forty years later, Felix Hoffman, a young chemist working at the Bayer Drug Company in Germany, stumbled upon M. Gerhardt's formula, and a thought struck him: This stuff just might ease his father's arthritis pain. He mixed up a batch and gave it to his dad. *Voilà*—it worked—something no drug on the market had done! By 1899, Bayer was manufacturing aspirin in powdered form. The tablets that we know today first appeared in 1915.

TIP Baby, it's cold outside! But what if you've got a chore to do out there, and you can't do it with gloves on? Protect your bare skin by massaging your hands with **BABY OIL** before you head out the door. It'll close up the pores and help prevent skin damage from the frigid air.

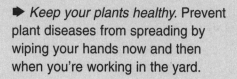

Baby Wipes

Baby wipes first hit the supermarket shelves in 1980 and quickly found their way into homes from coast to coast—even where there were no babies! These premoistened disposable towels have a zillion-and-one uses. Here are some of my favorites.

Around the House

➤ *Clean up spills.* Blot up coffee, soda pop, or other spilled liquids from carpets or upholstered furniture.

➤ *"De-art" your walls.* When young Georgia O'Keefe uses them as a vertical sketch pad, rub the marks off with a baby wipe.

➤ *Spruce up the bathroom—fast.* Just wipe down all the surfaces, and buff with a dry washcloth.

Out and About

➤ *Degrease your hands.* Wipe them after pumping gas, or after changing the oil in your car or lawn mower.

➤ *Degrease your vehicle.* Just wipe the gunk off with a baby wipe. It works like magic on cars, bikes, boats, and trailers—without damaging the paint job.

➤ *Keep your plants healthy.* Prevent plant diseases from spreading by wiping your hands now and then when you're working in the yard.

➤ *Say no to rust.* Periodically rub down metal tool parts to keep them clean and free of rust.

For You and Yours

➤ *Baby painful hemorrhoids.* Just use wipes instead of toilet paper. (But toss them in the trash afterwards—they're not flushable!)

➤ *Clean minor wounds.* Use a wipe instead of soap and water on scrapes and scratches.

➤ *Clean Fido's feet.* After a winter walk, wipe your dog's paws thoroughly to remove road salt and other ice-melting chemicals.

➤ *Deodorize your hands.* Rub them with a wipe after chopping garlic or onions.

➤ *Remove makeup.* (Keep the wipe away from your eyes, though!)

➤ *Shine shoes.* Swipe them with a wipe, and buff them with a soft, dry cloth.

➤ *Soothe burns.* Ease the pain of sunburn and other minor burns with a gentle rubdown.

And Don't Forget the Baby Wipes Boxes!

These babies can perform almost as many jobs as the wipes themselves. Just take a gander at these possibilities:

➡ *Building blocks.* Just collect 'em and let the kids build towers, bridges, and even whole towns.

➡ *Cleanser containers.* When you've whipped up a homemade cleaning formula (like the dozens of dandy ones you'll find in Chapters 4 and 5), store any leftover potion in a clean baby wipes box.

➡ *Clutter busters.* Use them as mini storage chests for all kinds of tiny odds and ends, such as hobby, craft, and sewing supplies, spare electrical parts, and small office gear.

➡ *Mini safes.* Leave the label on, insert your jewelry or other small valuables, and stash the box in the bathroom. Chances are, no burglar would think of "cracking" it. (It goes without saying—I hope—that this trick is not meant to replace your safe deposit box at the bank!)

➡ *"Piggy" banks.* Cut a slot in the lid, and drop in your pocket change at the end of every day. You'll be surprised at how fast it adds up!

➡ *Pitching-practice targets.* Stack 'em up outdoors, then wind up and let 'er rip. Three strikes and you win!

➡ *Seed-starting trays.* Sow your seeds in individual containers with drainage holes, and set two of the pots into each box.

➡ *Slug and snail traps.* Sink the containers in the soil, leaving about $1/8$ inch sticking up above the surface. Then pour in your bait of choice (you'll find some dandy ones throughout this book). The slimers will belly up to the bar, fall in, and die happy.

➡ *Treasure chests.* Give a box to a child who's collecting tiny treasures (as all kids seem to do at one time or another). Of course, you'll want to prime the pump, so to speak, by tucking in some stamps, marbles, mini toy animals, or whatever the future Smithsonian curator is gathering.

TIP When you've got a hangnail that's driving you nuts, soothe away the pain with this favorite Putt family remedy: Add 4 capfuls of **BATH OIL** (any kind will do) to 2 cups of warm water and soak your ailing fingertip in the solution for about 15 minutes.

TIP Like lots of other folks, Grandma Putt wore eyeglasses (spectacles, as she called them). But *unlike* most folks, she never had the lenses cloud over on her. How come? Because every morning, she'd wipe them with a few drops of **COLOGNE** on a soft, cotton cloth. (*Warning:* Never use paper tissues or paper towels on plastic lenses; they'll cause tiny scratches.)

TIP Having trouble getting a splinter out of your finger? Pour about 2 tablespoons of **EPSOM SALTS** into a cup of warm water, and soak the sore digit in the solution. The salts will draw the invading fragment right out. (It should take only a few minutes, depending on the depth of the splinter.)

TIP Sweaty feet and blisters tend to go hand in hand (or should I say, foot in foot?). My Uncle Art had that problem, big time, but Grandma taught him how to get rid of both those annoyances. You can do it, too. Before you go to bed at night, dissolve about 1 cup of **EPSOM SALTS** in a basin of warm water, and give your tootsies a five-minute soak. Then dry 'em thoroughly and say good night.

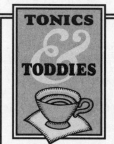

COOL-AID FOR BURNS

When you linger too long in the sun and your skin turns a painful shade of pink, reach for this cooling—and healing—remedy.

2 capsules of vitamin E
½ cup of aloe vera gel*
1 tsp. of cider vinegar
½ tsp. of lavender oil

Using sharp scissors, open the tip of each vitamin E capsule and squeeze out the oil into a bowl. Then mix in the other ingredients. Gently smooth the mixture directly onto your ailin' skin. Until the pain goes away, keep slathering on as much as you need to feel cool and comfortable.

* Grandma Putt took her aloe straight from the plants on her windowsill, but you can easily buy a tube at the drugstore and keep it stashed in your medicine chest.

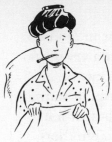

TIP When you're battling a sore throat, reach for good old **HYDROGEN PEROXIDE.** Gargle with it (don't swallow!) three times a day until you feel relief—which might be a lot sooner than you'd expect!

TIP Getting a splinter in your finger (or anyplace else) can be painful, all right—but when you can't even find the danged thing, it's also frustrating as all get-out. The next time that happens to you, apply a drop of **IODINE** to the general area. You'll locate the offending sliver in no time!

TIP The same **MENTHOLATED RUB** that's been easing chest colds since Grandma's day is also a terrific tick repellent. Just smooth the stuff onto your skin, and the tiny, disease-spreading terrors will give you the cold shoulder.

TIP Pour antiseptic **MOUTHWASH** over cuts and scrapes. It kills germs on your skin just as it does in your mouth.

TIP When mosquito bites have you itching like crazy, reach for a bottle of antiseptic **MOUTHWASH.** Moisten a tissue with it, hold it on the bite for about 15 seconds, and kiss that itch good-bye.

TIP Grandma Putt didn't have to worry about too much salt in her diet, but nowadays, lots of folks do. If you're one of them, here's a simple way to cut back: Paint over some of the holes in an empty salt-shaker with clear **NAIL POLISH.** Be sure to let the polish dry thoroughly before you fill the shaker.

TIP If you wear sterling silver earrings in pierced ears, paint the posts with clear **NAIL POLISH** to prevent tarnish from forming—and causing nasty ear infections.

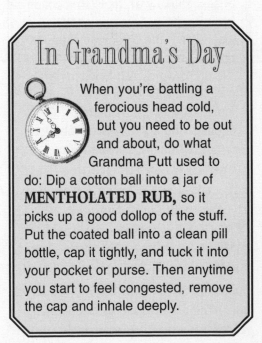

In Grandma's Day

When you're battling a ferocious head cold, but you need to be out and about, do what Grandma Putt used to do: Dip a cotton ball into a jar of **MENTHOLATED RUB,** so it picks up a good dollop of the stuff. Put the coated ball into a clean pill bottle, cap it tightly, and tuck it into your pocket or purse. Then anytime you start to feel congested, remove the cap and inhale deeply.

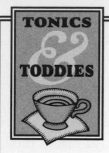

TONICS & TODDIES

No, No Nosebleed Tonic

Whenever I got a nosebleed as a youngster, Grandma Putt would sit me down and administer this tried-and-true remedy.

2 tbsp. of witch hazel
6 drops of cypress essential oil
    (available at health-food stores)
Cotton balls

Pour the witch hazel into a clean bottle with a tight-fitting lid. Add the cypress oil. Label the bottle with the contents, and store it in the medicine chest. Then, when the need arises, shake well, moisten a cotton ball with the potion, and gently insert it into the bleeding nostril. Sit up straight, with your head tilted just slightly forward. Within two or three minutes, the blood should stop flowing. To speed up the process, squeeze the soft tissue of your nose firmly, but gently, between your thumb and forefinger.

TIP What's more annoying than postnasal drip? Not a whole lot that I can think of! So here's a simple formula that'll end that hassle fast. Melt ¼ cup of **PETROLEUM JELLY** in a small saucepan. Remove it from the heat and stir in 10 drops each of peppermint, eucalyptus, and thyme essential oils. When the mixture has reached room temperature, spoon it into a clean glass jar for storage. Apply a small dab to the inside of each nostril one to three times a day. The secret to this trick: The petroleum jelly keeps the oils from being absorbed into your skin—thereby allowing you to inhale their drip-stopping essence over a prolonged period of time.

TIP Ouch! The doorbell rang, and when you jumped up from the couch to answer it, you banged right into the coffee table! Well, don't chew yourself out for your clumsiness (as Grandma Putt always said, what's done is done). Instead, just measure out 5 parts **PETROLEUM JELLY** to 1 part ground hot pepper, then melt the jelly in a saucepan, and stir in the pepper. Let the gel cool, spoon it into a clean glass jar, and apply it to the bruised area once a day. (Just be sure to wear rubber or plastic gloves when applying the gel, because this stuff is *hot*.)

TIP A case of pinkeye is no fun— to put it mildly. And neither is the yucky discharge that gums up your eyelashes. To nix that noxious goo, mix 1 part baby **SHAMPOO** to 10 parts warm water, dip a cotton ball into the solution, and clean the crud away.

TIP Cut yourself shaving? Stop the bleeding with the closest thing at hand—**SHAVING CREAM.** Grab the little drop that's always left on the nozzle, and dab it onto the nick. Let it dry, and rinse it off. (This stuff works its magic on any small cut, not just razor nicks.)

TIP If you suffer from asthma, relief is as close as your bathroom. Just turn on the shower and crank up the water temperature as high as it'll go. Let the room get good and steamy, then sit back and relax for 10 to 15 minutes. The **STEAM** will thin the sticky mucus that's clogging up your breathing passages.

TIP Before you head out to chop wood or dig in the garden, rub some **TALCUM POWDER** on your hands. It'll absorb excess perspiration and prevent blisters.

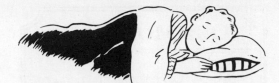

TIP A good night's sleep is important for good health, but on hot, humid summer nights, drifting off isn't so easy. What to do? Just sprinkle **TALCUM POWDER** between the sheets. It'll absorb moisture and help you feel cooler.

TIP If you have trouble falling asleep at night, here's an easy project that'll send you off to dreamland in a flash. Grab two **WASHCLOTHS** from the bathroom, and sew them together on three sides, front to front. Flip them inside out, and stuff the pouch with equal amounts of dried leaves of catnip, rabbit tobacco (a.k.a. pearly everlasting or, in scientific circles, *Gnaphalium obtusifolium*), mint, and sage. Sew the fourth side shut, and lay this little pillow beside your head at night. (Here's a tip for traveling insomniacs: Make an extra "sweet dreams" pillow, and tuck it into your suitcase, so you won't forget it on your next trip.)

ONE MORE TIME

Old cologne and perfume bottles make terrific containers for many of Grandma's homemade potions and lotions. But sometimes the original scent just won't go away. Before you give up, try this no-fail trick: Wash the bottle with soap and water, rinse well, and fill it with rubbing **ALCOHOL.** Let it sit for a couple of days, then empty out the alcohol, and rinse with clear water. Wait until the bottle dries out, then pour in your new, old-time creation.

TIP When you've been working or playing hard in the hot sun, give your aching muscles a nice, cooling treat. Here's how: Mix 2 cups of **WITCH HAZEL,** 2 teaspoons of light corn syrup, and ½ teaspoon of castor oil in a jar with a tight-fitting lid. Add a few drops of your favorite scented oil if you like. Shake well, and massage the potion into your sore body parts for almost-instant relief.

Your
GOOD LOOKS

TIP To Grandma Putt, "cleanliness is next to godliness" was more than just an old saying—she really lived by those words! Why, she even kept her combs so clean you could eat with them! How? Every now and then, she'd scrub them with a tooth-brush dipped in rubbing **ALCOHOL.**

TIP Are you prone to sweaty feet—and the aroma that often comes with them? Then this heirloom remedy's for you. Mix 1 teaspoon of alum (available at drug and health-food stores) and ¼ cup of rubbing **ALCOHOL** in 1 cup of water. Pour the mixture into a hand-held spray bottle, and spritz those wet dogs as needed.

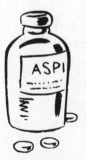

TIP If Grandma Putt could see the price tags on some of those fancy dandruff shampoos, she'd hit the roof! In fact, I still do, because for my money, this easy treatment beats 'em all, hands down. Just mash five **ASPIRIN** tablets and put them in a bottle with 1 cup of cider vinegar and ⅓ cup of witch hazel. Cap the bottle and shake it thoroughly to mix the ingredients. Shampoo as usual, then comb the solution through your hair. Wait 10 minutes, and rinse with warm water.

TIP Before you shave your legs with an electric razor, dust them with **BABY POWDER.** That way, you'll prevent painful (and unattractive) friction burns.

TIP Soothe sore, cracked cuticles and hangnails the way Grandma did—by rubbing **CASTOR OIL** into the skin around your nails every night at bedtime. Before you know it, you'll see—and feel—an amazing difference!

TIP Stop paying an arm and a leg for fancy skin exfoliators. Instead, use Grandma's favorite technique: Massage your wet skin with handfuls of **EPSOM SALTS,** starting with your feet and working up toward your neck. When you're finished, rinse off with a shower or bath.

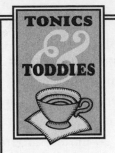

TONICS & TODDIES

PURE-AND-SIMPLE WRINKLE REMOVER

As we all know, life has its little ups and downs. And after a while, the accompanying smiles and frowns begin to leave their mark. Well, don't run out and pay megabucks for fancy cosmetics or painful Botox® treatments. Instead, erase those lines with this old-time formula.

Mild soap
Warm water
Milk of magnesia
¼ cup of virgin olive oil
Witch hazel (refrigerated)

Wash your face with the soap and water, dry it, and wait 10 minutes. Using a cotton pad, spread a thin layer of milk of magnesia on your face (making sure to keep it away from your eyes!), and let it dry completely. Apply a second layer of milk of magnesia; this will dissolve the first one. Wipe it all off with a warm, damp washcloth. Next, heat the olive oil in a small pan over low heat until it's just lukewarm. Apply it to your face with a cotton pad, leave it on for five minutes, and wipe it off with the witch hazel. Repeat this procedure twice a week. Within a couple of weeks, you'll be looking considerably less, um, experienced.

TIP Wash excess oil right out of your hair with good old **EPSOM SALTS.** Mix 1 cup of salts and 1 cup of lemon juice in 1 gallon of water, and let the mixture sit for 24 hours. Pour the solution onto your dry hair, wait 20 minutes, then shampoo as usual.

TIP Don't spend your money on pricey dandruff shampoos—use **MOUTHWASH** instead. Just mix 1 part minty mouthwash with 10 parts water, and apply it to your hair after shampooing. Massage it into your hair and scalp, but don't rinse. You'll have hair that's squeaky clean, flake-free, *and* minty fresh!

TIP Heading off on a trip? Before you pack your liquid cosmetics, seal the edges of the bottle caps with **NAIL POLISH** to keep the contents from leaking out all over your makeup kit. Remember to pack the nail polish, too, so you can reseal the bottles for the return trip.

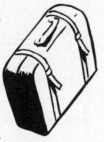

TIP To prevent costume jewelry from leaving green marks on your arms, neck, or ears, coat the parts that touch your skin with clear **NAIL POLISH.**

ONE MORE TIME

When you've just given yourself a **HOME PERMANENT,** and you have a bunch of those little papers left over, don't toss 'em in the trash. Instead, tuck 'em in your purse. They're perfect for blotting lipstick or absorbing excess oil from your face—without disturbing your makeup.

TIP Folks in Grandma Putt's time knew how to cope with emergencies—even minor ones, like running out of lipstick. They'd make a stand-in supply by putting a teaspoon or so of **PETROLEUM JELLY** in a small dish, and mixing in some red food coloring (how much you use depends on how dark you want the shade to be).

TIP If you dye your hair at home, keep the stuff from flowing into your eyes by rubbing a line of **PETROLEUM JELLY** above your eyebrows. (This trick also works for keeping shampoo out of a baby's or dog's eyes at bath time.)

TIP Here's a space-saving beauty tip to use on your next weekend jaunt or trek to the gym:

Instead of packing shampoo *and* your favorite soap, just toss a bottle of baby **SHAMPOO** into your bag. Use it all over to get squeaky clean and satiny soft from the tip of your nose to the tips of your toes!

TIP Who says **TOOTHBRUSHES** are only good for cleaning teeth? As Grandma knew well, those mini bristles are just the ticket for getting dirt out from under hard-working fingernails, prepping toenails for a pedicure, and even grooming unruly eyebrows.

In Grandma's Day

Nowadays, stores sell so many kinds of **ANTI-PERSPIRANTS,** Grandma Putt would be amazed. Well, can you believe it took mankind more than 5,000 years to come up with a no-sweat formula? The Sumerians launched the first recorded effort around 3500 B.C. The first successful brand, Mum®, hit the market in 1888. There was no big hoopla, though. In fact, folks were so embarrassed by perspiration, much less (heaven forbid!) body odor, that they asked for antiperspirants in drugstores in the same "this-is-our-little-secret" tones that a college student might use for you-know-what today. Not until 1914 did manufacturers begin touting their drying prowess in national magazines.

Family and
FRIENDS

TIP Help your dog's ears steer clear of infections by cleaning them every week or so with a mix of 1/4 cup of rubbing **ALCOHOL** and 10 drops of glycerin (available at the drugstore). Shake the solution well, dampen a cotton swab with it, and gently wipe out dirt and wax. *Caution:* If the pup shakes his head, immediately remove the swab to avoid damaging his eardrum.

TIP After you've pulled a tick out of a dog's or child's (or your own) skin, drop the foul thing into a jar of rubbing **ALCOHOL** to kill it instantly. Whatever you do, though, don't use the old-time trick of dabbing the tick with alcohol—or anything else—before you pull it out. That can cause the pest to regurgitate germs into the victim's skin.

ONE MORE TIME

Whenever you finish a bottle of **ROLL-ON DEODORANT,** pry off the roller ball, wash the bottle thoroughly, and fill it with tempera (poster) paint or fabric-painting ink. Then pop the ball back in, and give it to the kids—or use it for your own craft projects.

TIP Stick **BATHTUB APPLIQUÉS** on a child's schoolbag, so no one else grabs it by mistake. (This same trick will make your luggage stand out from the crowd on the airport baggage carousel.)

TIP Even when Grandma was a lass, no child's birthday party was complete without a game of Pin the Tail on the Donkey. But if your partygoers are too young to be trusted with pins, here's a safer way to play: Make the tails from **COTTON BALLS** with an inch or so of double-faced tape attached to each one. (If you think a donkey looks too weird with a puffy tail, let the kids play Pin the Tail on the Bunny instead!)

TIP On those unfortunate days when my dog had a run-in with the wrong end of a skunk, Grandma Putt used this time-tested formula to save the day: Mix 1 quart of 3 percent **HYDROGEN PEROXIDE,** ¼ cup of baking soda, and 1 teaspoon of liquid hand soap in a bucket. (Either hand soap or nondetergent dishwashing liquid will work.) Then corral your pal and soak him thoroughly with the solution. Rinse well, and towel him dry. Presto—no more *eau de skunk*!

TIP At one time or another, all kids seem to go through a "let's-be-spies" stage. So give your youngsters a helping hand by mixing up a batch of disappearing ink. Just mash a **LAXATIVE TABLET** in a bowl, add 1 tablespoon of rubbing alcohol, and mix until the tablet has completely dissolved. Then hand it over to the secret agents, who can write messages using a small, thin paintbrush or an old-fashioned fountain pen (still available at stationery and discount department stores). When the solution dries, the writing will vanish. To make it reappear, just lightly dampen a cotton ball in ammonia, and dab it over the text area.

TIP If your tiny tyke is dressing up as a furry critter (say a kitten or a bunny) for Halloween, put the finishing touch on her costume by dabbing a little pale pink **LIPSTICK** on her nose.

TIP Have your young artists run out of finger paint? Make a new supply by squirting **SHAVING CREAM** into small bowls, and adding a few drops of food coloring to each one (the more you use, of course, the darker the shade will be).

TIP For a small child, zipping up a jacket can be a daunting task. Make that job easier for the tyke in your life (as Grandma Putt did for me) by attaching a metal **SHOWER CURTAIN RING** to the zipper pull.

TIP Want to make bath time more fun for a child? Get a **SPONGE** in the shape of a boat, or a favorite animal, and cut a slit in one end. Then tuck in a tiny, hotel-size bar of soap, or some leftover soap slivers. Bingo—a soaping tub toy!

GRANDMA PUTT'S
Secret Formulas

GRANDMA'S CRYSTAL PALACE

When I was a lad, Grandma Putt helped me make these sparkly treasures. It was one of my favorite rainy-day projects, and my grandchildren still get a kick out of growing their own crystals.

½ cup of water
¼ cup of Epsom salts
1 sponge
Shallow bowl

Boil the water in a pan. Remove it from the heat, pour in the Epsom salts, and stir until they're completely dissolved. Put the sponge in the bottom of the bowl, and pour the Epsom salts solution over it. Put the bowl in a sunny spot, and keep a close watch on it. As the water evaporates, crystals will form all over the sponge, forming what looks like a miniature ice palace. Best of all, no two crystals are alike, so you'll get a new result each time.

Around the
HOUSE

TIP Make a terrific, streak-free window cleaner by mixing equal parts of rubbing **ALCOHOL** and nonsudsing ammonia in a hand-held spray bottle.

TIP Chrome was all the rage in Grandma Putt's day—on kitchen furniture as well as fixtures and appliances. Grandma kept that shiny finish spotless by rubbing it with a soft cloth dipped in rubbing **ALCOHOL.** (This trick works like magic on today's stainless steel appliances, too.)

TIP To remove the starch buildup from your iron (the kind with an old-time stainless steel bottom, *not* the nonstick kind!), dampen a soft, cotton cloth with rubbing **ALCOHOL,** and wipe the gunk away. Then gently go over the surface with extra-fine steel wool, and buff with a soft cloth.

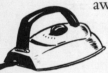

TIP When your television or computer screen gets grimy, don't reach for a spray cleaner (if the liquid seeps down into the edges, it can do major damage to the inner workings). Instead, put ½ cup of rubbing **ALCOHOL,** 1 tablespoon of baking soda, and ½ cup of cool water in a jar with a tight lid—an old mayonnaise jar is perfect. Mix the ingredients thoroughly, then dip a soft cloth in the mixture, and clean that screen. Store the remaining cleaner in a cool spot.

GRANDMA PUTT'S
Secret Formulas

GRANDMA'S ALL-PURPOSE CLEANER

Long before those fancy, multipurpose spray cleaners came on the market, Grandma Putt used this super-powered potion to keep her house spotless.

2 cups of rubbing alcohol
1 tbsp. of ammonia
1 tbsp. of dishwashing liquid
2 qt. of water

Mix all of the ingredients in a bucket, pour the solution into a hand-held spray bottle, and go to town. This concoction will clean glass, tile, chrome, and just about any other hard surface. (When in doubt, though, always test first in an inconspicuous spot.)

TIP Are aphids, mealybugs, or other teeny terrors buggin' your houseplants? Just dab each critter with a cotton swab dipped in rubbing **ALCOHOL,** and kiss those pesky pests good-bye!

TIP If the good, fresh coffee in your Thermos® bottle tastes like it's been sitting around for a month, it's time to give that flask a

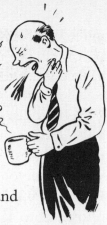

deep-down cleaning. How? Just fill the bottle with water, pop in four **ANTACID TABLETS,** and let the mix soak for an hour or so. Rinse well. Then wake up and taste the coffee!

TIP Grandma Putt had the happiest, healthiest houseplants. Her secret: She fed each of them once a month with an **ASPIRIN** tablet dissolved in 1 cup of water.

TIP Have you got paper stuck to a wooden tabletop? No problem! Just dampen the paper with **BABY OIL,** give it a few minutes to soak in, and you'll be able to pull it right off.

TIP To keep soap scum from building up on your glass shower door, rub it down once a week with a moist cloth dipped in **BABY OIL.**

TIP Before Grandma ironed a pleated skirt, she slipped a **BOBBY PIN** over each pleat (at the hem end). Then she pressed from the waist toward the hem, pulling out the pins to finish the job.

TIP Have you been using a commercial gadget to remove those annoying little "pills" from your sweaters? Well, stop that right now! The sharp blades in those things can damage delicate fibers. Instead, do the job with a fine-tooth **COMB.** Just lay the sweater on a table or counter, and holding the comb flush with the garment, move it gently across the surface. As the pills catch between the teeth, lift them away. Be sure to work carefully, so you don't snag the sweater itself.

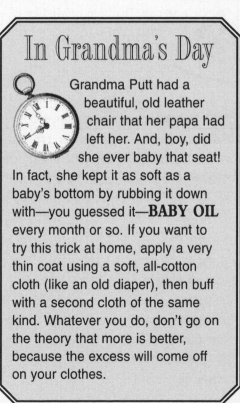

In Grandma's Day

Grandma Putt had a beautiful, old leather chair that her papa had left her. And, boy, did she ever baby that seat! In fact, she kept it as soft as a baby's bottom by rubbing it down with—you guessed it—**BABY OIL** every month or so. If you want to try this trick at home, apply a very thin coat using a soft, all-cotton cloth (like an old diaper), then buff with a second cloth of the same kind. Whatever you do, don't go on the theory that more is better, because the excess will come off on your clothes.

TIP A large **COSMETIC BRUSH** makes a dandy duster for your home office equipment. It's perfect for cleaning the nooks and crannies in your fax machine and your computer keyboard, as well as the computer's fan cover and that jungle of cable connections.

TIP If you're tired of having your long fingernails tear through rubber gloves, try this trick: Before you put on your next pair, push a **COTTON BALL** (or a piece of one) onto each finger.

TIP Most of Grandma Putt's pals kept **COTTON SWABS** in the bathroom. But Grandma didn't stop there; she also stashed a package in her cleaning closet, and used them for touching up chips, dings, and scratches on walls and furniture.

TIP Whoops! Your favorite bead necklace just broke! Don't run to the jewelry store; just restring those beads on **DENTAL FLOSS.**

TIP Need to get a stain out of a comforter or pillow? To avoid washing the whole, big thing, isolate the mark with **DENTAL FLOSS.** Just push the filling out of the way, gather up the soiled area, and tie it off tightly with the floss. Then proceed with the appropriate stain-removal treatment.

In Grandma's Day

When you're wearing **RUBBER GLOVES** to clean your bathroom—or any other area of your house—do you ever stop to wonder who invented these handy hand covers? Grandma knew, and now I'm going to tell you. It was Dr. William Halstead, chief of surgery at the Johns Hopkins University Hospital in Baltimore, back in 1890. His chief surgical nurse, Caroline Hampton, developed a rash on her hands every time she scrubbed up for an operation. To solve her problem, the doc made plaster casts of her hands, took them to a rubber-products manufacturer, and asked him to mold thin gloves from the casts. They worked so well, and were so much more sterile than even the best-scrubbed hand, that surgeons everywhere began ordering gloves for themselves. It wasn't long before their patients, knowing a good thing when they saw one, took the idea home.

ONE MORE TIME

 A traveler couldn't ask for handier holders than the tins and plastic boxes that **THROAT LOZENGES** come in. Hang on to your empties, then the next time you're ready to hit the road, gather up a few and turn them into these useful aids:

▷ **Car deodorizer.** Poke a dozen or so holes in the lid, and fill the bottom with your favorite potpourri or strongly scented soap. Snap the lid closed, and shove the container under a car seat.

▷ **Lipstick palette.** When you get close to the end of a tube, use a clean popsicle stick to scoop out whatever's left. Put several different colors in the lozenge box, and pack it (along with a lipstick brush) in your makeup bag.

▷ **Seed suitcase.** If you save seeds from your garden plants and want to share some with the folks you're visiting, use lozenge containers to convey the goods (one kind of seed per box, of course).

▷ **Sewing "basket."** Just toss in a tiny pair of scissors, needles, safety pins, a few bobbins of thread, and extra buttons to match the clothes you're packing.

▷ **Shoe-shine kit.** Fill an empty aspirin tin with shoe polish and tuck it into the lozenge container, along with a small cotton cloth (like a square cut from worn-out flannel pajamas).

▷ **Soap container.** Pop in either a small, travel-size bar of soap or a sliver of a large one.

On the home front, use lozenge containers to corral all those tiny odds and ends that tend to drift into the corners of drawers—like these, for instance:

▷ **Business cards**

▷ **Buttons**

▷ **Nails, screws, nuts and bolts**

▷ **Needles and pins**

▷ **Paper clips**

▷ **Pushpins and thumbtacks**

▷ **Rubber bands**

▷ **Small batteries**

▷ **Small drill bits**

▷ **Stamps**

▷ **Sticky-note pads**

▷ **Twist ties**

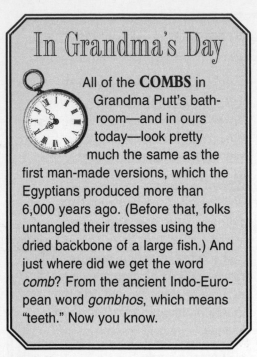
TIP When you want to hang a lightweight picture and you're fresh out of wire, use **DENTAL FLOSS** instead.

TIP Whenever twine was in short supply (as most things were in the war years), Grandma used unwaxed **DENTAL FLOSS** to truss poultry for cooking.

TIP Grandma Putt left me her mama's soup tureen and several other big, lidded serving dishes that live on a tippy-top shelf until we need them for Thanksgiving dinner or some other festive occasion. And I'm sure not about to risk having the two pieces come apart and break into shards when I pull the thing down! So I tie the top and bottom together with **DENTAL FLOSS.** If you try this trick, be sure to loop the floss around the knob on the lid handle, then run it in a figure-eight pattern through (or around) the handles on the base.

TIP Unwaxed—and unflavored— **DENTAL FLOSS** works great for slicing cakes, quick breads, and soft cheeses.

TIP We all know how gunk builds up in the bottoms of vases, cruets, and decanters. Instead of trying to scrub it out with a brush, take a tip from the folks who make Waterford® Crystal: Fill the vessel about halfway with water, and pop in two **DENTURE CLEANING TABLETS.** Let it stand for an hour or two, then rinse well.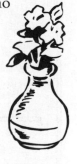

TIP You say you found a vintage glass pitcher at a flea market, but it's cloudy inside *and* out? No problem! Just set it in a bucket of water, pop in two or three **DENTURE CLEANING TABLETS,** and let it soak until the clouds drift by. (Two or three hours should do it.)

TIP Use **DENTURE CLEANING TABLETS** to wash super-grimy windows, indoors or out. Just dissolve several tablets in a bucket of water, dip a soft cloth in the solution, and wipe the glass clean. Then rinse with clear water, and dry with a second cloth.

TIP The commercial stain removers that we take for granted didn't exist in the days when Grandma Putt was doing load after load of laundry. Fortunately, she had a lot of spot-busters that were just as effective as those fancy sprays and gels (if not more so). One of the best was—and still is— **DENTURE CLEANING TABLETS.** To put these marvels to work on your clothes or table linens, just put the fabric in a container that's large enough to hold the soiled portion, fill it with warm water, and drop in

two tablets. Leave the material in the solution until the marks disappear, then launder it as usual. (*Caution:* Use this trick only on colorfast fabrics. To play it safe, test a hidden spot, like an inside seam, before you plunge ahead.)

TIP **DENTURE CLEANING TABLETS** are just the ticket for getting coffee and tea stains out of china teapots, cups, and mugs. Just fill the vessel with warm water, pop in a tablet, let it dissolve, and wait a minute or two. Pour out the water and eyeball the ceramic surface. If you still see marks, repeat the procedure.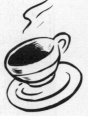

TIP If Mother Nature wouldn't cooperate and deliver frosted windowpanes in time for Christmas, Grandma knew how to make her own festive "frost," and you can, too. Mix 4 tablespoons of **EPSOM SALTS** in 1 cup of beer. Paint the solution onto the glass for an overall wintry effect, or use stencils to apply images of your choice—like snowmen or snowflakes. Want more color? Add a few drops of food coloring to get red for Santa's suit or green for holly branches. After the holidays, just wash the stuff off with clear water.

ONE MORE TIME

When your **HAIRBRUSH** gets too ragged to use on your hair, move it to the laundry or broom closet. Then use it to clean your vacuum cleaner, your dryer's lint trap, and other hard-to-get-at places.

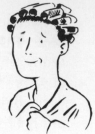

TIP Grandma kept the leaves of her houseplants shiny bright by squeezing a small dab of **HAIR CONDITIONER** onto a soft, cotton cloth, and gently wiping the leaves with it.

TIP If you have a hard time gripping a pen, say, because of arthritis or a hand injury, this trick will make it easier: Find a tube-shaped, foam **HAIR CURLER,** and shove the pen through the opening.

TIP To get pet hair off of upholstered furniture, spray a sponge with **HAIR SPRAY** (pump or aerosol), and while it's still tacky, run it across the fabric.

TIP When aphids start plaguing your houseplants, reach for the aerosol **HAIR SPRAY** and a plastic bag that's big enough to hold the plant and its pot. Spray the inside of the bag—not the plant! Then put the victimized plant inside, fasten the bag tightly with a twist tie, and set it in a spot away from direct sun (otherwise, the heat inside will build up and kill the plant). Wait 24 hours, and remove the bag. Those itty-bitty bad guys will be history! (*Note:* This trick works on outdoor container plants, too.)

TIP Before you hang a Christmas wreath outside, spray the ribbons and bows with super-hold **HAIR SPRAY** and let it dry. They'll stay clean and perky. (Just don't hang the wreath where it'll get rained on, or the hair spray will wash off.)

GRANDMA PUTT'S
Secret Formulas

CHRISTMAS TREE SURVIVAL TONIC

Every year, without fail, Grandma Putt poured this elixir into our Christmas tree stand to keep that ol' tree fresh and green throughout the year-end holidays. I still use it—I've never found a better formula!

2 cups of clear corn syrup
4 tbsp. of household bleach
4 multivitamin tablets with iron
1 gal. of very hot water

As soon as you bring your tree indoors and set it up, mix all of the ingredients in a bucket, and pour the mixture into the stand. Deliver a fresh dose whenever the water level starts going down, and your evergreen will stay as fresh as a daisy right into the new year.

TIP When I was growing up, satiny Christmas tree ornaments were the bee's knees (as Grandma Putt would say). Like lots of old-time treasures, these glittery orbs are staging a big-time comeback. But they still have the same old problem: After a few holiday seasons, the threads begin to unravel. I stop the fraying the same way Grandma did, by spritzing the balls with **HAIR SPRAY,** and pressing the stray ends back into place.

TIP Your Christmas tree will keep its needles longer if you spritz it from top to bottom with **HAIR SPRAY.**

TIP **HAIR SPRAY** will make cut flowers last longer. Just give the posies a spray after they've been in the vase for a day or so.

TIP Grandma Putt was not what you'd call the frilly type, but she did love her ruffled curtains and bedspreads. And to keep those ruffles stiff and perky, she sprayed them with aerosol **HAIR SPRAY** after every washing.

TIP If you do a lot of sewing by hand or cross-stitch embroidery, this tip's for you: You'll find it

In Grandma's Day

It's probably a safe bet that no bathroom in the country is without a box of **ADHESIVE BANDAGES.** Well, we owe these handy plasters (as Grandma called them) to a young Johnson & Johnson employee named Earle Dickson. In the 1920s, Mr. Dickson married an accident-prone young woman, who was forever cutting herself in the kitchen. The injuries were too minor to require the company's large surgical dressings (the product that had launched the Johnson brothers on the road to fame and fortune), so Mr. Dickson would simply snip off a piece of sterile gauze and stick it to a length of adhesive tape. Then one day, tired of making these blood-stoppers one by one, he found a way to produce them in quantity by covering the sticky portions with a temporarily clinging fabric. James Johnson, the company president, heard about this new technique and requested a demonstration. Mr. Dickson complied, and Band-Aids® were born!

easier to thread your needle if you stiffen the end of the thread with a spritz of **HAIR SPRAY** before you push it through the needle's eye.

TIP A light coat of **HAIR SPRAY** will keep newly polished brass from tarnishing.

TIP Like any red-blooded American kid, I rarely came home without dirt and grass stains on my clothes. Grandma never scolded me (remembering her own, much younger days). She just told me to go change my clothes and bring back the soiled duds so she could get the stains out. Then she put the soiled part of the garment in the bathroom sink, and poured in enough **HYDROGEN PEROXIDE** to submerge the spot. She let it soak for an hour (or longer if necessary), then laundered the clothing as usual.

TIP Treat bloodstains with the same **HYDROGEN PEROXIDE** formula as grass stains, but add ½ teaspoon of ammonia to the peroxide. (*Caution:* Don't use peroxide or ammonia on nylon.)

TIP **HYDROGEN PEROXIDE** gets coffee, tea, and wine spills out of marble—but you must act fast before the stain can seep into the porous stone. Rub the spot with a sponge dipped in a solution of 1 part peroxide to 4 parts water, and wipe it off pronto. Repeat as necessary until the mark is gone. (If you reach the scene after the stain has set, all is not lost. For Grandma Putt's simple remedies, see page 177.)

TIP If any of your dark-colored wooden furniture gets scratched, just reach into the medicine chest, and grab the **IODINE.** Dip a cotton swab into the bottle,

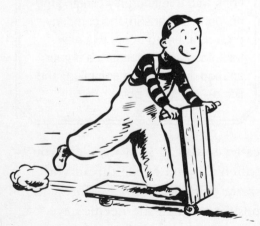

and dab that ding away. (Before you try this, test it first in a hidden spot to make sure the color blends in nicely.)

TIP Instead of struggling to get a paintbrush into tiny, tight crannies (like the space where a door frame almost meets a corner), use a wedged-shaped **MAKEUP SPONGE.**

TIP Use a clean **MASCARA BRUSH** to get lint or pet hair out of hard-to-reach places like pockets and hems.

TIP Like any grandmother, Grandma Putt treasured my childhood mementos—like the newspaper photos of me winning a blue ribbon for my giant pumpkin at the county fair. There were a lot of those clippings, and she knew how to make them last so long that I still have them to enjoy today. Before she put them into her scrapbook (using adhesive photo corners, *not* glue), she gave them a bath in this old-time preservative: Dissolve one **MILK OF MAGNESIA** tablet in a quart of club soda (make sure it's fresh and fizzy), and let it sit overnight. In the morning, mix thoroughly and pour the solution into a shallow pan. Insert your clipping, wait two hours, then *very gently* take it out and lay it on a soft towel to dry. That paper will stay as fresh as this morning's news for a good 20 years. Then you (or your grandchildren) will have to repeat the procedure.

GRANDMA PUTT'S
Secret Formulas

PIONEER PLANT FOOD

Are your houseplants looking less than their best? Give them a nutritional boost with this old-time chow.

¾ **cup of ammonia**
1 **tbsp. of Epsom salts**
1 **tbsp. of saltpeter (available at drugstores)**
1 **tbsp. of baking powder**
2 **multivitamin tablets with iron**
½ **tsp. of liquid hand soap**
½ **tsp. of unflavored gelatin**
1 **gal. of water**

Mix all of the ingredients in a bucket, pour the mixture into a container with a tight lid, and label it. (Use several jars if you don't have one that's big enough.) Then, once a month, use 1 cup of Pioneer Plant Food per gallon of water instead of your regular fertilizer. Your plants will perk up fast!

TIP When it's time to give your wooden cutting boards a rub-down, use **MINERAL OIL.** Unlike vegetable oil, it won't turn rancid, and it won't attract pesky pests.

TIP If your houseplants could do with a little more light, take a tip from Grandma Putt, and set each one on a **MIRROR.** Or line a whole windowsill (and maybe even the frame) with mirrors. The sun's rays will bounce off the glass and reflect onto the foliage.

TIP Once upon a time, what I wanted most in the world was a bird that would fill our house with tuneful melodies. Well, Grandma Putt got me a beautiful, yellow canary, but the little guy refused to perform. I was devastated, but Grandma knew just what to do. She hung a small **MIRROR** in the cage above a perch. When my feathered friend saw his reflection, he assumed it was another bird, and he started crooning up a storm to his new buddy.

TIP Rats! You took your favorite leather handbag out of stor-age, took one whiff, and said "P.U."—mildew! Don't despair. Just dampen a cotton pad with antiseptic **MOUTHWASH,** and gently rub the bag's surface thoroughly. Wipe it dry with a soft, cotton cloth, buff with a second cloth, then apply a commer-cial leather-nourishing cream. (This same trick works on any mildewed leather, including shoes, luggage, and furniture.)

TIP Keep a **NAIL BRUSH** in the laundry room and another one in your household cleaning kit—it's just the ticket for scrubbing away small stains.

TIP When you remove curtain or drapery hooks, mark their locations with a tiny dab of **NAIL POLISH.** That way, when it's time to put that hardware back on, you won't have to second-guess where it goes (or spend your precious time measuring).

ONE MORE TIME

When you need to paint screws or upholstery tacks to match a wall or complement your furniture, stick the pointed ends into an old **SPONGE.** Then spray or brush on the paint color of your choice.

In Grandma's Day

Like a whole lot of other bathroom products that we take for granted, Kleenex® TISSUES appeared on the scene when Grandma Putt was a girl. They started out as thin, gauzelike paper called Cellucotton that Kimberly-Clark produced as liners for GIs' gas masks during World War I. When the war ended, the company used the surplus to make "Kleenex Kerchiefs," which it heavily promoted as "the Sanitary Cold Cream Remover." Women all over the country scrambled to buy the handy things. (Until then, they'd used washcloths and towels to take off their makeup.) But they soon began writing to the company with a complaint: Their husbands and children were forever snatching the Kerchiefs to blow their noses! The folks at Kimberly-Clark took the hint, changed their marketing strategy, and the rest, as they say, is history.

TIP If the numbers on your dial thermostat seem to get smaller by the day, get out a bottle of brightly colored **NAIL POLISH** (and your reading glasses) and mark your usual temperature of choice. Then you'll find it in a snap every time!

TIP Over time, the gradation marks on measuring cups can fade almost out of sight. Grandma solved that problem by painting them with **NAIL POLISH.** (Just make sure you get them in *exactly* the right spots, or your recipes may not turn out quite the way you expected!)

TIP When you empty a bottle of **NAIL POLISH,** don't throw it away! Instead, clean it and the little brush with nail polish remover. Then use the bottle to hold home-made paint or stain for your budding artists (you'll find some dandy recipes in Chapter 4). Or, if you're about to paint a room or a piece of furniture, pour some of the paint into the bottle. It'll come in handy for touching up dings and scratches down the road!

TIP Anytime I got a new pair of shoes, or had my old ones reheeled, Grandma would hand me a bottle of clear **NAIL POLISH** and tell me to paint the backs of those heels before I set foot out of the house. She said it would keep my footgear scuff-free longer, and, as usual, she was right.

TIP Tired of losing the 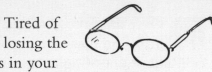 screws in your eyeglasses? Make sure the tiny things are screwed in tightly, then paint the ends with clear **NAIL POLISH.**

TIP Grandma Putt loved having folks over for supper. And she'd no more have set her table with paper napkins than she'd have dished up her favorite casserole on paper plates. So she had a *lot* of opportunities to use this little trick: To get lipstick stains out of cotton or linen napkins, cover the spot with a dab of **PETROLEUM JELLY,** then launder as usual. (This trick works on any washable fabric—for instance, that cotton turtleneck you pulled on *after* you'd applied your bright red lipstick.)

TIP Your shower curtain rings will glide more smoothly if you rub a thin coat of **PETROLEUM JELLY** onto the rod.

TIP If you have an artificial Christmas tree, you know how hard it can be to get the thing apart after the holidays are over. End that yearly struggle by dipping the end of each branch into **PETROLEUM JELLY** before you insert it into the tree trunk. When you're ready to "undecorate" it'll slide right out.

TIP Shine patent leather shoes, belts, and purses with **PETRO-LEUM JELLY.** Apply a thin coat with a soft cloth, wipe it off with another one, and buff with a third.

GRANDMA PUTT'S
Secret Formulas

INTO-THE-SHOWER CLEANER

Tired of battling the mildew that builds up on your bathtub, glass shower doors, or vinyl shower curtain liner? Here's a simple formula that'll stop that crud before it has a chance to form.

½ cup of rubbing alcohol
1 tbsp. of liquid laundry detergent with enzymes
3 cups of water

Mix all of the ingredients in a hand-held spray bottle, and keep it on the side of the tub. Then issue an all-points bulletin that says the last person out of the shower or bath each day must spray the solution on all of the wet surfaces. Follow up once a month by wiping down the walls with the same solution, and you can kiss mold and mildew good-bye.

ONE MORE TIME

 When the time comes to retire your old **SHOWER CURTAIN,** don't throw it away. Here's a tub full of good uses for that fabric or vinyl sheet.

Indoors

▷ **Temporary window covering.** Just thread a spring-tension rod through the holes in the top of a fabric shower curtain, and pop it into place in the window frame—no rings or brackets needed!

▷ **Packing "blanket."** Wrap a fabric shower curtain around furniture to protect it in the moving van (or the back of your minivan).

▷ **Painting drop cloth.** Spread vinyl shower curtains on floors and furniture to catch drips.

▷ **Child-size "construction material."** Give fabric shower curtains to the youngsters, and they'll have a field day using them to create forts, castles, and stage sets.

Outdoors

▷ **Pest-control aid.** Lay a fabric shower curtain on the ground under plants plagued by beetles or weevils, and gently shake the branches. When the bugs come tumbling down, gather up the trap, and dump the contents into a tub of water laced with a cup of liquid hand soap or rubbing alcohol.

▷ **Plant protectors.** Toss fabric shower curtains over plants when late or early frosts threaten. Or make a cold frame by draping a clear vinyl shower curtain over stakes pounded into the ground.

TIP Mend a leak in a plastic or lead pipe (temporarily) by squeezing **PETROLEUM JELLY** into the crack and wrapping waterproof tape around the pipe. That'll stem the drip until the plumber arrives.

TIP Coat the insides of candle holders with **PETROLEUM JELLY.** That way, the hardened wax drips will come off lickety-split.

TIP Grandma always kept a can of **SHAVING CREAM** in the kitchen so she could grab it in a snap when any food spilled on the dining room carpet. She'd spray enough of it on the area to cover the stain completely, let it soak in for a few minutes, and blot it up with a sponge dampened in cold water or club soda.

TIP A can of **SHAVING CREAM** belongs in your workshop, too, because it's great for cleaning grimy or paint-spattered hands. Just squirt the foam on, and wipe it off with a paper towel—no water needed!

TIP When Grandma's fingers started getting a little less agile, she had a hard time grabbing hold of the tiny rings in her rubber drain plugs. What did she do? She thought big! She just slipped a **SHOWER CURTAIN RING** through the little ring on each of the plugs. Bingo—no more fumbling!

TIP Pop **SHOWER CURTAIN RINGS** over the rod in your closet and use them to hang belts, costume jewelry, and handbags.

TIP To keep clothes and linens smelling fresh as a daisy, stash bars of scented **SOAP,** minus the wrappers, on shelves and in drawers (lavender was Grandma's favorite). But wait—there's 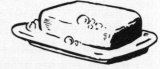 more! Besides sharing its nice aroma, the unwrapped soap will harden and, therefore, last longer when you use it.

TIP Fresh out of your favorite bathroom cleanser? Don't run to the supermarket. Instead, grab that bottle of liquid hand **SOAP** that's sitting on the sink (the standard 10-ounce size), and mix the contents with a pound of baking soda in 1 cup of warm water. Then scrub-a-dub-dub!

TIP Make a reluctant drawer glide smoothly by rubbing the runners with a bar of **SOAP.** If that doesn't do the trick, sand the runners with fine-grit sandpaper, and reapply the soap.

TIP Balky curtain rings will move right along if you rub bar **SOAP** on the rods.

TIP Do you have some old lace that's gotten mildewed (say, an heirloom wedding veil, or a pair of antique curtains you picked up at a flea market)? Send the mildew packin' by rubbing the lace with a bar of mild **SOAP** until a visible film develops. Set the piece in the sun for several hours, then rinse in cold water.

TIP In the entry hall of Grandma Putt's house, she had a big, ceramic umbrella stand. I have it now, and I still use her trick for keeping it fresh and dry. I cut a large **SPONGE** to fit inside the base, and it catches the drips.

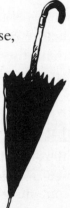

TIP When something greasy lands on your upholstered furniture, don't panic. Here's a simple solution: Sprinkle a thick layer of **TALCUM POWDER** over the mark, and let it stand for about 10 minutes. Then brush off the powder. If the spot is still visible, repeat the procedure until all the grease has been absorbed.

OLD-TIME BOARD CLEANER

You've found some beautiful old wood boards that you want to recycle into paneling or furniture. There's just one problem: The things are filthy! Well, don't fret about it. Just mix up a batch of this power-packed cleaner. It—and a little elbow grease—will make that vintage lumber sparkle.

3 parts sand
2 parts liquid hand soap
1 part lime

Mix all of the ingredients together in a bucket, and scour the boards using a stiff scrub brush. Rinse with clear water, and rub dry with a clean towel. Then pat yourself on the back for your lucky find, because new wood could never look this good!

TIP Grandma Putt knew that **TALCUM POWDER** could do a lot more than soak up grease and moisture. For one thing, it silences your squeaky floorboards. Just sprinkle a little powder along the edges, and those boards will be as quiet as a mouse.

TIP Ants won't cross a line of **TALCUM POWDER.** Use it at the entrance to your pantry, or wherever you don't want the tiny troublemakers to roam.

TIP You've just hand-washed your best sweater, and now you've got a sink brimming over with suds. Make those bubbles disperse by sprinkling **TALCUM POWDER** over them. Then your wash water will flow right down the drain, without the need to chase it with gallons of fresh water.

 TIP Wipe playing cards with **TALCUM POWDER** to keep them free of grease and dirt.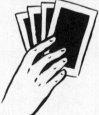

TIP Whenever Grandma cleaned her jewelry or other small, delicate treasures, she used an extra-soft **TOOTHBRUSH** (like the kind made for baby's first teeth).

TIP Keep a **TOOTHBRUSH** in the kitchen, and use it to scrub cheese graters, can openers, strainers, waffle irons, and other gadgets with tiny nooks and crannies. To keep the brush itself spic and span, just run it through the dishwasher with your regular load. Or do what

---

ONE MORE TIME

Don't toss out those empty **TALCUM POW-DER** containers—or baby powder, either! Instead, wash them and turn them into mini sprinkling cans for your houseplants or seed-starting flats, or use them to dispense homemade powdered cleansers. (You'll find scads of great ones in Chapter 4.)

Grandma Putt did in the days before dishwashers came along: Just dunk the bristles in boiling water after every use.

TIP A **TOOTHBRUSH** makes a dandy substitute for the mushroom-cleaning brushes they sell in fancy kitchenware stores.

TIP When you load up a picnic basket or road-trip cooler, pack a paring knife in a plastic **TOOTHBRUSH HOLDER.** The knife will stay clean and sharp, and you won't get a nasty surprise when you reach for a sandwich!

TIP If the back of your chair leaves a scuff mark on the wall, scrub it off with **TOOTHPASTE**

(the old-fashioned white variety, not the gel kind). This trick will work even better if you use an old, clean toothbrush.

TIP Long ago, piano keys were made of real ivory, instead of the plastic that's used today (much to the relief of this old elephant lover!). If you have one of those old-time keyboards, clean it the way Grandma did, by rubbing the keys

---

In Grandma's Day

Giving your **TOOTH-BRUSH** early retirement leads to healthier teeth and gums and gives you a steady supply of cleaning aids. But did you know it can also help you lick a cold or the flu? That's because germs linger on a wet brush, and when you use the same one over and over, you keep reinfecting yourself. So the next time you come down with a sore throat, runny nose, fever...the whole nine yards...do what Grandma Putt always made me do: Get yourself a fresh toothbrush, and put the old one to work elsewhere. (Just dip it in boiling water first, or run it through the dishwasher.)

---

gently with **TOOTHPASTE** on a soft, cotton cloth. Then rinse with milk, and buff with a fresh cloth.

TIP Clean the base, a.k.a. soleplate, of your iron with **TOOTH-PASTE** applied with a soft cloth. Just a couple words of caution: Don't try this trick on a nonstick iron, and be sure to use white toothpaste—not the gel kind or one of the potent abrasive types. (Of course, you *will* remember to unplug the iron before you clean it, won't you?)

TIP Time to polish some silver that has intricate engraving? Rub it with a dab of white **TOOTH-PASTE** on a soft, cotton cloth. Then wipe off the paste, and buff with a fresh cloth.

TIP What's that? Company's coming for supper tomorrow, and your best tablecloth is wrinkled? Well, don't bother to iron it. Just grab a clean **TOWEL** from the bathroom, and lay it on the table (use two or more towels if one isn't big enough to cover the whole table). Spread the cloth on top of the towel, and lightly spray it with water. Then toddle off to bed. While you're snoozing, gravity will smooth out all the creases in the fabric.

TIP Any time Grandma Putt ironed hand-embroidered fabric of any kind (like her favorite tablecloths and pillowcases), she'd lay it face down on a **TOWEL,** and iron the reverse side. This way, the stitchery didn't get flattened.

TIP To safely store your good table linens or out-of-season curtains, first pad the bar of a cedar suit hanger (the cedar will repel moths) with a cotton hand **TOWEL.** Cover it with a piece of acid-free tissue paper (available at craft shops),

and drape your folded fabric over that. *Hint:* If the pieces will be in long-term storage, take them off their hangers and refold them every month or so, as I do with Grandma Putt's special Christmas tablecloth. This will prevent discoloration and wearing along the creases.

TIP When you need to move a heavy piece of furniture across a wood or tile floor, reach for a couple of thick, clean **TOWELS** (dirty ones could scratch the floor). Fold them over, and shove one

ONE MORE TIME

Whenever you use the last square of toilet paper on a roll, think twice before you toss that **TOILET PAPER TUBE** in the trash. You may be able to give it a second career as one of these handy household helpers:

▷ **Cat toy.** Just give it to Fluffy, and she'll frolic for hours on end!

▷ **Cord corral.** Fold up an appliance cord until it's just long enough to reach from the gadget to the wall outlet (or surge protector), then stuff the excess into the tube. To make the cardboard look less, um, utilitarian,

cover it with fabric, wrapping paper, or wallpaper scraps that complement your decor.

▷ **Dollhouse furniture.** Cut the tubes to the appropriate length, cover them with paper or fabric, and presto—you've got all-but-instant end tables or ottomans.

▷ **Party favor.** Stuff the tube with candy, small toys, or other tiny treasures; wrap it with colorful paper, and tie the ends with ribbon.

▷ **Ribbon reel.** When you save ribbon from packages, twirl it around a tube to keep it neat and unwrinkled.

TIP It happens to all of us now and then: We put a load of clothes in the dryer and go about our business. Hours later, we come back to find a pile of wrinkled duds. Well, don't pull 'em out and start ironing! Instead, get those creases out the easy way: Dampen a large bath **TOWEL,** toss it into the dryer with the clothes, and let the machine run for about 15 minutes. And this time, unload it promptly!

The great
OUTDOORS

TIP Send bad bugs to their just rewards with this bathroom-variety weapon. Mix ½ cup of rubbing **ALCOHOL,** ½ teaspoon of mild liquid hand soap or dishwashing liquid, and 1 cup of tap water in a hand-held spray bottle. Then take aim and let 'er rip. (*Caution:* Some plants are extra-sensitive to alcohol, so test-spray a few of the leaves first—and be sure to aim very carefully, because this potent potion will kill garden-variety heroes right along with the villains.)

under each end. Then slide that baby right along. (Use four towels, one under each leg, if a single one won't span the distance.)

TIP Before Grandma washed her heirloom crystal (or any treasured breakable) in her porcelain sink, she'd create a safety cushion by covering the bottom and sides of the sink with a clean bath **TOWEL.**

DEER DAMAGE PREVENTION POTION

When deer are dining on everything in sight, whip up a batch of this potent repellent.

¼ **cup of Dr. Bronner's Peppermint Soap®***
¼ **cup of liquid kelp (from the garden center)**
2 **tbsp. of cayenne pepper**
1 **qt. of warm water**

Mix all of the ingredients in a bucket, and pour the mixture into a hand-held spray bottle. Then spritz your deer-plagued plants thoroughly. (Just remember, though— this stuff will taste as bad to you as it does to the deer, so don't use it on anything you intend to eat!)

* Or substitute ¼ cup of liquid hand soap and 1 teaspoon of peppermint extract.

TIP If you need to do battle with bugs on a large scale (for instance, beetles that are gobbling up your roses or ticks that are hanging out on your shrubs), mix 2 cups of rubbing **ALCOHOL** and 1 tablespoon of liquid hand soap in 1 gallon of water in a bucket. Then pour the solution into a 6 gallon hose-end sprayer jar, and spray your plants from top to bottom—and make sure you get under all the leaves.

TIP Make a potent weed killer by mixing 2 tablespoons of rubbing **ALCOHOL** and 1 pint of water in a hand-held spray bottle. Then fire away. (Just aim carefully to avoid killing plants you want to keep.)

TIP Before you wash a painted porch or deck that's really grimy, wipe it with a soft cloth or mop that's been dipped in rubbing **ALCOHOL.** It'll dissolve the greasy dirt so the detergent can really get in there and do its job.

TIP Grandma Putt was crazy about her big old pine trees. But they sure made a mess when the sap dripped all over her metal lawn chairs (not to mention her wheelbarrow)! To get the goo off, she just dampened a soft, cotton cloth with rubbing **ALCOHOL,** and buffed the sticky stuff away.

TIP Want to get moss off of a brick, stone, or concrete walkway? Spray that green fuzz with a solution of 2 tablespoons of rubbing **ALCOHOL** per pint of water, then rinse it away with the garden hose.

Great Garden Chow

Grandma Putt always said that one of the best garden helpers she had was sitting right in her medicine chest. This miracle worker is none other than good old Epsom salts, which goes by the scientific moniker of *magnesium sulfate heptahydrate*. And therein lies the secret to its success: Magnesium supplies the oomph that makes any plant's metabolism hum right along. Here's how to serve up that super chow to your garden plants.

Plants	Feeding Instructions
Annuals and perennials	Put a pinch of Epsom salts in the bottom of each planting hole.
Bulbs (both spring-mer-blooming)	Mix $1/2$ cup of Epsom salts and $1/2$ bushel of wood ashes, and sprinkle this mixture around the plants when the sum-foliage first appears.
Flowering shrubs	In spring and fall, sprinkle Epsom salts around the root zone at a rate of $1/4$ cup of salts per 9 inches of shrub circumference.
Herbs	Every few weeks, water the plants with a solution of 2 tablespoons of Epsom salts per gallon of water.
Roses, bare-root	Before planting, soak the roots for 24 hours in a solution made from 1 tablespoon of Epsom salts, 1 vitamin B_1 tablet, and 1 teaspoon of baby shampoo mixed in 1 gallon of water.
Roses, established	In May and again in June, give each shrub 1 tablespoon of Epsom salts with its regular feeding (to get your roses off to a rousing start in the spring, see Grandma Putt's "Wake Up and Smell the Roses Tonic" on page 39).
Turf grass	In spring and fall, mix 3 pounds of Epsom salts per 50-pound bag of dry, natural/organic lawn food, and apply the mixture at half of the recommended rate going east to west, then apply the other half going north to south with your broadcast or drop spreader. If you use a synthetic/chemical fertilizer, spread the fertilizer first, clean your spreader to remove any residue, then follow up with the salts.
Vegetables (especially tomatoes and peppers)	Dissolve 3 tablespoons of Epsom salts in 1 gallon of warm water, and give each plant 1 pint of this mixture just as it starts to bloom.

TIP You left your favorite leather gardening gloves out in the rain, and now they're stiff as boards. Don't fret: Just dip them in a sink full of warm water, squeeze them dry in a towel, and then rub **CASTOR OIL** into the leather. Those gloves will be as soft as they were on the day you bought them!

TIP Tie vines to their supports with green, mint-flavored **DENTAL FLOSS.** The green color makes the floss less noticeable and the mint scent helps repel pests.

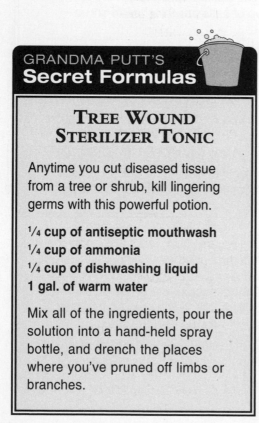

**GRANDMA PUTT'S
Secret Formulas**

TREE WOUND STERILIZER TONIC

Anytime you cut diseased tissue from a tree or shrub, kill lingering germs with this powerful potion.

1/4 **cup of antiseptic mouthwash**
1/4 **cup of ammonia**
1/4 **cup of dishwashing liquid**
1 **gal. of warm water**

Mix all of the ingredients, pour the solution into a hand-held spray bottle, and drench the places where you've pruned off limbs or branches.

TIP When you get a tear in your favorite leather work gloves, do what Grandma did: Stitch it up with **DENTAL FLOSS.**

TIP Grandma Putt used to save all of the **HAIR** from her brush—and mine and our pets' too—and tuck a handful into each hole at planting time. She told me that the prickly texture would discourage insect pests, and it did. But now I know that it does more than that: Hair is chock-full of minerals that make plants grow stronger and healthier.

TIP Keep the wooden handles of all your tools smooth and splinter-free by applying a thin coat of **HAIR SPRAY.** (Either pump or aerosol will do the job.)

TIP Use aerosol **HAIR SPRAY** to kill flying insects on contact.

TIP Pruning shears will work better, longer, if you lubricate the moving parts with a little **LIP BALM.**

TIP Does your yard or driveway have low spots where water collects after a rain? Stop those puddles from becoming mosquito maternity wards by pouring a little

MINERAL OIL into each one. (A tablespoon to half a cup will do the trick, depending on the size of the pool.) The oil will spread across the surface and smother any eggs or larvae.

TIP Sometimes, Grandma knew that some tiny terrors were lurking on the undersides of her plants' leaves, but she wasn't sure what kind. Fortunately, she knew an easy way to make a positive ID: She'd just glue or tape a small **MIRROR** on the end of a yardstick, and shove it under the foliage.

TIP Feed your lawn with this mixture: 1 cup of antiseptic **MOUTHWASH,** 1 cup of Epsom salts, 1 cup of dishwashing liquid, and 1 cup of ammonia in your 20 gallon hose-end sprayer. Fill the balance of the sprayer jar with warm water, and let 'er rip.

TIP Tired of mixing, mingling, and then losing your golf, tennis, or squash balls? Mark your own with a tiny drop of **NAIL POLISH.**

TIP When I was a boy, I loved to go fishing with my pals. But you can bet Grandma Putt wasn't about to let me take precious earthworms from her garden! Instead, she

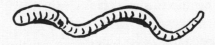

showed me how to make fish-egg bait. It's simple, too. You just coat small pieces of sponge (about ½ inch across) with **PETROLEUM JELLY.** (Any color sponge will lure 'em to your hook.)

ONE MORE TIME

When you replace your **TOOTHBRUSH** every three months (as dentists advise), the old ones can pile up fast. It's a good thing, too, because you couldn't ask for a handier cleaning aid. They're perfect for getting dirt out of hard-to-reach places like the crevices in garden tools, your lawn mower's engine, and the treads in work shoes and sneakers—not to mention the grime under your fingernails!

TIP Protect your plants from snails, slugs, and other slithery thugs by coating the stems with a mixture made from 1¼ cups of **PETROLEUM JELLY,** 1 cup of castor oil, and 3 tablespoons each of cayenne pepper and hot sauce. Just mix everything together in a bucket, and smear it on the stems (or trunks if the victims are trees or shrubs).

TIP Before you put your garden tools away for the winter, guard them against rust by rubbing down the metal parts with a little **PETROLEUM JELLY.**

TIP There was nothing Grandma Putt loved better than birds. She had birdhouses and nesting boxes all over her yard. To prevent wasp invasions, she smeared a coat of **PETROLEUM JELLY** on the inside top of each box.

TIP When a bird leaves a "present" on your leather bag, jacket, or (yikes!) your convertible's leather upholstery, don't panic. Just rub the stain away with **PETROLEUM JELLY** on a soft cloth.

TIP Lubricate the wheels of garden carts, lawn mowers, and wheelbarrows by smearing **PETROLEUM JELLY** around the cylinders.

TIP Are anthills making a mess of your lawn? Use Grandma's favorite anti-ant solution to bid 'em *adieu.* Simply mix ¼ cup of liquid hand **SOAP** and 1 gallon of water in a bucket, and pour the solution on the mound. Repeat the procedure about an hour later to make sure the liquid penetrates to the queen's inner chamber.

Hair Dryers

Electric hair dryers have been around since the roaring twenties. But not until the swingin' sixties did the familiar, pistol-grip blow dryer become a fixture in bathrooms all across the country. But these gadgets can do a lot more than dry hair. In fact, I know a lot of folks who don't even have hair (at least not much) who keep a few dryers around the house. Here's a sampling of what they do with them—and you can, too!

▶ *Clean jewelry.* Fill a bowl—*not* a sink—with lukewarm water and stir in a few squirts of mild dishwashing liquid. Put the jewelry in the bowl, let it soak for a few minutes, and scrub each piece very gently with a soft toothbrush. (One made for baby's first teeth is perfect.) Rinse with clear water, lay the pieces on a towel, and dry them on low. *Caution:* Don't use this trick on soft stones such as opals, pearls, turquoise, or jade. When in doubt, check with a jeweler before you proceed.

▶ *Defrost dinner.* Set the dryer on hot, and unfreeze meat or vegetables, or soften ice cream. Immediately cook any defrosted meat.

▶ *Defrost your freezer.* Blast the ice with your hair dryer, and it'll melt away before your very eyes. Just be sure you never lay the thing down inside the freezer or refrigerator—even if the dryer's turned off!

▶ *Defrost frozen pipes.* Set the dryer on warm and hold it close to the frozen section. Use caution with plastic pipes—if you get too close, the pipe may melt along with the ice!

▶ *Dry-food storage tins.* After you wash and towel-dry them, finish the job with a hair dryer set on low. This way, you know the metal won't rust, and you've eliminated any lingering moisture that could be absorbed by the grub you stash inside (like cookies, rice, or pasta).

▶ *Dust your stuff.* Use the coolest setting, take aim, and blow the dust away. This trick is just the ticket for lampshades, fabric hangings, artificial flowers, and anything with intricate carving or relief work—like wooden furniture or ceramic pieces. You can even blow the dust out from behind radiators, bookcases, and refrigerators!

(continued)

FAST FORWARD

(continued from page 41)

▶ *Get crayon marks off of wallpaper.* Set the dryer on high, and hold it on the marks until the wax softens. Then wipe off the wax with a few drops of Murphy's Oil Soap® on a damp cloth.

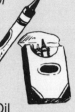

▶ *Get to work (or play) on time.* When time's a-wastin' and the pantyhose you need to wear are still damp, hang them on the shower rod and blow them dry.

▶ *Loosen up a pan-bound cake.* If you've baked a cake in a pan lined with wax paper and let it sit too long, unstick it by running a hair dryer, on high, over the bottom of the pan. Then turn the pan over very carefully, and ease the cake out.

▶ *Make bandage removal ouchless.* Blow hot air onto the ends for a few seconds. You'll soften the adhesive, so the tape will lift right off.

▶ *Reshape stretched sweater cuffs.* Just dip each cuff in hot water, then dry it on high.

▶ *Remove Contact® paper from shelves and drawers.* Use the warm setting, and heat up one small section at a time, gently lifting up the edges, and cutting off the paper as you go.

▶ *Remove hardened wax from candlesticks.* First put the candlesticks in the freezer for half an hour or so. Chip off as much wax as possible with your fingers, then set your dryer on low and blow the air over the drips until the wax melts. Then just wipe it away with a paper towel or soft, dry cloth.

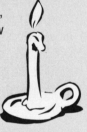

▶ *Shrink-wrap windows.* If you seal out Old Man Winter by taping plastic sheeting to your windows, a hair dryer can increase its protective powers. After you've attached the plastic, just turn the dryer dial to high and blast away. The covering will shrink to fit the glass.

CHAPTER TWO

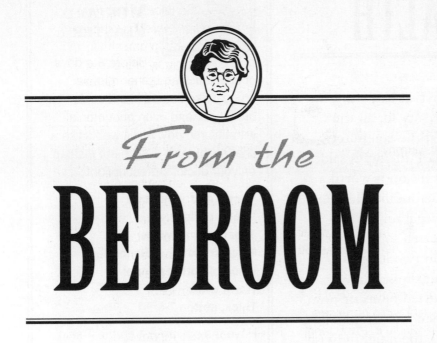

From the

BEDROOM

To your HEALTH

TIP Are your wrists beginning to pay the penalty for all the time you spend at the computer? Well, as Grandma Putt always said, an ounce of prevention is worth a pound of cure. Before that discomfort turns into carpal tunnel syndrome, make yourself some wrist supports. Just grab two long tube **SOCKS** from your dresser drawer, stuff them with dried beans or peas, and stitch the open ends closed. (Or, if you'd rather, tie them tightly with shoelaces.) Then put one tube in front of your keyboard, and the other at the front edge of your mouse pad. Now you can surf the Web to your heart's—and your wrists'—content!

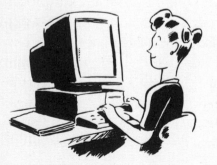

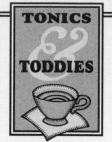

TONICS & TODDIES

GRANDMA PUTT'S OLD–TIME MUSTARD PLASTER

Before the days of antibiotics and other miracle drugs, folks treated chest colds, flu, bronchitis, and even pneumonia with this remedy. It still works like a charm—but use it *with*, not *instead of*, your doctor's prescription!

¼ **cup of dry mustard**
¼ **cup of flour**
3 tbsp. of molasses
Thick cream or softened lard
Piece of cotton flannel
Warm water
Thick, cotton T-shirt

Have the patient put on the T-shirt and lie down. Then mix the mustard and flour together, and stir in the molasses. Add enough cream or lard to get an ointment consistency. Dip the cotton flannel in the warm water, wring it out, and lay it on the patient's throat and upper chest, on top of the T-shirt. Apply the mustard mixture to the damp cloth, and leave it on for 15 minutes, or until the skin starts to turn red. *Caution:* This stuff is *hot*, so wear rubber gloves as you work with it, and make sure none touches the patient's bare skin.

TIP A pair of thick, cotton **SOCKS** can be the best pals your feet ever had—that is, if those dogs are prone to getting either dry and cracked, or tired and achy. I keep a couple of pairs close at hand, so when the need arises, I can whip up one of Grandma Putt's special tootsie treats, pronto. Then I spread the potion on my feet, put on the socks (to protect my sheets from the usually greasy ingredients), and hop into bed. (For a whole lot of foot-friendly treatments, see Chapters 3 and 4.)

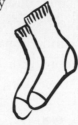

TIP Before you use a prepackaged ice pack to soothe a headache or muscle pain, cushion the cold slab by popping it into a soft, thick **SOCK.**

TIP When a chest cold, flu, or bronchitis strikes, pull a clean, thick **T-SHIRT** out of the drawer, and put it on (or have the patient in your care put it on). Then administer relief in the form of "Grandma Putt's Old-Time Mustard Plaster" (at left). You'll find more of Grandma's home remedies in Chapters 3 and 4.

Your GOOD LOOKS

TIP If you color your tresses and you do the job at home, here's a helpful hint: Before you begin, put on a stretchy, terry-cloth **HEAD-BAND,** and tuck cotton balls or pads inside. It's a more efficient way to catch drips than the usual method of "pasting" cotton to your head with petroleum jelly. (*Note:* This headband trick also works to keep home-permanent solution out of your eyes.)

TIP Before you treat yourself to any old-time beauty routines—or even a home permanent—protect your clothes from spills by making a smock, like the ones they give you at the beauty parlor. That's what Grandma did, and the process couldn't be simpler: Just grab an old **SHEET,** cut a head hole in the center, and a slit on each side for your arms. Then you're good to go. (In Chapters 3 and 4, you'll find a spa's worth of recipes for lotions, potions, creams, and masks.)

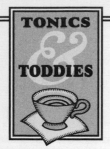

TONICS & TODDIES

CEREAL SCRUBBER

Here's an easy, and gentle, way to soften up rough heels, knees, and elbows—your whole body, for that matter.

1 part dry oatmeal
1 part baking soda
3 parts water

Mix the ingredients together in a bowl. Then use a cloth to apply the mixture to your body in a circular motion, paying special attention to areas that are rough, dry, or cracked.

fabric is cool, comfortable, and much wider than regular dressmaking material—so even if you're using fancy designer sheets, it's likely to cost you a lot less than you'd pay for similarly patterned cotton in a fabric store. (For a rundown on standard sheet sizes, see page 60.)

TIP If your bathroom is short on storage space, hang a **SHOE BAG** on a wall or door to hold cosmetics, toiletries, and other grooming tools.

TIP Need still more room for all your makeup gear? Take a tip from Grandma Putt: Put a plastic or cardboard **SHOE HOLDER** (the kind with separate, boxlike compartments) in the vanity cabinet under the sink, and stash small jars, bottles, and tubes in the cubbyholes.

TIP In Grandma's day, bed sheets were white—period. But if she could see the bright colors and pretty designs on **SHEETS** today, you know what she'd do? She'd get herself a few all-cotton sheets, cut 'em up, and sew herself some summer dresses or skirts using the colorful fabric. It's a great idea because the

TIP Turn a white cotton **SOCK** inside out, slip it over your hand, and bingo—you've got an exfoliating bath mitt—the perfect tool for applying my Cereal Scrubber (above). (There are a lot more remarkable recipes where this one came from, and you'll find 'em in Chapters 3 and 4.)

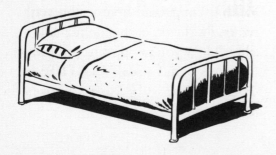

Around the
HOUSE

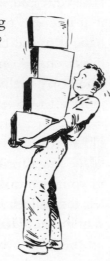

TIP Are you getting ready to move? Before you run out and buy packing material, "shop" first in your bedroom. **BLANKETS,** sheets, comforters, bed- spreads, and clothes will protect your household goods as well as bubble wrap and foam "peanuts" can. They won't leave smudges behind, as newspaper does. Best of all, they're free—and you have to move them anyway!

TIP You're about to start a wood- working project, and you know the dust is going to fly like crazy, but you don't want to spend time running out to buy a dust mask. So don't. Run to the bed- room, and pull out a padded **BRA** that's seen better days. Then cut off one of the cups, put it over your nose and mouth, and secure it with a headband or an old pantyhose leg. (The padding in many bras is made of the same stuff used in the disposable masks they sell in hard- ware stores.)

TIP Whenever I'd come home on a rainy day with my sneakers sopping wet, Grandma Putt would reach for a wire **CLOTHES HANGER** and bend the corners straight up. Then she'd tie one shoe to each side, and pop the hanger hook over the shower rod. (Or, if the rain had stopped by then, she'd hang it outside on the clothesline.)

TIP Turn a wire **CLOTHES HANGER** into a bunny hunter—dust bunnies, that is (like the ones that hide out under your furniture and refrigerator). Just bend the hanger into a long loop, and tie about half a dozen strips of old pantyhose onto the wire. Then, get down on your hands and knees, and go for it!

TIP Don't bother to take down the curtains before you wash your windows. Instead, just pull them as far to the side as you can, drape the ends over a **CLOTHES HANGER,** and pop the hook over the curtain rod.

Like many of the appliances that we take for granted today, **ELECTRIC BLANKETS** first hit the retail stores when Grandma Putt was getting on in years. But the basic concept goes back to her girlhood—1912, to be precise—when S.I. Russell patented an electric heating pad to warm the chests of tuberculosis patients. Almost immediately, inventors all over the country grabbed the idea and ran with it. Experiments went on through the 1930s, but no one could overcome two obstacles to public acceptance. One was price: Even Mr. Russell's little square pads sold for $150 each (more than most folks made in a month). Then there was the, um, disquieting fact that the wires frequently overheated and burst into flames.

Fast forward to World War II, when the Army wanted heated flight suits for its Air Corps pilots. Using good old Yankee ingenuity, military contractors found a way to surround heating elements with nonflammable plastics, and enclose them between two layers of fabric. When the war ended, that technology found its way into blanket makers' workrooms, and from there to bedrooms from coast to coast.

TIP As all of you costume-jewelry collectors know, bracelets and necklaces that "live" in a drawer can turn into a knotted mess in no time flat. But I know an easy way to keep them tangle-free and ready to wear. Just get a wooden **CLOTHES HANGER** and screw cup hooks into it at intervals of 1 inch or so. Then hang it in the closet, and drape your beads, chains, and pendants over the hooks. By the way, this also works great for organizing belts.

TIP You say you still have your grandma's wooden **CRADLE** in your bedroom, and your "baby" left for college last month? Here's a way to keep that beautiful heirloom on the job: Tote it into the living room, and use it to hold firewood or magazines (that is, until your first grandchild is ready to rock).

TIP If you're flying off on vacation and taking along some fragile items, then this tip's for you: Instead of packing those goodies in your regular carry-on tote, use a **DIAPER BAG.** It's the right size, it's lightweight—and it's padded. On the other hand, maybe you're starting out empty-handed, but you expect to come back with a few breakable treasures. In that case, fold up the bag and tuck it into your suitcase, so you'll have it for the return trip.

TIP Long after her children were grown and gone, Grandma Putt kept right on buying cloth **DIAPERS.** I still do. How come? Because there simply are no better cloths for polishing fine furniture, cars, and anything else that you want to keep smooth and gleaming.

TIP Do you have some post **EARRINGS** that you rarely, if ever, wear? If so, haul 'em out of your jewelry box and pull off the backs. Then use those little baubles as pushpins in a bulletin board.

TIP If you're like most women I know, you have two or three **HANDBAGS** that you use all the time, and several more that just sit on the closet shelf. But they don't have to. For instance, move one to your craft or sewing room to hold yarn, quilting templates, and other small gear. Use another to corral tools or emergency supplies in the car. Hang a rectangular purse by the door and make it the designated "outbox" for the family mail. The list could go on and on—if you just think outside the box, er, bag!

ONE MORE TIME

Got some **GLOVES** that have seen better days? Or maybe one of a pair has gone astray? That's too bad, but don't fret—there's gold in them thar fingers (that is, once you've cut 'em off of the hand part). Here's a handful of terrific ways to use those dandy digit covers:

▷ **Curtain protectors.** When you have to put curtains (especially sheers) on a metal rod, cover the end of the rod with a glove finger, so the fabric doesn't catch and fray.

▷ **Wall guards.** Pop glove fingers over the tips of broom and mop handles, so they don't leave marks when you lean them against walls.

▷ **Finger puppets.** Paint faces on them using markers or fabric paint. Or go whole hog, and sew or glue on the facial features, using tiny buttons for eyes and noses, and snippets of fabric for ears.

▷ **Thimbles.** Use a finger of an unlined leather glove to protect your own digit when you're sewing or doing needlework.

In Grandma's Day

Like a lot of folks I know, Grandma Putt just *loved* **BUTTONS.** But she didn't let them pile up in a jewelry box or a dresser drawer. She put those tiny trinkets to good use—even when she didn't have any clothes that needed them. You can, too. Here's a quintet of examples. (And I'm sure you can come up with a whole lot more!)

● Use tiny buttons to stuff "bean-bag" toys for the kids. Or, if your creations are small enough, sew a ribbon on top, and hang 'em on the Christmas tree.

● Glue decorative buttons of all sizes onto a plain wooden box or mirror frame. Presto—a useful work of folk art!

● Recycle big buttons as markers for board games.

● Make a one-of-a-kind vest or jacket by sewing fancy buttons all over the front. (Don't put 'em on the back, or you'll get a rather uncomfortable surprise the first time you lean back in a chair!)

● String big metal or plastic buttons together. Then hang them in fruit trees and bushes. The noise they make as they jangle in the wind will discourage hungry birds.

TIP Some **HANDKERCHIEFS,** especially the ones from Grandma Putt's era, seem too darn pretty and delicate to blow your nose with. So don't! Instead, do what a friend of mine did with her Grandma's hankies—turn them into pillows. Use a single one to make a mini pillow, or piece four or more together for a larger one. And, to make the most of a good thing, use your treasured textiles for the front of the pillow, and find coordinating fabric for the back.

TIP If you have a **JACKET** that's seen better days, give it—or at least the sleeves—a useful retirement. Just cut them off below the shoulders, stuff them with old socks or pantyhose, and put them to work blocking drafts under doors.

TIP When Grandma Putt got a new **JEWELRY BOX** for Christmas one year, she moved her old leather one from her bedroom to the living room, and used it to hold coasters, fireplace matches, and other small odds and ends. (You could even stash your TV and stereo remotes inside.)

TIP With just a **PANTS HANGER** (either the clamp or clip type) and a transparent plastic sleeve (available in office-supply stores), you can make quite a statement! What kind of statement, you ask? That's up to you. For instance, you might photocopy the ingredient-substitution chart on page 176, slide it into the sleeve, and hang it on the back of a cupboard door in your kitchen. Or copy the stain-removal chart on page 160, and suspend it from a hook by the washing machine. I could go on, but you get the idea.

TIP Make a laundry bag by running a drawstring through the top of a **PILLOWCASE.** In fact, if you know a youngster who's headed off to college, make three bags—color-coded for what Grandma called "the patriotic sorting method." That way (with luck), the young scholar will remember to keep her red shirts, white socks, and blue jeans separate in the wash!

TIP Here's the simplest way I know of to clean the crystals on a chandelier: Remove the glass baubles from the fixture, and very carefully put them into a clean **PILLOWCASE.** Then tie it closed, set the bundle on the top rack of your dishwasher, and run it through with the rest of your load. Those tiny treasures will come out sparkly bright!

TIP Instead of carrying a basket of laundry down the stairs, stuff those washables into a **PILLOW-CASE**—even if it's not one you intended to wash—and toss it down ahead of you. (After all, it's a lot more pleasant to wash and fold an extra pillowcase than it is to trip and take a tumble!)

TIP Prevent sock loss by binding each pair together with a **SAFETY PIN** before you toss them into the washing machine. (On pages 54 and 55, you'll find tons of terrific things to do with the socks that were orphaned *before* you read this tip.)

TIP When the time came to untrim our Christmas tree, Grandma Putt always spread a **SHEET** around the base. That way, any loose needles fell onto the fabric. When we'd taken off all of the ornaments, we'd wrap the sheet around the tree, haul 'er outside, and deck 'er out with edible treats for the neighborhood birds.

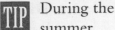 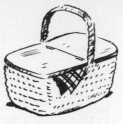

TIP During the summer, when all the fresh vegetables were coming in from the garden, we had a lot of picnics at our place. And Grandma always covered her rectangular picnic table with a fitted, twin-size **SHEET**—it was a perfect fit! What's more, the stitched corners kept the cloth in place whenever a breeze came up.

TIP If you need a 90-inch round tablecloth, but just can't find the color or pattern you want, make your own from a king-size **SHEET.** It's so big, you can cut your whole circle from one piece of fabric—no seams necessary!

TIP As you know if you've shopped for comforter covers lately (or duvet covers as the fancy catalogs call them), these things can cost a small fortune. If Grandma could see those price tags, she'd say, "Land sakes, that's highway robbery! After all, they're nothing more than two **SHEETS** stitched together!" Then she'd get herself two sheets, in the size and color(s) she wanted, and sew 'em together herself! You can, too—just turn the sheets front-to-front, and sew around both sides and one end. At the second end, attach your choice of fasteners. Snaps, buttons, ribbon ties, or Velcro® tape will all hold that comforter inside, where it belongs.

TIP Hang a **SHOE BAG** in the hall closet or mudroom to hold gloves, scarves, earmuffs, and other small outdoor gear.

ONE MORE TIME

Do you need **TIEBACKS** for some curtains you've just made (from sheets, perhaps)? Or maybe you'd just like to replace your plain, old fabric ties with something a little snazzier. Well, Grandma would give you this piece of frugal—and creative—advice: The first place to shop is your (or your spouse's) dresser. Chances are, those drawers hold a few things you haven't worn in donkeys' years, but will give you the best-dressed windows on the block. Here's a handful of suggestions:

▷ **Chain belts**

▷ **Fabric belts and sashes**

▷ **Leather shoelaces**

▷ **Necklaces**

▷ **Neckties**

▷ **Scarves**

TIP Pens, notepads, ink-jet cartridges, envelopes... In a home office, all those small supplies can add up to big-time clutter. Here's a simple solution to that problem: Just hang a **SHOE BAG** on the back of the closet door, or on the wall by your desk. Then stash your gear in the pockets.

TIP To save space in your kitchen cupboards, hang a clear, plastic **SHOE BAG** in your pantry, or on the back of a cupboard door. Then stash your dried herbs, spices, nuts, and other small, packaged foods in the pockets.

TIP Grandma Putt stored her **SHOE POLISH** in her bedroom, because (of course) that's where her shoes were. But she used it all over the house to patch up dings and scratches in her wood floors and furniture. Natural-color polish is perfect for any light-colored wood like pine or pecan. For darker woods, use tan, brown, or oxblood—experiment in a hidden spot until you find the shade that works the best. Then, just push the polish directly into the scratch, and watch it vanish!

TIP When Old Man Winter arrived at Grandma's place, we always set a freestanding **SHOE RACK** inside a boot tray, and used it for drying hats and mittens.

TIP Whenever you tumble-dry pillows or washable down jackets, toss a clean **SNEAKER** into the dryer. It'll balance the load and puff up the stuffing.

TIP Anytime she needed to keep a tablecloth in place, indoors or out, Grandma borrowed a pair of **SUSPENDERS** from Uncle Art or Grandpa Putt. She'd crisscross them under the table, clip them to the edges of the cloth, and adjust the suspender tabs to pull the cloth taut across the top.

TIP Wooden hangers put a lot less strain on clothes (especially delicate silks and lightweight cottons) than wire or plastic hangers do. There's just one problem: A lot of garments tend to slide off that slick, wood surface. Fortunately, there's a simple solution: Just slip a cotton **T-SHIRT** onto the hanger, then put your blouse, dress, or whatever on top.

ONE MORE TIME

 Have you ever wondered what becomes of all the single **SOCKS** that go astray between the laundry hamper and the end of the drying cycle? Well, I've never solved that mystery, but I do know a gazillion great uses for the lonely left-behinds. Here's a small sampling:

▷ **Baby-size knee guards.** Cut the tops off of a child's tube-type socks, and use them as knee pads for a crawling infant.

▷ **Back savers.** Instead of lifting heavy furniture to move it around a room, slip a soft, thick sock over each leg, and glide that piece to its new location.

▷ **Bird chasers.** Clip brightly colored socks to fruit-tree branches, your garden fence, or posts that you've stuck in the ground. When the birds see those mini banners waving in the breeze, they'll go elsewhere for dinner. (The secret to this trick lies in the vibrant color, which birds find scary, so save the pastels and earth tones for other purposes.)

▷ **Car window defogger.** Carry an orphaned sock in your car, and slip it over your hand when you need to wipe fog from the windows.

▷ **Cold-drink holders.** Cut the foot off of a clean sock and slip the ankle part over a glass. Then add ice, and pour in your cooling beverage.

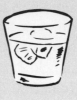

▷ **Dust cloths.** A cotton sock, pulled over your hand, is just the ticket for dusting knickknacks, mini or venetian blinds, or anything else, for that matter! To extend your reach, or to get into tight places (say, under the couch or clothes dryer), slip the sock over a yardstick or broom handle.

▷ **Exfoliating bath mitts.** Just turn a clean, white sock inside out, shove your hand inside, and use it in the bath or shower. It'll slough off those dead skin cells every bit as well as a store-bought cloth or loofah.

▷ **Hand puppets.** Paint or sew faces on plain-colored socks. Then call the kids together and say, "Let's give a puppet show!"

▷ **Jewelry holders.** Toss a sock into your gym bag. Then, when you take off your jewelry at the pool or health club, tuck it into the sock and knot the sock closed. You'll be able to retrieve your treasures quickly.

▷ **Junior-size shoe bags.** Pack children's shoes in grown-up socks when you're traveling.

▷ **Moth chasers.** Fill 'em with cedar shavings, or bug-repelling herbs (see Chapter 3 for some dandy choices), and tie the tops shut. Then, tuck 'em among your clothes and linens to fend off moths and silverfish.

▷ **Paintbrushes.** When you need to paint hard-to-reach places, like the inside edges of a radiator, or the back of a pipe that's close to the wall, use an old—but hole-free—sock. First, 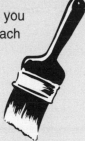 put on a rubber glove (in case the paint soaks through the sock), and slip the sock over that. Then dip your hand into the paint, reach for the object of your painting spree, and slide that slender "brush" right along.

▷ **Siding protectors.** Before you lean an extension ladder up against a wall, pop a thick sock over the tip of each side rail.

▷ **Sponge-mop extenders.** When your last mop head is on its last legs, and there's no time to go buy a new one, cover the old-timer with a thick, cotton sock (a puffy sneaker sock is perfect).

▷ **Tiny-dog sweaters.** Cut off the toe, and make two holes for the front legs. If you want the sweater to last for more than a wearing or two, hem or stitch around the "arm" holes so the fabric doesn't fray.

What *Not* to Do with Old Socks (or Shoes)

▷ *Never* recycle cast-off socks or shoes as puppy toys—or, if you do, don't blame young Rover if he chews up your good ones. To a dog, a threadbare sock or a battered loafer looks and smells *exactly* the same as your brand-new cashmere socks, your favorite slippers, or your fancy designer pumps.

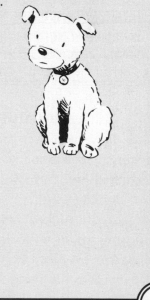

retain. Then cut the same size from the back. Put the back and front together, with the outsides facing each other, and stitch around three sides. Turn this "envelope" inside out, and fill it with the stuffing of your choice, such as old socks, pantyhose, cotton batting, or a premade pillow form. Then stitch the fourth side closed. A single pillow commemorating your visit to Yankee Stadium will be a conver-sation starter when folks come to visit. But a whole couch or porch swing filled with your gathered treasures will be an ever-growing, three-dimensional scrapbook!

Family and
FRIENDS

TIP Calling all **T-SHIRT** collectors! Have you ever thought of turning all those soft souvenirs into throw pillows? No? Well, maybe you should—especially if the color-ful gems are tucked away, unseen and unworn, in your dresser draw-ers. Just cut a piece from the front that includes the design and as much background as you'd like to

TIP A **BELT** can come in handy at the supermarket when you need to keep a toddler safely inside the seat of a shopping cart.

TIP A fabric **BELT** (the kind with metal D rings) is a dandy device for keeping toddlers and pets from exploring forbidden territory—like the cabinets in your kitchen, bathroom, or workshop. Just loop the belt around two of the knobs or handles on the doors, and pull it tightly through the rings.

TIP When my Uncle Art outgrew his high chair (long before I came on the scene), Grandma Putt stashed it in the attic, so she'd have it on hand when tiny tykes came to visit. At some point, the restraining strap had gone astray, but that was no problem: Grandma just used one of her elastic **BELTS** to hold the youngster in place. (If you don't have an elastic belt, any fabric or soft leather one will work just fine.)

TIP Baby the horse in your life by giving him a baby **BLANKET.** No, I don't mean you should put it in his stall so he can cuddle up with it at night! Just spread it across his back before you put on his saddle pad. The blanket will feel soft against his skin, and it'll be a darn sight easier for you to wash than that bulky pad.

TIP In the summer, Grandma Putt used to make me a giant bubble blower by bending a wire **CLOTHES HANGER** into a circle (more or less), leaving the hook in place to use as a handle. Then she'd pour Bombastic Bubble Solution (see page 58) into a shallow pan, dip the loop into the "drink," and draw it gently through the air—making the biggest bubbles I'd ever seen.

TIP Turn a fabric or lightweight leather **GLOVE** into a super-duper cat toy. First, sew a 10-inch length of ribbon to each fingertip. (Anywhere from ½- to ¾-inch ribbon will work.) Then, at the ends of the ribbon, tie, glue, or sew on pompoms, lightweight toys, empty thread spools, or tiny bags of catnip. At playtime, just pull on the glove, wave your hand around at Puffy's eye level, and watch her light up!

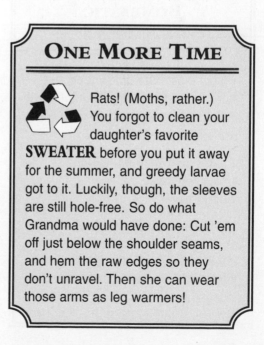

ONE MORE TIME

Rats! (Moths, rather.) You forgot to clean your daughter's favorite **SWEATER** before you put it away for the summer, and greedy larvae got to it. Luckily, though, the sleeves are still hole-free. So do what Grandma would have done: Cut 'em off just below the shoulder seams, and hem the raw edges so they don't unravel. Then she can wear those arms as leg warmers!

TIP Whenever you bathe an infant, do what Grandma always did: Wear cotton **GLOVES.** They'll give you a better grip than you'd have with bare hands, and they'll feel a whole lot better on the baby's skin than rubber gloves would.

TIP Here's an idea for all those snackers on your Christmas and birthday gift lists: Find a plastic **JEWELRY BOX** that has several partitions, and fill each cubbyhole with a different tiny treat. For instance, put raisins in one, miniature jelly beans in another, M&M'S® in a third, and so on.

TIP A lot of youngsters seem to go through a stage when they love playing pirate. (I know I did.) So Grandma gave me a **JEWELRY BOX** to use as a treasure chest. She even jump-started my hoard by tucking in some booty like marbles, coins, and shiny baubles.

TIP A **LINT-REMOVING ROLLER** (which you probably have in your bedroom) can help detick a short-haired dog or cat. Just roll that sticky tube over your pet's body; it'll pick up speck-size nymphs that you can barely see, much less grasp with tweezers.

TIP Turn a **NECKTIE** into a sea serpent. Just paint or sew a face on the wide end, stuff the "body" with old pantyhose or cotton batting, and stitch the whole thing shut. If you want to go all out, cut triangles out of felt, and glue or sew them in a line along the back to form the monster's dorsal fins.

GRANDMA PUTT'S
Secret Formulas

BOMBASTIC BUBBLE SOLUTION

Just like any other kid, I loved blowing bubbles, but I didn't need a store-bought solution. Grandma Putt made me a never-ending supply using this simple recipe.

2 parts dishwashing liquid
1 part vegetable oil
2 parts water

Mix the ingredients together in a shallow bowl or tub. Then dip your bubble blower into the fabulous fluid, and make marvelous, miraculous bubbles.

Then give your creation to your favorite dragon-loving child, or use it as a draft-stopper under a door.

TIP When a genuine emergency strikes, and you need to vacate your house *fast*, don't waste time looking for your cat's carrier. Just grab the kitty, pop her into a **PILLOWCASE,** and make tracks! (This is also a great way to corral a tiny dog or puppy.)

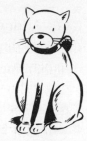

TIP Grandma made my very first Halloween costume from (can you believe this?) a white **PILLOWCASE.** She cut arm- and eyeholes in the appropriate places, and there I was—the scariest, tiniest ghost on the block! If you'd like to try something a little more elaborate, just paint, sew, or glue on the design of your (or the trick-or-treater's) choice. For instance, add eyes, ears, and a nose to a white case, and you've got a polar bear cub!

TIP You can also turn a **PILLOWCASE** into a small child's painting smock (another of Grandma's favorite tricks). Simply cut openings for the youngster's arms and head, and he's ready to get creative.

ONE MORE TIME

Before you toss your threadbare **CLOTHES** in the ragbag or (heaven forbid!) the trash can, think twice. As Grandma Putt knew well, even when clothes are too far gone for anyone to wear, there can still be a lot of life left in the fabric. Offer it to a scout troop, senior center, quilters' group, or an artist who works in mixed media. Here's a sampling of possible second "careers" for those duds:

▷ **Appliqués or patches for other clothes**

▷ **Collage makings**

▷ **Decorative coverings for shoeboxes and other homemade storage containers**

▷ **Doll and teddy bear clothes**

▷ **Dollhouse upholstery, rugs, or linens**

▷ **Pillows**

▷ **Quilt squares**

▷ **Rag rug strips**

TIP To add real pizzazz to a present, wrap it in a pretty **SCARF** instead of paper. Or, for the young cowboy or cowgirl in your life, use a big bandanna instead.

Sheet Sizing

As Grandma Putt knew, sheets can do a lot more than just cover a bed. But, whether you're using them to wrap a present, cover a picnic table, or make a summer frock for yourself (or your granddaughter), it helps to know what size sheet you'll need. The exact measurements vary somewhat from one manufacturer to another, but here are the general guidelines.

Sheet Size	Measurements in Inches (width x length)
Twin	66 × 96
Twin, extra-long	66 × 102
Full (a.k.a. double)	81 × 96
Queen	90 × 102
King	108 × 102
California King	108 × 110

TIP When you hit the road with children or pets, drape a king-size **SHEET** over your car's backseat and floor. Then, when you come to a rest stop, pull it out and shake off all the cookie crumbs or pet hair.

TIP If your children or grandchildren sleep in bunk beds, as I did at Grandma's house, here's a simple way to give the kid on the bottom a better view: Just put a colorful, fitted **SHEET** on the bottom of the top mattress. Better yet, use a plain white or light-colored sheet, and let the bottom-dweller paint his own design, using markers or fabric paint.

TIP When Christmas or a birthday rolls around, and you have a really big present to give, do what Santa Claus did the year I got my first sled: Wrap that bulky treasure in a **SHEET.** (Back then, of course, the only color choice was white, but nowadays, you have a rainbow of shades—and even seasonal patterns—to choose from.)

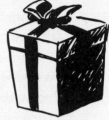

TIP Heading off on a long road trip with a young child? Relieve his boredom—and save your sanity—by making him a portable "playroom." First, find a **SHOE BAG** (the kind that fastens to a wall or door), and hang it over the back of the front seat. Then fill the pockets with an assortment of small toys, games, and books, as well as some nonmessy snacks. Or, if you want to block the hot sun, and the youngster doesn't mind losing the view, fasten the bag from the hook above a backseat window.

TIP Whenever one of Grandma Putt's young grandchildren came for a visit, she had a terrific way to keep him or her amused for hours: She'd hang a **SHOE BAG** in the playpen, so the tot inside could practice putting toys in the pockets.

TIP A young mother I know is a lawyer who has to buy a lot of "court-appropriate" business suits and dresses. They all seem to come with **SHOULDER PADS,** which she doesn't care for, so she takes them out—and tapes them onto the corners of tables, so her toddler won't get hurt when he waddles into them!

TIP Here's a clever tip for all you Santas (right out of Grandma Putt's idea bank): Wrap small Christmas presents in red or green **SOCKS,** and use white sneaker laces as "ribbon."

TIP Moving to a new house is even more stressful for dogs and cats than it is for us humans. To keep your critters from running off in confusion and panic, put them in a securely closed room while the furniture is being moved in. And give them an unlaundered **SWEAT-**SHIRT or T-shirt of yours to snuggle up to. The familiar scent will help ease their fears and steady their nerves.

TIP Give young Rembrandt or Georgia O'Keefe a grownup's **T-SHIRT** to wear as a painting smock.

In Grandma's Day

Grandma never owned more than a few pairs at a time, but she would have been fascinated to learn that folks have been wearing **SHOES** for at least 4,000 years (the earliest known example is a woven-papyrus sandal found in an Egyptian tomb built in 2000 B.C.). But footgear was not made in standard sizes until the early 1300s. King Edward I of Britain realized that his empire needed an accurate system of measurement. So, in 1305, he decreed that the length of three contiguous dried barleycorns would be considered 1 inch. British cobblers adopted the system, using barleycorns as their guide. Customers began requesting shoes that measured, say, 30 barleycorns, and before long, "size 10."

The great
OUTDOORS

TIP When you're just learning to play golf, one of the hardest techniques to grasp is moving your arms in unison when you swing. It was *murder* for me—until a golf pro taught me this practice trick. Get a **BELT** (either fabric or leather will do), and fasten it around both arms at your biceps. Then grab a club, and swing. You'll be forced to move both arms as a single unit. Eventually, your muscles will get in the habit of working that way, even without their training "wheels."

TIP Grandma Putt was not an expert on cars, but she gave me what may be the best automotive advice ever I've ever heard: Always keep a **BLANKET** in the trunk. That way, you're prepared if you decide to stop for an impromptu picnic, get stranded in the cold, or encounter accident victims who need help.

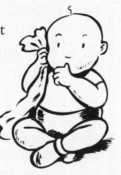

TIP A **BLANKET** comes in handy when you need to load or unload the trunk and your car's exterior is less than spotless. Just drape it over the back of the trunk and the bumper, and proceed with your task—confident that you won't mess up your clothes in the process.

TIP As I imagine you know by now, there's nothing my Grandma Putt loved better than puttering in her garden. She even enjoyed getting down on her knees and pulling weeds. In fact, she could spend hours doing that—thanks to the knee protectors she made by cutting the cups off of an old padded **BRA!**

TIP Turn a wire **CLOTHES HANGER** into a debris-skimmer for a garden pond or child's wading pool. Just bend the hanger into a circle (more or less), and cover the loop with an old pantyhose leg. For more great uses for pantyhose, see page 64.

TIP As far as Grandma Putt was concerned, nothing said "summertime" like a garden full of sweet corn, growing as high as an elephant's eye and headed straight for the moon. Unfortunately, the neighborhood raccoons, birds, and squirrels shared her taste in food. But they didn't get the goodies at Grandma's place, because she knew just what those critters *didn't* like: **PERFUME.** Every year, just after the corn pollen had dropped, she'd put a little cloth cap over each ear, tie it on loosely with string, and touch the top with a dab of fragrance (usually from a sample she'd gotten for free at the local department store). Those rampaging robbers got their kicks—and their corn—in somebody else's garden! Instead of pieces of cloth, you can make your ear-toppers from pantyhose toes. For a gazillion other great ways to use pantyhose, see page 64.

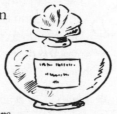

TIP Grandma Putt always kept several big compost piles cookin' at her place. You can't very well do that if you garden on a balcony or patio, as lots of folks do these days. But that doesn't mean you have to buy your "black gold" at the garden center. A plastic **SWEATER BOX** (like the ones you probably have in your closet or under your bed) makes a great mini compost bin. Just drill holes in the bottom, set the box on strips of wood, and tuck it out of sight behind a planter or trellis.

TIP You can also turn those plastic **SWEATER BOXES** into Lilliputian storage "sheds." A friend of mine, who gardens on a tenth-story balcony in Manhattan, uses them to store hand tools, potting soil, organic fertilizer, and all sorts of other horticultural helpers.

TIP Even if your garden covers acres, plastic **SWEATER BOXES** can come in mighty handy as terrific seed-starter flats. You can approach the project in one of two ways. Either fill the box with individual, draining containers, or drill holes in the bottom, fill the whole thing with starter mix, and sow your seed. Then invert the lid for a nifty drainage tray, and set the box in that. Now you're good to grow!

Pantyhose

It's too bad that Grandma Putt didn't live to see the debut of pantyhose, in 1958. In fact, she was already a grandma when nylon stockings came on the market in 1940. Throughout the war years, they remained in such short supply that nobody could buy many of them—certainly not enough to build a stockpile of oldies the way folks can nowadays. I'll tell you one thing, though: If Ethel Grace Puttnam were with us today, she'd have a ball inventing "second careers" for these gauzy marvels. "Just think of the possibilities!" she'd say. Like these, for instance.

Around the House

▶ *Ah, dry up!* Fill a pantyhose foot with a few sticks of chalk, or a lump or two of charcoal, and tie it shut. Then hang it in your basement, or anyplace else where dampness is a problem.

▶ *Clean dust magnets.* It's no secret that metal mini blinds and computer and television screens attract dust like there's no tomorrow—and so does pantyhose!

▶ *Dry a sweater without stretching.* Instead of clipping it directly to the laundry line, string a pair of pantyhose through the sleeves, and clip the toes to the line.

▶ *Dust in those hard-to-reach places.* Shove a yardstick or a thin strip of wood partway down one pantyhose leg, leaving the foot and lower leg empty. Then reach behind the dryer, under the fridge, up to the top bookshelf—or anyplace else dust clouds are gathered.

▶ *Hang your onions.* And garlic, too. Just drop a bulb into a pantyhose leg, tie a knot, drop in another one, and so on. When you want to use one of the bulbs, cut just below the knot above it.

▶ *Hold that soil.* Before you put a plant in a pot (indoors or out), lay a square of pantyhose over the pot's drainage hole to keep the potting mix from leaking out.

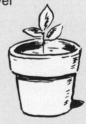

➤ *Mend a window screen (temporarily).* Cut a patch of pantyhose that's about half an inch larger all around than the tear in your screen. Then brush rubber cement over the tear, and press the patch into place. Later, if you want to make a permanent repair (rather than replace the whole screen), peel off the patch, and rub the cement away with your finger.

➤ *Polish your floor.* Pull a pantyhose leg over your mop, and proceed as usual with the shiner-upper of your choice (perhaps one of the super-duper ones in Chapters 3, 4, and 5).

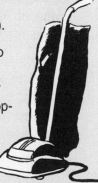

➤ *Save your stuff.* To vacuum dust from drawers, counters, or shelves without swooping up the contents, cover the cleaner's nozzle with a pantyhose leg.

➤ *Scrub walls.* Also windows, furniture—and even nonstick cookware. Just wad the pantyhose into a ball, and use it as you would any sponge or scrub pad.

➤ *Simplify post-Christmas cleanup.* After you haul the tree outside—and *before* you start cleaning up the aftermath—put a pantyhose leg over the vacuum cleaner nozzle. The needles will stick to the nylon instead of being swooshed inside to clog up the vacuum. When you've finished the job, just peel off the stocking over a wastebasket, and drop it inside.

➤ *Stuff stuff.* Use old pantyhose as stuffing in toys, throw pillows, and draft-stoppers.

Out and About

➤ *Block chilly winds.* When a cold snap strikes, either at the beginning or end of the growing season, cover small plants with pantyhose. Just cut off a piece, knot the top, slip it over a plant, and pull the bottom closed.

➤ *Collect seashells.* On your next trip to the beach, take along a pair of old pantyhose, and use the legs to hold the shells you pick up. Then, before you head for home, just dunk the whole shebang in the water to rinse off the sand.

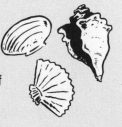

(continued)

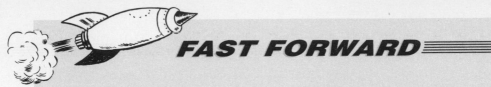

FAST FORWARD

(continued from page 65)

▶ *Give your garden a drink.* Of compost tea, that is—it's the healthiest libation a plant could ask for. Just fill a pantyhose leg with "black gold" and let it steep in 5 to 10 gallons of water for three or four days. Then pull out the "tea bag," and serve up the brew. (You can make manure tea—another bracing garden beverage—the same way.

▶ *Guard your garbage.* To keep raccoons, dogs, and other roving rascals out of your trash can, secure the lid down with a pair of old pantyhose. Just loop them through the handle on top, and tie one leg to each of the side handles.

▶ *Hold the odor.* Use pantyhose legs to hold aromatic critter deterrents, like deodorant soap, bloodmeal, or hair (from either humans or pets).

▶ *Keep debris out of a rain barrel.* Put a piece of pantyhose over the end of the downspout, and fasten it with a rubber band.

▶ *Prevent pest damage.* Cover ripening fruits, vegetables, and sunflower heads with pantyhose to protect them from nibbling insects, rodents, and birds.

▶ *Put your plants on the up-and-up.* Tie up vines and floppy plants with strips of pantyhose. Besides supporting the stems, the nylon will attract static electricity, which will give your plants added get-up-and-grow power.

▶ *Scrub up.* Cut off a pantyhose leg, tuck a bar of soap into the toe, and hang it up near your handiest outdoor faucet. Then clean the dirt off *before* you head inside.

▶ *Store bulbs for the winter.* When you dig up gladiolus and other tender bulbs, dust them with medicated baby powder, drop them into a pantyhose leg, and hang in a cool, dry place.

▶ *Wash your car.* Scrunch pantyhose into a ball, and use the wad to polish the old jalopy without harming the finish.

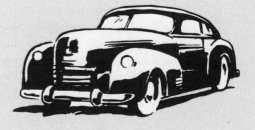

For You and Yours

▶ *Brew a relaxing bath.* Cut off a pantyhose leg about halfway up, put one of Grandma's bath-time "teas" into the toe, and knot the top. Toss this "tea bag" under running water in the tub, then sink in and soak your cares away. (See Chapters 3 and 4 for some oh-so-soothing Tonics & Toddies.)

▶ *Captivate your cat.* Stuff a panty-hose toe with catnip, and tie it shut. Then toss the toy to Fluffy and watch her jump for joy!

▶ *Clean and soften your skin.* Follow the directions for the "tea bag" described in "Brew a relaxing bath" above, but substitute cleansing grains for the "tea." Then, step into the tub or shower, and scrub-a-dub-dub! (Chapters 3 and 4 are also chock-full of recipes for skin-softening cleansers.)

▶ *Keep wet shoes in shape.* Just stuff them with pantyhose, so they'll hold their shape as they dry.

▶ *Make pony- and pigtail holders.* Cut across a pantyhose leg to make rings that are about an inch wide. Then roll them up, so they're rounded, like the ones you buy in stores.

▶ *Muzzle a frightened or injured dog.* Cut off a pantyhose leg, and tie it gently around Rover's snout to keep him from snapping in panic or pain.

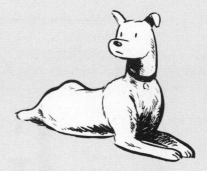

▶ *Remove nail polish.* Just cut pantyhose into 1-inch rings, dampen them with polish remover, and rub off the polish.

▶ *Scrub your back.* Cut off a panty-hose leg, put a bar of soap inside, roughly at the center of the length of the leg, and tie a knot at each side of the soap. Then, just grasp one end of the hose in each hand, and glide the soap holder back and forth across your back.

CHAPTER THREE

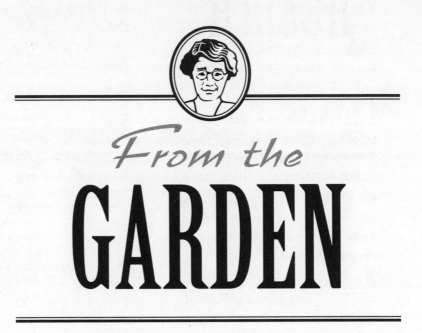

From the

GARDEN

To your
HEALTH

TIP Grandma Putt always kept an **ALOE VERA** plant growing on a sunny windowsill in her kitchen. And I'll tell you, that plant was a regular first aid kit! Grandma used it to treat everything from kitchen burns, cuts, and scratches to sunburn, frostbite, poison ivy, insect bites—and even skin that was simply dry or irritated. To put this miracle stuff to work, just snap off a lower leaf near the center stalk. Remove any spines, and then split the leaf in half lengthwise. Scrape out the gel and apply it directly to the affected site.

TIP Anytime I'd come down with a bout of stomach flu, Grandma would hand me a big glass of **APPLE** juice, and tell me to drink up. It nearly always sent the nasty tummy bug packin', and now I know why: Apples contain compounds that act very much like penicillin to fight flu and other viruses.

TIP **APPLES** also fight tooth decay. So, to help keep the dentist away (as well as the doctor), just munch a slice or two of apple after each meal or snack.

TIP Are you trying to lose weight? Then wake up and smell the **BANANAS!** Studies have shown that dieters who sniffed a banana whenever they felt like munching lost an average of 30 pounds in 6 months.

TIP When you're battling a headache that just *won't* go away, try this old-time remedy: First, put a bottle of witch hazel in the refrigerator to chill for an hour or two (better yet, keep a bottle stashed there). Then, put 1 teaspoon of dried **BASIL** into 1 cup of hot (not boiling) water, and let it sit for 10 minutes. Strain it into a large bowl, let it cool, and add 2 tablespoons of cold witch hazel. Soak a cotton washcloth or hand towel in the tea, wring it out, and lay the compress over your forehead and temples. Before you know it, you'll feel blessed relief! (If, no matter what you do, your headache persists for more than a day, get yourself to the emergency room, pronto.)

them aside. Put 1 quart of water in a pan, bring it to a boil, and reduce it to a simmer. Add 3 tablespoons of the bark, cover, and let it simmer for about 10 minutes. Remove the pan from the heat, and let the contents steep for an hour. Strain out the solids, soak a clean, cotton cloth in the tea, wring it out slightly (you want it to be wet, but not dripping), and lay it on the affected skin. Repeat the procedure as often as you like to bring relief from pain and itching. (*Note:* If you don't have any birch trees growing nearby, you can order bark from many herb shops and some botanical gardens.)

TIP Grandma also made an antiseptic solution from **BIRCH BARK,** and used it to treat cuts and wounds of all kinds. To mix up your own supply, pour 1 pint of vodka into a jar with a tight-fitting lid, and add ½ cup of dried birch bark (either ground or broken into small pieces). Let it sit for two weeks or so, shaking the jar once a day. Strain the liquid into a clean bottle, through fine cheesecloth; old, clean pantyhose; or a coffee filter. Put a lid on the bottle, and store it in the

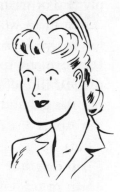

TIP When Grandma Putt was just a little girl, growing up on her Grandpa Coolidge's farm, she learned how to make a powerful **BIRCH BARK** poultice for treating nasty skin conditions like acne, eczema, and psoriasis. If you want to try this trick at home, it's easy. Just peel off a patch of birch bark, and let it dry in the sun. Then break or grind it into small pieces, and set

medicine chest. Use it whenever you need to disinfect cuts, scrapes, or sores of any kind.

TIP Boils can be as painful as all get-out, and the very dickens to heal. But Grandma Putt knew a lot of garden-variety cures for the nasty nuisances. One of the simplest was to cover the spot with a raw **CABBAGE** leaf. Hold it in place with a bandage or strip of cotton cloth, and leave it on for about half an hour. Repeat several times a day, waiting two or three hours between treatments.

TIP If you suffer from arthritis, or know someone who does, this tip has your name on it: Pull a few sturdy, outer leaves from a head of **CABBAGE,** blanch them until they're soft (but not falling apart), and apply them to the inflamed joints. Secure them with a gauze wrap or elastic bandage, and leave them in place for half an hour or so.

TIP Blanched **CABBAGE** leaves can also reduce facial inflammation caused by burns, acne, or surgery. Once or twice a day, apply the wet leaves to your face, and keep them on for 5 to 10 minutes. (This will take close attention, because the leaves will be slippery!)

TIP When Grandma was a youngster, no one thought it was odd to see someone walking around with a raw **CABBAGE** leaf under his hat—it was a favorite way to cure headaches.

TONICS & TODDIES

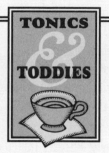

HEIRLOOM FLU STOPPER

When Grandma was growing up, antibiotics were few and far between—and a vaccine lay decades ahead. Getting the flu was serious business. That's why, when anyone in the family showed signs of coming down with the Big F, Grandma pulled out the big guns, in the form of this powerful potion.

1 large, tart, juicy apple
1 qt. of water
2 shots of whiskey
½ tsp. of lemon juice
Honey (optional)

Boil the apple in the water until the apple falls apart. Strain out the solids, and add the whiskey and lemon juice to the remaining liquid. Sweeten to taste with honey, if you like. Then get in bed and drink the toddy. If you've acted in time, by morning, those germs will be history!

TIP **CARROTS** and their juice are loaded with germ-killing chemicals that make them perfect for fighting infections, and for reducing swelling and inflammation. To treat sunburn and other minor burns, first sponge the skin with ice water. Then, dip gauze in fresh carrot juice (either made in your home juicer, or bought at your local organic market), and squeeze it out so it's wet, but not dripping. Put this dressing over the affected area, and secure it lightly with more gauze or lightweight fabric. Repeat several times a day until the pain and swelling are gone.

TIP Drinking lukewarm **CARROT** juice was one of Grandma's most effective methods for relieving asthma symptoms.

TIP When a sore throat strikes, douse the flames with a **CARROT** poultice. Just grate a large carrot and spread it on a soft, clean cloth. Wrap it around your throat (with the gratings against your skin, of course!) and cover it with a scarf to keep it in place. Leave it until the gratings lose their cool feeling, and repeat every few hours, as needed.

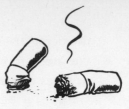

TIP Trying to quit smoking? Do what Grandma Putt recommended: Whenever you get the urge to light up a cigarette, reach for a raw **CARROT** instead. I'll bet gold bricks to bunny rabbits that before long, your craving for "cancer sticks" will be history.

TIP Of all the plants in Grandma's garden-variety medicine chest, **CATNIP** was one of the most versatile. She used catnip tea for everything from reducing fevers to

ONE MORE TIME

The next time you chop the tops off of your home-grown **CARROTS,** don't toss 'em—turn 'em into mouthwash. Those frilly greens are chock-full of antiseptic compounds that kill germs and sweeten your breath. Here's all you need to do: Boil 3 cups of water in a pan, add ½ cup of chopped carrot tops, and simmer for 20 minutes. Remove the pan from the heat, and let it sit for another half hour. Strain, and store the potion in a tight-lidded glass container in the refrigerator. Then use it to rinse and gargle each morning, as you would with any mouthwash.

relieving nausea and nasal-allergy symptoms. And, of course, a nice, strong "cuppa" was just what Dr. Grandma ordered whenever she or Grandpa had trouble sleeping at night—or when I just didn't want to settle down and go to bed. She made it using the simple, all-purpose herb tea recipe in "Tea Times Two" on page 78.

TIP When a cold, flu, allergy attack, or (gasp!) a night on the town leaves your eyes swollen and inflamed, treat those peepers to a **CATNIP** eyewash. To make this restorative elixir, bring 3 cups of water to a boil, and add 2 tablespoons of fresh catnip leaves. Reduce the heat setting to low, and simmer for three minutes (no more!). Remove the pan from the burner, and let the brew steep for another 50 minutes. Then strain out the solids, pour the liquid into a clean glass jar, and store it in the refrigerator. When the need arises, either fill an eyecup with the elixir and bathe your eyes several times a day, or 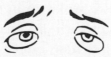 soak a terry-cloth towel in the solution and put it over your eyes for half an hour—repeating the process until you feel relief.

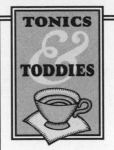

TONICS & TODDIES

REMEDY FOR THE RUNS

Diarrhea is no fun now, and it was no more amusing in Grandma's day. Fortunately, she had a great-tasting cure that was as close as one of her backyard apple trees.

1 apple, peeled and cored
1 tsp. of lime juice
1 tsp. of honey
Pinch of cinnamon

Puree all of the ingredients in a blender or food processor, pour the mixture into a bowl, and eat up. Just a few words of caution: Never give this concoction—or anything containing honey—to a baby under one year of age. And, if the diarrhea lasts more than a day or two, call your doctor.

TIP Sore gums or aching teeth called for **CATNIP** leaves, straight from one of Grandma's plants. She'd just pop a leaf into her mouth, and hold it against the painful area until the hurt went away—which was nearly always faster than you can say, "Here, kitty, kitty!"

TIP After a long, hectic day, calm your frazzled nerves with a **CELERY-CARROT** cocktail. Just mix equal parts of celery and carrot juice, and add honey to taste, if you'd like. Then sit back, relax, and drink up!

In Grandma's Day

Most folks think **DANDELIONS** are nothing but nasty old weeds. But to Grandma Putt, having a patch of those golden flowers growing in her yard was like having a drugstore right on her doorstep! She said every part of the plant was good for you—and it was especially effective against indigestion, and kidney and liver problems. She tossed the young leaves in salads, steamed the older ones just as she did spinach, and roasted the roots to make coffee. But that's not all! Every night before dinner, she had a small glass of dandelion wine (see her recipe on page 76), and throughout the day, she sipped two or three cups of her dandelion tea. (You'll find that recipe in a tip on page 75.) It must have worked: Grandma was the healthiest woman in town!

TIP One time, Grandpa Putt came down with a case of the gout, and Grandma advised him to eat 15 to 20 sweet **CHERRIES** a day until the pain and swelling went away. It sounded like a good idea to him, so he gobbled up his full ration, and before we knew it, he was back on his feet, as good as new.

TIP That same sweet **CHERRY** remedy works wonders to ease arthritis pain and stiffness.

TIP Sprained ligaments are no bed of roses. But a stroll (or hobble) into the herb garden can speed up the recovery process. Just pluck two to four leaves from a **COMFREY** plant, blanch them, and put them over the sprained body part. Cover the leaves with an elastic bandage, and go about your business. Renew the dressing every day, and you'll be back in the running before you know it.

TIP What's that? You say you woke up in the middle of the night with dry, chapped lips, and you're fresh out of lip balm? Well, don't run out to the all-night convenience store—that is, not if you have a store-bought **CUCUMBER** in the kitchen. Just wash the cuke, dry it with a clean towel, and run your lips back and forth over the waxy peel several times. This veggie stand-in will never replace ChapStick®, but it *will* let you snooze in comfort until you can get to the store the next morning!

TIP **CUCUMBER** juice also helps relieve the pain and itch of eczema. Just dab it onto your skin once a day with a cotton pad.

TIP Whenever I spent too much time at the ol' swimming hole and came home with a painful 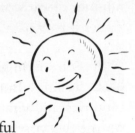 sunburn, Grandma Putt knew exactly what to do: She had me soak in a tepid bath with a few tablespoons of **CUCUMBER** juice added to it. (To make cucumber juice, just puree a cuke, strain out the seeds and pulp, and pour the juice into a bowl.)

TIP When your feet feel so tired and achy that you don't think you can stand up for another minute, reach for three or four **CUCUMBERS.** Chop them up, toss the pieces into your blender or food processor, and whirl them into a thick pulp. Put an equal amount into each of two pans that are big enough to hold your feet. Then sit

back in your easy chair, put a tootsie into each pan, and think lovely thoughts. The next thing you know, you'll be ready to go out and dance the night away—or at least take Rover for a stroll around the block.

TIP To cure whatever ails you— or to keep away anything that might—follow Grandma's lead and sip a cup of **DANDELION** tea every now and then. To make it, just put 2 teaspoons of fresh, chopped dandelion roots and leaves in a pan, pour in ½ cup of spring water, and bring it to a boil. Remove the pan from the heat, and let the mix steep for 15 minutes, then strain and enjoy the hot liquid. Make a cup two or three times a day, and drink to your health.

TIP Some of the best-looking plants in Grandma's garden were also the most powerful. Take **EVENING PRIMROSE,** for instance. You couldn't ask for a prettier flower, and the leaves are a potent remedy for boils. Just crush them, so they release their volatile oils, put them directly on the boil, and cover them with a gauze pad. Add a strip of gauze or a bandage to hold the pad in place, and leave it on for 30 minutes or so. Repeat every two to three hours, several times a day.

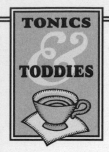

TONICS & TODDIES

GRANDMA PUTT'S DANDELION WINE

Grandma swore that a nightly glass of this golden vino kept her in the pink of health all her life. I don't know whether that's what did the trick—but it sure didn't hurt!

4 lemons
4 oranges
1-gal. bucket of dandelion blooms (no stems)
2 gal. of water
8 cups of sugar
1 pkg. of baker's yeast

Juice the lemons and oranges, and put the citrus rinds, juice, and dandelion blooms in a pan with the water. Bring the mixture to a boil, and continue boiling for half an hour. Remove the pan from the heat, and let it sit for 24 hours. Strain the mixture into a crock or large glass jar, and stir in the sugar and yeast. Cover the container, and leave it in a cool, dark place for two weeks. Then strain the elixir again, and pour it into wine bottles.

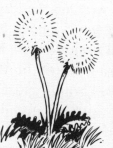

TIP If you're allergic to bee stings, here's a tip that could make your backyard a safer and more pleasant place: Grow plenty of **FEVERFEW** in your outdoor living areas—the buzzers won't go anywhere near it. (P.S. This old-time perennial is also one great-looking plant. It reaches about 2 feet tall and has lacy, light green leaves and delicate, daisylike flowers from early summer to early fall. It's hardy in Zones 5 to 9.)

TIP Folks have known about the healing powers of **GARLIC** for centuries, and Grandma Putt sure was a believer—she grew enough of the pungent bulbs to kill off all the vampires in Hollywood! One of the simplest ways she put it to work was to ease the pain of a toothache. Anytime I got one, she'd just peel a garlic clove, crush it, and apply it directly to the gum above or below the affected tooth. Then I'd hold it there until the ache subsided. The relief generally lasted long enough for me to get into town to see the dentist (who would promptly hand me a big glass of mouthwash!).

TIP Scientific studies have shown that eating just one fresh **GARLIC** clove a day can reduce your bad cholesterol levels by 17 percent, thereby lessening your heart attack risk by 25 percent—proving once again that Grandma really *did* know a thing or three about maintaining good health!

TIP When you feel like you've got a four-alarm fire blazing in your throat, put out the flames the way Grandma Putt did. Mix 1 crushed **GARLIC** clove, 1 teaspoon of salt, and a tiny pinch of cayenne pepper in a glass, fill it with warm water, and stir. Gargle with the solution, and repeat as needed. (But if your throat doesn't feel better in a day or so, call your doctor.) This same potion will speed the healing of a chest cold or bronchitis. Massage the fiery solution onto your chest several times a day.

TIP You can also treat a sore throat with **GARLIC** oil. Make it the way I describe in the tip on page 78, and rub it on the front and sides of your neck. Then breathe deeply. The volatile compounds will be absorbed right through your skin to the source of the pain.

TIP Here's an old-time method for lowering blood pressure: Soak $\frac{1}{2}$ pound of peeled **GARLIC** cloves in 1 quart of brandy for two weeks, shaking the mixture a few times a day. Then strain it, pour the liquid into bottles with tight stoppers, and take up to 20 drops a day.

TIP If you act fast, **GARLIC** can even help fend off a cold. The minute you feel one coming on, start eating a whole clove every couple of hours. You won't win any popularity contests around the office, but you may avoid a lot of uncomfortable days and nights!

TIP You say you've already *got* a nasty head cold? Just do what Grandma did to send it packin': Several times a day, crush a **GARLIC** clove, put your nose up close to it, and inhale deeply. You might not like what you're smelling—but neither will the cold germs!

TIP As a boy, I was prone to lots of earaches, as many kids are. Grandma treated them by putting a few drops of warm **GARLIC** oil in my ear. To make the oil, she sliced one garlic clove, added about 2 teaspoons of olive oil, and heated it for a minute or two. Then she'd strain it, and let it cool to lukewarm before she used it.

TIP If you're suffering from rheumatism or sprained ligaments, this healing potion of Grandma's belongs in your medicine chest. Put 1 cup of high-quality olive oil into a glass jar that has a tight lid. Peel and crush four cloves of **GARLIC,** and add them to the oil. Cover the jar, and leave it in a warm place for a full week. Strain it into a clean bottle, and store it in a cool, dark spot. Then, once or twice a day, massage a teaspoon or two of the oil into your achin' body parts.

TIP Attention, Snow-belt dwellers! You know those days when you get so cold outdoors that, after you come inside, you just can't stop shivering, even though the room is toasty warm? The next

time that happens, try Grandma's warmer-upper. Just peel and grate two **GARLIC** cloves, and mix the pulp with a pinch of cayenne pepper. Divide the mixture into two portions, and wrap each half in a

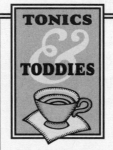

TONICS & TODDIES

TEA TIMES TWO

An herbal infusion is simply an extra-strong tea that's ideal for topical use—although you can also drink it, provided the herbs are edible (and you prefer your tea on the strong side). This recipe makes 1 cup of brew, but you can double, triple, or even quadruple the recipe if you need more for a particular use (like soaking your feet), or if you simply want to keep a supply on hand.

1–2 heaping tbsp. of dried herbs
8 oz. of fresh spring water

Put the herbs in a ceramic or glass mug, jar, or pitcher. Boil the water, and pour it over the herbs. Let the mixture steep for 10 to 15 minutes, strain, and pour the tea into a clean container. Allow it to cool before you use it on your skin, or drink it at whatever temperature suits your fancy.

piece of muslin, or old, clean panty-hose. Then put one of these little pouches on the base of each heel. You should feel toasty warm all over within minutes.

TIP You say your tootsies are nice and warm, but painful corns are driving you nuts? No problem! Just slice off a sliver of **GARLIC** the same size as the corn, put it on top of the blasted bump, and secure it with a bandage. Replace the mini poultice every day until the corn drops off.

TIP As Grandma knew, you don't have to be a jock to get athlete's foot. If this nasty fungus has attacked your tootsies, chase it off the way she would. Steep half a dozen **GARLIC** cloves in a bowl of hot water for an hour. Then soak your feet in the "tea" for 20 minutes. When the fungus takes a more aggressive approach, reach for even stronger medicine. Crush six garlic cloves, put them in a jar with a tight lid, and add enough olive oil to cover them by half an inch or so. Put the lid on, shake the container, and let the mix sit in a dark place

for a few days. Then, shake it again, and brush the oil onto your clean, dry feet with a soft brush or cotton pad. Just one word of caution: This potent stuff can burn sensitive skin, so use it with care, and don't get it on open cuts or sores.

TIP Rheumatoid arthritis is no match for **GINGER.** Steam a few chunks of the fresh root until they're soft, and mash them with a teaspoon or two of olive oil. Wrap the mix in a slightly dampened cloth, and lay this poultice over the painful area. Repeat the procedure anytime you feel the need.

TIP Sluggish bowels may not be one of life's major ills, but they sure are a nuisance! So rev 'em up the way Grandma did—with a warm

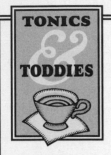

TONICS & TODDIES

GILLY-FLOWER SYRUP

As early as Mr. Shakespeare's time, the sweet-smelling blooms that we call pinks, carnations, and sweet William were all known as "gillyflowers," or sometimes "gilloflowers." And, like most other plants back then, they earned their keep. For instance, they formed the prime ingredient in this headache remedy from Grandma's youth.

½ **lb. of gillyflower blossoms (any kind will do)**
5 cups of water
5 cups of sugar

Put the flowers in a heat-proof container. Bring the water to a boil, pour it over the blooms, and let it sit for 12 hours. Strain the liquid into a pan, and heat it on low, mixing in the sugar until it's thoroughly dissolved. Store the syrup in a tight-lidded container in a cool, dark place (or in the refrigerator), and take a teaspoon or two at the first sign of a headache.

GINGER poultice. Put 2 gallons of water in a pot, and bring it to a boil. Grate 4½ tablespoons of fresh ginger into a cheesecloth bag, dunk it in the water, and remove the pot from the heat. Let the pouch steep until the water cools to a comfortable (but still warm) temperature. Then dip a clean towel into the brew, and lay it over your abdomen until the compress cools. Repeat the process four more times, reheating the water and applying a fresh compress each time. You'll find that things will soon be on the move again.

TIP Grandma also used fresh, grated **GINGER** to help clear up—or even prevent—migraines. Just brew it into a tea following the recipe on page 89, and drink a cup of it every few hours.

TIP Looking for a new deodorant? Don't peruse the miles of aisles at the drugstore— "shop" in your own back-yard instead. Just cut enough **GRASS** clippings to loosely pack a large canning jar, and pour in enough vodka to cover them completely. Close the jar tightly, and set it in a cool, dark place for 7 to 10 days, shaking it every couple of days. Strain out the clippings, and pour the liquid into a clean bottle with a tight lid. Now you've got liquid chlorophyll, which is one of the best odor-stoppers around. Just dab it onto your underarms with a cotton ball, and you'll feel baby-fresh all day. (*Note:* Don't use clippings from any lawn that's been treated with chemical herbicides or pesticides.)

TIP When clogged sinuses are driving you to drink, clear 'em up with Grandma's time-tested trick: Take 1 teaspoon of grated, fresh **HORSERADISH** daily (or as needed) until your symptoms subside. Just how do you take this fiery stuff? Any way you like! It works whether you spread it on a sandwich, mix it in tomato juice, or eat it straight from the spoon. After you're breathing freely again, a few teaspoons a month should help prevent another attack.

TIP Before antibiotic ointments came along, **JUNIPER BERRY** tea was often just what the doctor ordered to treat burns, scrapes, and even infected wounds. It still works (of course), and it's a snap to make. Just put 4 cups of water in a pan,

and bring it to a boil. Stir in ½ cup of juniper berries, remove the pan from the heat, and let the mix steep for one hour. Strain out the berries, and wash the affected area with the brew several times a day.

TIP Whenever I got a bout of hiccups, Grandma Putt would hand me a slice of **LEMON.** She didn't have to tell me what to do, because I had the routine down pat: I'd stick the lemon under my tongue, suck it once, hold the juice for 10 seconds, and then swallow. It worked like a charm every time!

TIP To soothe the itch of insect bites, poison ivy, or skin allergies, make a paste of **LEMON** juice and cornstarch, and rub it gently onto the problem areas.

TIP When a bee stings you, get the stinger out, then squeeze **LEMON** juice onto the spot to head off pain and swelling.

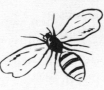

TIP Relieve constipation with this simple remedy: Before breakfast, drink four tablespoons of **LEMON** juice and a little honey (to your taste) mixed in one cup of warm water.

TIP Stop a throbbing headache by rubbing half of a fresh-cut **LIME** across your forehead.

TIP When you've been on your feet all day, pamper those tired dogs by massaging **LIME** juice into the skin.

TIP Ease the pain of a sore throat by drinking the juice of one **LIME** mixed with 1 tablespoon of pineapple juice and 1 teaspoon of honey in a glass of lukewarm water.

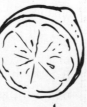

TIP Grandma used to make a salve that she kept on hand for soothing all sorts of aches and pains, including bruises; tired, burning feet; and varicose veins. If you want to make your own supply, just mix 1 cup of **MARIGOLD** petals and ½ cup of petroleum jelly in a pan, and cook it on low heat for about 30 minutes. Strain the mixture through cheesecloth or old, clean pantyhose until it runs clear, and store in a glass jar with a tight lid. Massage this salve into the affected skin before you go to bed at night. Then, to keep the grease from staining your sheets, put on old, soft, cotton pajamas. Or, if you don't have any expendable jammies, simply wrap any kind of soft, cotton fabric around your legs. (Strips cut from an old sheet, or a couple of old T-shirts would be perfect.)

TIP Grandma grew one of the best bronchial medicines you could ever ask for: **ONIONS.** The pungent bulbs are a rich source of quercetin, a chemical that helps relieve chest colds, bronchitis, and even asthma attacks. Eat them raw in a salad, stir-fry them with other vegetables, or make yourself a big bowl of onion soup. No matter how you eat them, you should soon feel your airways clearing up.

TIP Even when you're feeling so lousy you don't want to eat *anything*, **ONIONS** can still break up lung congestion. Just cut a large onion into thin slices, and cook them in a little water until very soft. Wrap the cooked onions in a clean towel, and lay it over your chest for 20 minutes.

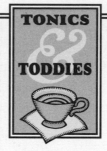 **TIP** Silence a cough with one of Grandma Putt's favorite remedies, honey-**ONION** syrup. Just put one finely sliced onion in a pot, and add enough honey to cover the slices completely. Simmer, with the lid on, over very low heat for 40 minutes, watching carefully so the honey doesn't burn. Let the syrup cool, and pour it into a bottle with a tight stopper. Take a teaspoonful every hour until your cough subsides.

TIP Here's a little trick that will unclog your sinuses fast. Just cut an **ONION,** hold it cut side up under your nose, and take a big whiff. Those nasal passages will be free and clear in no time flat!

TIP The next time you bang your leg on the coffee table (or maybe on your way down the stepladder), grab an **ONION.** The same chemicals that make your eyes water also flush excess blood. Immediately after the unfortunate encounter, cut a slice of raw onion (the stronger the better), put it over the bump site, and leave it on for 15 minutes. If you've acted fast enough, no bruise should develop.

TONICS & TODDIES

ALL-PURPOSE COUGH SYRUP

Grandma Putt used this old-time elixir to quiet any cough that came her way—including my childhood case of whooping cough.

2 large, sweet onions
2 cups of dark honey
2 oz. of brandy

Peel the onions, cut them into thin slices, and spread them out in a single layer in a shallow bowl. Pour the honey over them evenly, and cover the bowl with wax paper or anything else that fits (for instance, a pot lid, or a wooden cutting board). Let the bowl sit for eight hours or so, strain off the syrup, and mix it with the brandy. Give the patient 1 teaspoon every two to three hours, or as needed, to stop the coughing.

TIP Grandma often cleared up an earache with an **ONION** poultice. To make one, just heat half an onion in the oven until it's warm (not hot). Wrap it in cheesecloth, and hold it against your sore ear. The chemicals in the onion will help increase your blood circulation, and flush away the infection.

TIP **PARSLEY** can work wonders on existing bruises. Just chill a handful of fresh sprigs, crush them, apply them to the bruise, and cover it with a bandage. Within 24 hours, those blues and purples will start to lighten up.

TIP Nothing puts a damper on a good meal like a bout of indigestion. But you 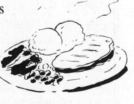 can ease the discomfort in a flash, the way Grandma did—by eating a few sprigs of fresh **PARSLEY.** When there's no fresh parlsey on hand, scoop ¼ teaspoon of the dried version out of the jar, mix it into a glass of warm water, and drink up. Your tummy will feel better in no time.

TIP Grandma never went in much for store-bought mouthwash. She had several breath-freshening

tricks, but most often, she simply chewed on a sprig of **PARSLEY** that she plucked off of a plant as she puttered among her herbs.

TIP Winter can be rough on your skin, indoors or out. Hot, dry indoor air can leave your skin feeling dry and irritated. And on sunny days, cold, dry breezes outdoors can deliver a nasty windburn before you know it. To ease both kinds of discomfort, cut a fresh **PEACH** in two, and rub the juicy surface over the ailin' skin. You'll feel better in no time!

TIP I learned this simple headache remedy from Grandma Putt, but it actually goes back to ancient Greece. When you feel that old, familiar throbbing, pluck a handful of **PEPPERMINT** leaves, and press them against your temples. Soon, your head will be throbbin' no more!

TIP Refresh your tired tootsies by soaking them in a **PEPPERMINT** infusion. Use the Tea Times Two recipe on page 78, but increase the amount by enough to fill two shallow, foot-size pans.

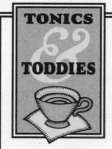

TONICS & TODDIES

FAREWELL FROSTBITE FORMULA

If you live in cold-winter territory and spend a lot of time outdoors, make up a batch of Grandma's trusty frostbite remedy, and keep it close at hand.

1¼ cups of white wine
2 tbsp. of whole black peppercorns
1 tbsp. of horseradish root, coarsely grated
1 tbsp. of fresh gingerroot, coarsely grated

Pour the wine into a clean glass jar that has a tight lid, and add the pepper, horseradish, and ginger. Let it sit for one week, then strain out the solids, using very fine cheesecloth or a coffee filter. Keep the liquid in a tightly closed bottle in a cool, dark place. Then anytime Jack Frost bites your fingers, nose, or other tender body parts, apply a generous coat of the solution to your affected skin, using a cotton ball or a very soft, clean paintbrush. You'll feel instant relief from the burning pain.

TIP If you're an asthma sufferer and you like spicy food, here's a piece of news that should make you stand up and cheer: hot chili **PEPPERS** help to thin mucus and reduce inflammation in your bronchial passages. So what are you waiting for? Eat up!

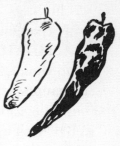

TIP When painful cold sores break out in your mouth, they can make you feel like climbing the walls. Get relief fast with this classic remedy. Just soak a piece of cotton pad in fresh **PLUM** juice, press it against the sore, and hold it in place for 10 minutes, or as long as you can. If you need to, repeat the procedure until the nasty little bump is gone.

TIP As we all know, **POTATOES** are one of the healthiest foods you can put inside your body. But, as Grandma Putt knew well, the common spud can also do terrific things for the *outside* of your body. For instance, it's perfect for easing the pain and itch of eczema. Just grate a raw potato, dip a cotton pad in the shreds to absorb some of the juice, and gently dab all of the trouble spots.

TIP Grandma also used peeled **POTATOES** as a remedy for hemorrhoids. She just grated 1 to 2 tablespoons of raw potato, wrapped it in cheesecloth, and put it in the icebox until it was nice and chilled.

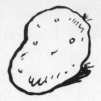

Then she pulled the pouch out, gave it to the hemorrhoid sufferer, and instructed him to go to his room, pull down his pants, and sit on the spuds.

TIP Coax a splinter out of your skin by taping a slice of **POTATO** onto the affected site, or if the sliver is in your finger or toe, hollow out a space that's just the right size, and slip the digit into the tater. (Hold it in place with a sock if you need to.) Leave it on overnight, and by morning, you'll be able to pluck the splinter right out.

TIP Got a minor burn? Grab a raw **POTATO,** slice the end off, and rub the burn gently with the cut surface. You'll feel almost instant relief.

TIP To relieve a headache, Grandma recommended this routine: Soak three or four thin **POTATO** slices in vinegar. Then, tie a bandanna around your head, and tuck the potato slices into it at your temples and forehead. Leave it on for a few hours. When you take it off, the spuds will be hot and dry— and your head should be ache-free!

In Grandma's Day

For centuries before Grandma Putt was little more than a gleam in her daddy's eye, **YARROW** was famous as a blood-stopper. Just about everyone kept a few bunches hanging in the toolshed, where they could reach it quickly if they cut themselves. In fact, it was such a widespread habit that, to this very day in France, yarrow is known as "the carpenters' herb."

TIP Whenever anyone in our family came down with a cough or sore throat, Grandma Putt would make a batch of her **RADISH** syrup. The recipe couldn't be simpler. Just cut six or eight radishes into thin slices, spread them out on a plate, and sprinkle them with a tablespoon or so of sugar. Cover them loosely with wax paper or aluminum foil, and let them sit overnight. In the morning, you'll find the slices swimming in a rich syrup. Drain it off into a glass bottle or jar, and take a teaspoonful whenever you feel the need.

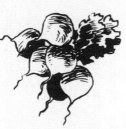

TIP Few skin afflictions are more painful than shingles. But this truly ancient remedy can help ease the discomfort. Put about a cup of **RASPBERRY** blossoms in a mortar and crush them with a pestle (or use your newfangled food processor), and blend in enough honey to make a paste (a tablespoon or so should do the trick, but let your eye be your guide). Apply it very gently to the afflicted skin. Then, to keep the sticky stuff from getting all over your sheets or furniture, put on loose, clean, all-cotton pajamas or a cotton T-shirt.

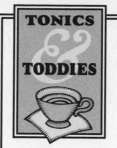

TONICS & TODDIES

MAGICAL MARIGOLD OIL

Grandma Putt always grew plenty of pot marigolds (a.k.a. calendulas), which she used to make this powerful, but oh-so-gentle potion. It's terrific for healing minor cuts, scrapes, and burns; soothing the pain and itch of insect bites; and even massaging tired, achy muscles.

5 cups of wilted calendula blossoms*
Extra-virgin olive oil

Put the blossoms in a 3-quart pan, and add enough olive oil to reach 2 inches above the flowers. Heat the mixture on low until it *almost* simmers. Let it steep over low heat, uncovered, for six to eight hours, or until the oil has turned a deep, golden-orange color, and has a strong herbal aroma. (Test for "doneness" every hour or so, and make sure the oil doesn't start to simmer.) Remove the pan from the heat, and let the brew cool to room temperature. Strain it through cheesecloth or a sieve, and store it in a tightly capped bottle in the refrigerator. It will keep for a year.

*Pluck them from the plant, and let them sit in the shade for a couple of days.

TIP Grandma used a **RASPBERRY** elixir to treat bloodshot eyes. Just boil 1 cup of water, add 1 teaspoon of chopped raspberry leaves (not the fruit), and remove the pan from the heat. Steep the mixture for 10 minutes, strain, and let it cool to a temperature that's comfortable to touch. Soak a soft, clean cloth in the solution, lie down in a comfortable spot, and lay the cloth over your closed eyes. Relax for 10 minutes or so. If your peepers are still red, repeat the procedure.

TIP Prevent tartar buildup on your teeth by rubbing your choppers every few days with the cut side of a **STRAWBERRY.** Wait at least half an hour before you rinse.

TIP For an even more thorough approach to dental hygiene, do what Grandma did: Mash a **STRAWBERRY,** dip your toothbrush in the pulp, and brush as you would with your regular toothpaste. As advised above, hold off rinsing as long as you can, because the longer the berry juice remains on your teeth, the more effective it will be at removing tartar.

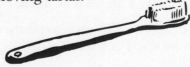

TIP For those times when you don't have fresh **STRAWBERRIES** on hand, keep a supply of strawberry-leaf mouthwash in the refrigerator. (The leaves contain many of the same plaque- and germ-fighting chemicals that make the fruits so good for your teeth and gums.) To make the brew, put 1 cup of fresh strawberry leaves into a heat-proof glass or ceramic bowl, and cover them with 1 cup of boiling water. Let the mix steep until

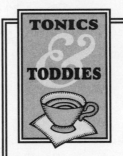

TONICS & TODDIES

HEARTBURN RELIEF REMEDY

This tasty juice will ease heartburn pain and give you a dose of nutritious garden veggies at the same time!

2–3 sprigs of parsley
2 garlic cloves, peeled
1 angelica stalk
1 medium carrot
1 celery stalk
Water

Put all the solid ingredients in a blender or food processor, and liquefy. Add enough water to get the consistency you prefer. Pour the potion into a glass, and sip it slowly. You'll soon be feeling better.

the water has reached room temperature, strain it into another bowl, and mix in 2 teaspoons of either vodka or lemon juice (not both). Store it in the fridge, and use it as you would any other mouthwash.

 TIP Soothe inflamed eyes with a cup of Grandma's **STRAWBERRY** tea—made from the leaves, *not* the fruit. Boil 1 cup of water, add 1 teaspoon of chopped strawberry leaves, and remove the pan from the heat. Let the mix steep for 10 minutes, strain, and let it cool to a temperature that's comfortable to touch. Then, use it in one of two ways: Either soak a soft cloth in the solution, lie down, and put the compress over your eyes for about 15 minutes; or pour the solution into an eyecup, and rinse your eyes with it once or twice a day.

TIP **SUNFLOWER** seeds are not *only* for the birds. They're also a terrific headache remedy for humans. Just munch on a handful the next time the throbbing starts, and it should fly away fast.

TIP Brushing up against poison ivy or poison oak is no fun now, and it wasn't exactly a picnic when it happened to Grandma Putt and me, either. But she knew how

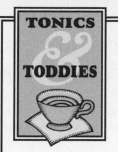

TONICS & TODDIES

GRANDMA PUTT'S HERB TEA

This was the simple recipe Grandma used to make both medicinal and cosmetic teas. It makes one cup. (For some of Grandma's favorite ingredients, see "Herbal Soothers" on page 90.)

1–2 tsp. of herbs (dried or fresh)
1 cup of fresh spring water
Honey (optional)

Put the herbs into a ceramic teapot or mug that you've preheated by pouring boiling water into it, then dumping it out. In a pan or teakettle, bring 1 cup of spring water to a boil, and pour it over the herbs. Let the mix steep for three to five minutes, and strain it into a fresh cup or mug. Add honey to taste, if you'd like, and drink a toast to good health!

to prevent a rash from breaking out if we acted fast enough. The only catch was that we had to be in the right place at the right time, because we needed to rush to the garden and pluck a green **TOMATO.** Then she'd cut it open and squeeze the juice onto the affected skin. (Fortunately, Grandma also knew a lot of great ways to ease the pain and itch if a rash *did* appear.)

Herbal Soothers

To Grandma's way of thinking, there was almost nothing that a cup of herbal tea couldn't cure. You'll find her easier-than-pie tea recipe in "Grandma Putt's Herb Tea" on page 89. And here's an inventory of her fresh-from-the-garden—or sometimes dried-from-the-garden—medicine chest. *Note:* If you're pregnant, on medication of any kind (even aspirin), or suffering from high blood pressure, diabetes, or any other chronic condition, check with your doctor before you dose yourself with any of these herbs.

Healing Herb	How It Helps
Angelica	Aids digestion, reduces gas, eases menstrual cramps, relieves cold and flu symptoms
Anise hyssop	Clears up sore throats and congestion, fights indigestion
Basil	Fights cold and flu infections, sharpens mental alertness, eases migraines, relieves stress, helps cure depression, stimulates the flow of milk in nursing mothers
Bay	Eases the pain of headaches and stomachaches, fights tooth decay
Bee balm, a.k.a. bergamot or Oswego tea	Helps ease nausea, vomiting, and flatulence
Borage	Acts as a gentle laxative and blood cleanser, relieves the pain and swelling of insect bites
Chamomile	Relieves muscle spasms and allergy symptoms, soothes upset stomachs, kills germs that produce gingivitis, relaxes tense nerves, aids liver health
Dill	Soothes upset stomachs, eases muscle spasms, freshens breath, and (for all you nursing moms) stimulates the flow of breast milk
Feverfew	Eases dizziness, tinnitus, and arthritis pain; relieves menstrual cramps; cures headaches
Garlic	Kills bacteria, clears lung congestion, lowers blood sugar and cholesterol levels, boosts circulation, and acts as an antihistamine
Ginger	Boosts immune system activity, helps fight colds and flu, relieves nausea and upset stomachs

Healing Herb	How It Helps
Lavender	Relaxes body and mind, eases stress
Peppermint	Stimulates mind and body, relieves nausea and upset stomachs
Rosemary	Stimulates memory, boosts energy, relieves the blues
Sage	Restores vitality and strength, fights fevers, and soothes mucous membrane tissue—thereby curing mouth ulcers, sore gums and throats, and even laryngitis

Your
GOOD LOOKS

TIP When Grandma Putt and her friends wanted to pamper their faces, they didn't run off to a fancy spa, or even the local beauty parlor. They made their own skin cleansers and softeners using ingredients fresh from their gardens and kitchens. This was one of the simplest—and it still works as well as it did decades ago. Mix ¼ cup of grated **CARROTS** with 1½ teaspoons of mayonnaise. Spread the mix on your face and neck, wait 15 minutes, and rinse with lukewarm water.

TIP When your skin is sunburned or irritated, whip up this super-simple soother. Puree half a **CUCUMBER** in a blender, and mix in 1 tablespoon of plain yogurt (*not* the nonfat kind). Spread the mixture on your face and neck, wait 30 minutes, and rinse with lukewarm water.

TIP Here's the simplest way I know of to lighten dark circles under your eyes—and soothe eyestrain at the same time: Just cut two **CUCUMBER** slices, lie down in a comfortable place, and put one slice over each eye. Relax for 10 minutes or so, and (as Grandma Putt would say) you'll be bright-eyed and bushy-tailed!

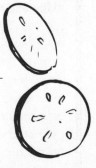

TIP Here's a **GRAPE** way to minimize those tiny lines that Father Time leaves around your eyes and mouth. Just cut green, seedless grapes in half, and squeeze the juice right onto the little creases. (This treatment is especially good for dry, sensitive skin.)

In Grandma's Day

In her later years, Grandma Putt's hands began to sport those brown souvenirs we call "liver" spots. They didn't stay around long, though, because Grandma knew exactly how to send 'em packin'. You can do it, too. Just pick some **DANDE-LIONS,** break the stems open, and squeeze a generous amount of the milky sap onto the blotches. Then rub with a circular motion until the fluid vanishes into your skin. Repeat the process two or three times a day until the marks fade. (If they're very dark to begin with, they may never vanish entirely, but they will become so light you'll hardly notice them.)

P.S. You can use the same dandelion treatment to get rid of warts—and in this case, the unsightly bumps *will* completely disappear.

TIP Make an anticellulite wrap using **GRAPEFRUIT** juice. (It works just like the ones used in fancy spas.) Mix ½ cup of fresh grapefruit juice, 1 cup of corn oil, and 2 teaspoons of dried thyme. Massage the mixture into hips, thighs, and buttocks, and cover the area with plastic wrap. Hold a heating pad over each body section for five minutes.

TIP Clear up blackheads and blemishes by rubbing them with **LEMON** juice several times a day.

TIP To polish dingy fingernails, cut a fresh, juicy **LEMON** in half, and dig your fingers into the flesh. Hold them there for one minute, then rinse in clear water. (Just make sure your fingers are free of cuts or scrapes, or you'll get a stinging surprise!)

TIP Make your fingernails stronger and whiter by soaking them in **LEMON** juice for 10 minutes, once a week. Then brush them with a half-and-half solution of white vinegar and warm water, and rinse with clear H_2O.

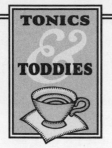

TONICS & TODDIES

HEIRLOOM HAIR LIGHTENER

If you want to make your hair a few shades lighter, don't rush off to the beauty parlor. Just mix up this old-time concoction.

Juice of 2 limes
Juice of 1 lemon
2 tbsp. of mild shampoo

Mix the juices and the shampoo in a container, pour the solution onto your hair, and massage it in. Sit in the sun for 15 to 20 minutes. Then rinse thoroughly, and apply a good conditioner. Repeat the process until you think you're blonde enough to have more fun!

TIP Soften your elbows, heels, and feet by rubbing half a **LEMON** on the skin. (This trick even works on calluses.)

TIP To fade freckles and age spots, dissolve a pinch of sugar in 2 tablespoons of **LEMON** juice, and dab the mixture onto each blotch with a cotton ball. Repeat the procedure every day or two until the spots have lightened.

TIP Treat your cracked, dry feet to Grandma's favorite moisturizing routine. Just combine 1 tablespoon of **LEMON** juice with 1 ripe, smashed banana, 2 tablespoons of honey, and 2 tablespoons of margarine. Stir the ingredients until creamy, then massage the mix onto clean, dry feet. Pull on a pair of cotton socks, and go to bed for the night.

TIP When you're in the mood for a soothing facial, just use your head—of **LETTUCE,** that is. Here's the simple procedure. Separate the leaves from a small head of lettuce (preferably Boston or Bibb, but iceberg will work, too). Wash them, and cook them in boiling water for five minutes. Remove them from the water, let them cool, and apply them to your face. Leave them on for 5 to 10 minutes, or as close to it as you can—they'll be slippery! Pat your face dry without rinsing. Store the leftover cooking water in a covered jar in the refrigerator, and use it as a toning lotion for your face and neck. (For more great ways to recycle cooking water, see the One More Time box on page 126.)

TIP Whip up a triple-treat face cream that will remove makeup, and clean and soften your skin by mixing the juice of one **LIME** with ½ cup of mayonnaise (the real kind, made with eggs and oil) and 1 tablespoon of melted butter (not margarine). Store the cream in a tightly closed glass jar in the refrigerator. Use it as you would any facial cleanser, and rinse with cold water.

TIP Sweeten your breath by drinking the juice of one **LIME** and a teaspoon or so of honey mixed in a glass of water.

TIP When Grandma's women friends wanted to lighten their hair, they'd go about it this way—and you can, too. Just stir 3 tablespoons of chopped **RHUBARB** stems into 3 cups of hot water. Simmer for 10 minutes, strain, and cool. Use the solution as a rinse after each shampoo.

TIP Grandma Putt made her own perfume by packing a glass jar with **ROSE** petals and pouring in as much glycerin as the container would hold. She let it sit for three weeks or so, then strained the liquid into a clean bottle with a tight stopper. (If you don't have roses in your garden, you can use any sweet- or spicy-smelling flower you like.)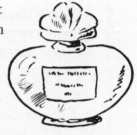

TIP Make a soothing facial cleanser by mixing 1 tablespoon of dried **ROSEMARY** in ½ cup of safflower oil. Let it sit in a covered container in the refrigerator for three days. Then take it out, and use it once or twice a day. (Just smooth it onto your face, rinse with lukewarm water, and pat dry.)

If you've got more freckles than you'd like to have, try this beauty tip. Cut a fresh **STRAWBERRY** in two, and rub the cut side over the spots. Repeat the procedure every day or two until the speckles disappear, or at least become less noticeable.

Invite Your Face to Tea

Not all of Grandma's herbal teas were meant for sipping. She also made a stronger version (technically called an infusion) that can work the same wonders for your skin that herb tea does for your innards. Any of these brews works as either a stand-alone treatment, or as a prep for your skin before applying one of the fruit-and-vegetable masks on page 96. Whichever way you use the tea, just dab it onto your face with a cotton pad, and let it dry. Or, to give your whole body a teatime treat, pour the potion into your bathwater. These were some of Grandma's favorite cosmetic tea "flavors." (To make your infusion, see "Tea Times Two" on page 78.)

Beautifying Herb	How It Helps
Chamomile (flowers)	Reduces inflammation, soothes, cleanses, supplies antifungal agents
Elder (flowers)	Cleanses, tones, acts as a gentle astringent
Lavender (flowers)	Soothes, cleanses, reduces inflammation
Linden (flowers)	Supplies the same benefits as chamomile (above), but in a milder form that's especially good for aging skin
Mallow	Soothes irritated skin
Mint	Tones and refreshes
Pot marigold, a.k.a. calendula (flowers)	Cleanses, soothes, reduces inflammation; often used in a half-and-half mix with chamomile or lavender
Rosemary	Tones, revitalizes, improves blood circulation to the capillaries
Thyme	Fights bacteria; is especially effective on acne and eczema
Yarrow	Tones, cleanses, heals; is particularly good for aging or damaged skin

TIP When it comes to cleaning, toning, and moisturizing your skin, this mask is the berries (as Grandma would say). Mash four medium-size, ripe **STRAWBERRIES,** and puree them in a blender or food processor with 1 tablespoon each of heavy cream and organic honey. Spread the mixture on your face and neck, keeping it away from your eyes. Wait 10 minutes, then rinse with lukewarm water.

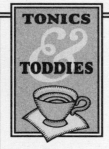

TONICS & TODDIES

TUTTI-FRUTTI FACIAL

Here's a fresh-from-the-garden formula that will soften your face, invigorate your senses—and smell like a yummy fruit salad.

6 strawberries
½ of an apple
½ of a pear
4 tbsp. of orange juice
Honey

Puree the fruits with the orange juice in a blender or food processor. Apply a thin layer of honey to your face, then smooth on the fruit mixture. Leave it on your skin for 30 to 40 minutes, rinse with warm water, and pat dry.

TIP Here's a mild, garden-fresh astringent for your face. Boil a few sprigs of fresh **THYME** in 2 cups of water. Remove the pot from the heat, and let the thyme steep for five to seven minutes, or until the water cools to room temperature. Take out the thyme, and add 2 teaspoons of fresh lemon juice. Pour this concoction into a glass bottle with a top and store it in the refrigerator. Apply it with a cotton ball or pad after washing your face.

TIP If you have oily—but not sensitive—skin, this cleanser is just for you. Puree a very ripe, medium-size **TOMATO** in a blender or food processor, strain out the solids, and mix the juice with an equal amount of fresh, whole milk. Apply the solution to your face and neck with cotton pads, wait 10 minutes, and rinse with lukewarm water.

TIP There was nothing Grandma Putt loved more than the sweet scent of violets. That's why, every night, she washed her face with this simple cleanser. Put 2 tablespoons of sweet **VIOLETS** (*Viola odorata*) in the top half of a double boiler with ¼ cup of evaporated milk and ¼ cup of whole milk. Simmer for about 30 minutes. Don't let the milk boil! Turn off the heat, let the mixture sit for two hours or so, and strain it into a bottle with a tight stopper. Store it in the refrigerator. To use, pat it onto your face with a cotton ball, massage gently with your fingers, and rinse with cool water.

TIP When it's summertime and the livin' is not so easy, take a little time away from the daily grind, and treat yourself to a **WATERMELON** facial. Just peel a slice of the fruit, and mash it in a glass or ceramic bowl until it's about the consistency of thin applesauce. Wash your face so it's squeaky clean. Spread the melon over your face, lie down, and put a piece of gauze or cheesecloth over the fruit (otherwise, it will probably slide off). Relax for 20 to 30 minutes, then rinse well and pat dry.

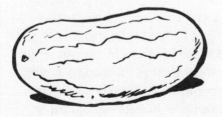

Around the
HOUSE

TIP One Christmas (after saving up all year), I gave Grandma small pewter candlesticks. Boy, did she treasure those! She used them on the dinner table every night. And to give them a classic, old-time sheen, she rubbed them every now and then with **CABBAGE** leaves.

TIP "Polish" your houseplants the old-fashioned way, with **CITRUS** juice (any kind will do). Just wipe the juice onto the leaves with a clean, soft cotton cloth, leaving the foliage sparkling, and better able to absorb carbon dioxide from the air.

ONE MORE TIME

After you've planted flats of annuals or groundcovers from the garden center, don't throw away the **PLASTIC TRAYS!** They're just the right size to hold papers in your home office, or outgoing mail on a hall table.

TIP When it came time to store our winter clothes and blankets for the summer, Grandma never used smelly old mothballs. Instead, she fastened pouches of dried **HERBS** to the hangers, and tucked them onto shelves or into blanket chests. She used individual types or a blend of several, depending on what she had growing in the garden at the time. These were her favorite moth-chasers: lavender, santolina, southernwood, tansy, thyme, and wormwood. (For several easy herb-drying methods, see "How Dry They Are" on page 105.)

TIP When spring-cleaning time rolled around—or whenever any bed in our house smelled less than springtime fresh—Grandma sprinkled the mattress with dried **LAVENDER,** let it sit for 10 to 15 minutes, then vacuumed. (If you prefer another scent, feel free to make substitutions. Any aromatic herb, or a blend of several, will perform the same odor-removal feat.)

TIP To get strong cooking odors 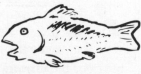 (like fish, onions, or garlic) off of knives, cutting boards, and your hands, rub them with the cut surface of a **LEMON** or **LIME.**

TIP Grandma Putt made her own furniture polish, and you can, too. Just mix 1 teaspoon of **LEMON** juice with 2 cups of olive or vegetable oil. Wipe it onto your wooden treasures with a soft, cotton cloth, then buff with a second cloth.

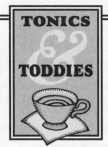

TONICS & TODDIES

GRANDMA PUTT'S LEMONADE

For my money, nothing says "summertime!" like a big glass of lemonade—but not just *any* lemonade. It has to be the genuine article, made from scratch the way Grandma did, using this simple recipe.

2 cups of water
$\frac{1}{2}$ cup of sugar
$\frac{1}{2}$ cup of fresh-squeezed lemon juice
Ice (and lots of it!)

In a saucepan, bring the water to a boil. Stir in the sugar, reduce the heat, and continue to stir until the sugar dissolves completely. Remove the pan from the heat and let it cool. Add the lemon juice, stir well, and refrigerate until the mixture is cold. Pour it into ice-filled glasses, add cold water to taste—and drink to those lazy, hazy, crazy days!

TIP Brighten up dingy, white cotton clothes or sheets by adding 1 cup of **LEMON** juice to the wash water.

TIP Clean silver by pouring **LEMON** juice onto the piece, and polishing with a soft, cotton cloth. Rinse with cool water, and wipe dry.

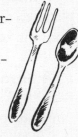

TIP Keep copper pots and pans sparkling bright by rubbing them with half a **LEMON** dipped in salt. Then wash them in warm, soapy water and rinse thoroughly. (Any trace of the fruit's acid on the metal, can cause pitting or etching.)

TIP Use a paste made of **LEMON** juice and cream of tartar to clean lacquered brass. Apply the paste with a soft, cotton cloth, let it sit for about five minutes, and wash the piece in warm, soapy water

TIP To clean your microwave oven, add 4 tablespoons of **LEMON** juice to 1 cup of water in a bowl (microwave-safe, obviously!). Boil the mixture inside the microwave for five minutes, or until the steam has condensed on the inside walls of the oven. Then wipe with paper towels.

GRANDMA PUTT'S
Secret Formulas

OLD-TIME EASTER EGG DYE

When it was gettin' on time for Peter Cottontail to come hoppin' down the Bunny Trail, Grandma and I would gather our dye makings from the garden, and spend a nice Saturday coloring eggs. Here's the simple formula.

Eggs
1 tsp. of vinegar
2½ cups of plant-dye material
Water

Put the eggs in a single layer in a pan with just enough water to cover them completely. Add the vinegar and your chosen fruits, vegetables, or leaves. (See "Produce to Dye For" on page 101.) Bring the water to a boil, reduce the heat, and simmer for 15 to 20 minutes. Remove the eggs promptly if you want lighter shades. For darker colors, strain the dye into a bowl with the eggs, and let it sit in the refrigerator overnight.

TIP Remove rust stains from your bathtub or shower by making a thin paste of **LEMON** juice and borax. Spread it on the stains and scrub lightly with a scouring sponge. Let the paste dry, then rinse.

TIP Whenever Grandma wanted to bleach linen or muslin, she'd dampen the cloth with some **LEMON** juice, and lay it flat on the ground in direct sun until it reached the degree of whiteness she wanted. Then she'd rinse it with clear water, and hang it on the clothesline. (But you can use your dryer if the fabric label says that's okay.)

TIP Polish dark-colored leather by dabbing a few drops of **LEMON** juice on a soft, cotton cloth, and rubbing it on. Then buff with another soft, clean cloth.

TIP Before you water your container plants—indoors or out—add a few drops of **LEMON** juice to the watering can. It'll lower the water's pH, thereby allowing the plants to take up more nutrients from the soil.

TIP If you've just moved into a house that was formerly inhabited by heavy smokers, clean the smoke film off of the windows with a solution of 2 tablespoons of **LEMON** juice per quart of water.

TIP Grandma had a collection of pretty wooden boxes. She gave them a glow, and a lemon-fresh scent, by rubbing them with **LEMON BALM** leaves.

TIP Outdoors, ants are regular Superbugs, breaking down organic material, fending off termites, and even eating mosquito eggs. But I'm sure you don't want the little guys traipsing through your house! So keep them out the way Grandma Putt did, by laying sprigs of fresh **MINT** in front of your doors, windows, and any cracks or holes that the ants could sneak through.

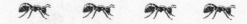

TIP Got ants in your house? No problem! Just used dried **MINT** to brew up a batch of strong tea, and spray it on the ants' pathways. The little rascals will turn right around and go back where they came from! (For my simple methods for drying mint and other herbs, see "How Dry They Are" on page 105.)

TIP To freshen the air in your kitchen fast, heat the oven to 300°F and set a whole, unpeeled **ORANGE** inside. Bake it for about 15 minutes with the oven door slightly ajar, then turn off the oven. Let the fruit cool before you take it out of the oven.

TIP Our house smelled like Christmas all winter long, thanks to an extra-simple potpourri that Grandma made by mixing 1 cup of orrisroot and 1 tablespoon of pine oil (both available at most craft-supply shops), then tossing that combo with 8 cups of fresh **PINE** needles.

Produce to Dye For

Dye *with*, I should say. Grandma Putt went all out for holidays, and Easter was no exception. Every year, we colored dozens of eggs to put in baskets for family, friends, and neighbors. The eggs came from Grandma's hens, of course—and the dyes came right from her yard and garden. If you'd like to try your hand at making natural dyes, see "Old-Time Easter Egg Dye" on page 99. Here's your color palette.

To Get This Color	Use These Materials
Blue	Blackberries, blueberries, chestnuts, red cabbage leaves
Green	Bracken, coltsfoot, spinach
Orange	Yellow onion skins
Purple	Blackberries or purple grapes
Red	Beets, cranberries, frozen raspberries, red onion skins
Yellow	Shredded carrots, carrot tops (the green part), lawn grass, lemon or orange peels

When Grandma peeled fruits or vegetables, she tossed most of those skins onto the compost pile. But for a few of them, she had other plans in mind. Here are some of the ways she put produce "packages" to work (and you can, too).

Apple Peels

▷ **Boost the bloom.** Bury apple peels in the soil around flowering shrubs.

▷ **Make dye.** The skins of Golden Delicious apples produce a green-gold color. (For more on fruit and vegetable dyes, see "Produce to Dye For" on page 101.)

▷ **Make aluminum sparkle again.** Fill a discolored aluminum pan with enough water to cover the stains, toss in a handful of apple peels, and boil it for two or three minutes. Then rinse and dry with a dish towel.

Banana Peels

▷ **Remove a plantar wart.** At bedtime, tape a piece of banana peel, inner side down, over the wart. Cover the peel with a large bandage or tight sock, and leave it on overnight. Repeat the procedure each night until the wart is gone—three or four nights, total, should do the trick.

▷ **Polish your leather shoes.** Just rub the inside surface of a banana peel over the leather, and buff with a soft, cotton cloth. Good-bye, scuff marks!

▷ **Repel aphids.** Scatter banana peels on the soil near your roses or other aphid-prone plants.

▷ **Make phosphorus- and potassium-rich fertilizer.** Let banana peels air-dry until they're crisp, then crumble them up, and store the pieces at room temperature in a sealed container. When a plant needs a jolt of either nutrient, work a handful of crumbles into the soil, and water well.

▷ **Catch garden pests.** Wasps, mosquitoes, and codling moths will fall for this banana-peel trap: Put one peel into a clean, 1-gallon milk jug with 1 cup of vinegar and 1 cup of sugar. Pour in enough water to almost fill the bottle, put the cap on, and shake well to mix the ingredients. Tie a cord or piece of wire around the handle, remove the lid, and hang the bottle from a tree limb. (*Note:* If your target of choice is codling moths, hang the trap in your apple tree before the blossoms open.)

Cucumber Peels

▷ **Call in the subs.** Use cuke peels instead of cabbage strips in slug and snail traps. (See my simple instructions in the tip on page 112.)

▷ **Repel ants.** Lay cucumber peels in their pathways.

Onion Skins

▷ **Keep whiteflies away.** Chop the skin of one medium onion, and let it steep overnight in 2 cups of water. Strain out the skin, add 1 quart of warm water, and spray your houseplants with the brew once a month.

▷ **Tint natural-fiber cloth or yarn.** Just use onion skins in the recipe on page 99 ("Old-Time Easter Egg Dye"), doubling or tripling the quantity if you need a bigger supply. Then, strain the liquid into a container that's big enough to hold your material. The exact color will vary with the type and texture of the cloth, but generally speaking, the skins of yellow onions will produce gold to yellow tones; red ones will give you (no surprise here) shades of pink and red.

Pineapple Rinds

▷ **Remove corns.**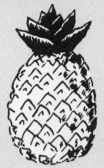
Tape a piece of pineapple rind, inner side down, over the bump, and leave it on overnight. In the morning, remove the covering and soak your foot in hot water for about an hour. The corn should come away fairly easily. If it doesn't, repeat the procedure for a few more nights.

Potato Peels

▷ **Return the sparkle to cloudy glassware.** Cover the hazy areas with wet potato peels. Leave them in place for 24 hours, then rinse with cold water, and dry with a soft cloth.

▷ **Trap wandering pill bugs.** When they stray from the compost pile, where they belong, and start munching on your living plants, send them back to work this way: Set out handfuls of potato peelings, covered with upside-down flowerpots. Check your traps every couple of days, and take the "prisoners" back to the pile.

TIP America's most-eaten vegetable can also remove stubborn scuff marks from shoes and boots. Just rub your footgear with a raw **POTATO,** and follow up with your usual polish.

TIP When you spend as much time in the old garden as Grandma and I did, you're bound to wind up with a lot of mud on your clothes. Grandma got the spots out by rubbing them with a

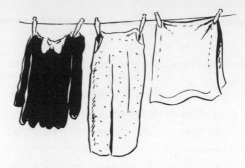

slice of raw **POTATO** before tossing the duds into the washing machine. They always emerged spotless.

TIP We've all been faced with this frustrating puzzle: You've just broken a lightbulb that's still in its socket, and you have to get the danged thing out without cutting yourself. How on earth do you do it? The way Grandma Putt did—that's how! First, make sure the power to the fixture is turned off! Next, push half of a raw **POTATO,** cut side first, against the broken bulb. Turn the spud just as you would to unscrew a whole lightbulb. It'll come right out. Then, toss the whole thing in the trash (don't try to separate the bulb from the tater).

TIP To deodorize your refrigerator, cut a raw **POTATO** in two, and set both halves inside, cut sides up. When the surfaces turn black (as they will in a week or so), just shave off the discolored layer, and put the clean sections back on the job.

In Grandma's Day

Like most gardeners, Grandma Putt was none too happy to see weeds growing in her lawn or garden—with a few exceptions. For instance, she almost jumped for joy in the spring, when **LAMB'S QUARTERS** and **PURSLANE** began appearing. So did I, because I knew what was coming next: Grandma would pluck off individual leaves from small purslane plants, and clip off the top 2 or 3 inches of lamb's quarters when the plants got to be 3 to 4 inches tall. Then she'd toss 'em all in a big salad with an oil-and-vinegar dressing. I'll tell you, boy, that was mighty fine eatin'! (In fact, it still is. Try it—you'll like it!)

How Dry They Are

Grandma Putt dried her home-grown herbs in her attic, which had the conditions herbs need to retain their volatile oils (the secret of their health-giving, house-cleaning, pest-defying power). What are those conditions? Low humidity, good air circulation, and near-total darkness. But you don't need an attic in order to dry herbs. Here's the rundown.

If You're Drying Your Herbs Here	Go About It This Way
In a dark room	Set old window screens or hardware cloth on bricks or other supports, and spread the herb stalks on top. Leave a door or window open a crack, and turn on a fan or two so that air circulates through the room.
In a room where light penetrates	Gather the sprays into bunches of five or six stems each, and tie the stems together with twine. Then put each bunch upside down in a brown paper bag (making sure the herbs aren't touching the bottom), fasten the top with a rubber band, and hang the bundles.
In an electric oven*	Heat the oven to 200°F, then turn it off. Spread your herbs in a single layer on a baking sheet, set them in the oven, and leave them for six to eight hours, or until crisp.
In a gas oven*	Spread your herbs in a single layer on a baking sheet. Then, turn the oven to its lowest setting, and heat it, with the door open, for two to three minutes at the lowest temperature that will keep the pilot light on. (This will get rid of any moisture.) Turn off the oven, set the herbs inside, and close the door. They should be dry in six to eight hours.
In a microwave oven*	Put a single layer of herbs between two paper towels, and nuke 'em for two to three minutes. Give them additional 30-second jolts as necessary until they're crisp. (But keep a close watch to make sure they don't burn!)
In a food dehydrator*	Set the temperature between 95°F and 100°F. Spread your herbs in a single layer on a tray, and put them in the dehydrator. Depending on the fleshiness of the leaves, the drying process can take anywhere from 4 to 18 hours, so be patient, and keep checking!

* To keep flavors and scents from mixing and mingling, dry only one type of herb at a time.

TIP When I was a boy, we all had inkwells on our desks at school, and we did all of our lessons with old-fashioned fountain pens. Although I loved writing with those things, I was not, shall we say, the most careful kid on the block. I was forever coming home with ink stains on my shirt, and sometimes even my pants. Fortunately, as usual, Grandma knew exactly what to do: She'd make me change into my play clothes, pronto. Then she'd lay the stained fabric on a flat surface, and put a slice of raw **TOMATO** on each ink blotch. When the tomato had absorbed all the ink, she'd launder the garment as usual.

TIP If you like your home decor on the rustic side, replace your traditional curtain rods with **TREE BRANCHES.** Just find or cut straight, slender branches to the length you need, and cut off any protrusions that could snag the fabric. (Depending on your taste and the type of tree, you can either strip off the bark or leave it on.) Then slide your curtains onto the branch, and rest your curtain rod on store-bought wood or metal rod mounts. *Note:* This trick works best with curtains that hang by tabs or rings, rather than those with rod pockets.

Family and FRIENDS

TIP Keep your canine and feline friends flea-free with this simple rinse. Just cut an **ORANGE** into thin slices, put them in a quart of hot water, and let the brew steep overnight (or for eight hours during the day). Then, once a day during the flea season, groom your dog or outdoor-roaming cat with a flea comb, and sponge on the orange rinse. (*Note:* Test it on a small patch of your pet's skin first, because some dogs and cats are allergic to the oils in citrus fruits.)

TIP When Grandma Putt went on a picnic, or took a walk in the woods, ticks could put a damper on the fun, all right. But nowadays—as we all know too well—they do a lot worse than that. These vile villains can also spread dreaded diseases to you and your four-footed pals. Fortunately, one of Grandma's most effective tick repellents still does a first-class job. (It repels fleas, too.) What is it? **PENNYROYAL,** a small-leaved, low-growing perennial herb that makes a terrific groundcover for shady spots. What's more, it has spikes of fragrant lavender flowers, it's a snap to grow, and it's hardy from Zones 4 to 10. To use it in your war against ticks, just dry the leaves, and grind them up in a blender. Then, rub the powder into your pets' fur; and sprinkle it around in their (and your) outdoor play spaces.

TIP If your children or grandchildren suffer from car sickness, as a lot of youngsters do, here's an easy way to make their road trips more fun: Five or 10 minutes before you head out, serve them each a cup of **PEPPERMINT** tea. You'll find Grandma Putt's Herb Tea recipe on page 89.

TIP Grandma Putt had several big, old **PINE** trees growing in her yard. Every year at Christmastime, she brewed gallons of what she called her Piney Woods Bath Tea, and sent bottles of it to her friends who lived where they couldn't grow these fragrant evergreens. It's a snap to make. For each one-bath "serving," put 1 cup of fresh pine needles in a pot on the stove, and add 2 cups of water. Bring it to a boil, and remove the pan from the heat. Let the mix steep for about half an hour, or until the water reaches room temperature. Strain off the pine needles, and pour the water through a funnel into a pretty bottle with a tight stopper. At bath time, pour the whole contents into a tub of water, at whatever temperature you prefer.

TONICS & TODDIES

LAVENDER BATH BLEND

Grandma Putt used to make nearly all of the Christmas and birthday presents that she gave her friends and family. One favorite of all the female recipients was this simple concoction.

1 part lavender blossoms (fresh or dried)
1 part comfrey leaves (fresh or dried)
1 part Epsom salts
Lavender oil

Mix the blossoms, leaves, and salts in a bowl. Add a few drops of the oil (let your nose be your guide), and blend the ingredients well with your hands or a wooden spoon. Store in a decorative jar or other lidded container. Use a handful per bath to relax tired, achy muscles.

ONE MORE TIME

The outsides of citrus fruits have almost as many uses as the innards. Just take a gander at these a-peeling possibilities (sorry—I couldn't resist).

Indoors

▷ **Asthma-relief aids.** Studies show that the limonene in **CITRUS** peels seems to neutralize inhaled ozone, which often triggers asthma attacks. So if you're troubled by this nasty condition, grab one of these colorful skins, and sniff early and often!

▷ **Corn removers.** Before you go to bed, press a piece of fresh **LEMON** peel—inner side down—to the top of the corn—and tape it on with a bandage or adhesive tape. Leave it on overnight, and repeat each night for a week.

▷ **Facial cleansers.** Grind **ORANGE** or **LEMON** peels in a blender or coffee grinder until they're about the consistency of cornmeal. Then mix about 1 tablespoon of the ground peels with enough plain yogurt to make a paste. (If you have dry skin, substitute vegetable oil for the yogurt.) Wash your face with the mixture, rinse with cool water, and pat dry. If you have "citrus grounds" left over, spread them out on a plate to air-dry for an hour or so, or nuke 'em in the microwave for about two minutes. Then store them in a clean glass jar until you're ready to make another batch of cleanser, or put them to another good use.

▷ **Garbage-disposal fresheners.** Every now and then, after you've squeezed the juice out of a **CITRUS** fruit, cut the rind into chunks, and run it through your disposal to prevent unpleasant odors from forming.

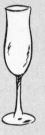

▷ **Glassware brighteners.** Put pieces of **LEMON** peel into the water you use to rinse glassware (including candlesticks and other decorative pieces). They'll come out crystal clear and shiny bright!

▷ **House sellers.** Real estate surveys show that this elixir is one of the two most likely aromas to make potential buyers say, "This is the place!" To make it, just bring 3 to 4 quarts of water to a boil, and add the shaved rind of one **ORANGE,** 1/4 cup of whole cloves, and four or five cinnamon sticks. Let the brew simmer until the scent has wafted through the house—or at least the kitchen. Then turn off the heat, and get outta Dodge while your agent guides the tour. (P.S. The other scent with top-class sales appeal is that of fresh-baked bread.)

▷ **Potpourri ingredients.** Dry an assortment of slivered **CITRUS** peels, then use them in a potpourri recipe, or add them to a store-bought blend to give it an extra kick.

▷ **Room fresheners.** Throw pieces of dried **CITRUS** peel (your choice of flavors) into the fireplace. They'll fill the whole house with a wonderful fragrance.

▷ **Tooth "brushes."** Wipe the inside of a slice of **LEMON** or **LIME** peel over your teeth and gums. Both fruits contain chemicals that whiten choppers and fight gum disease.

Outdoors

▷ **Cat repellents.** Scatter ground-up **GRAPEFRUIT, ORANGE,** or **LEMON** peels on freshly tilled soil to keep Fluffy from using it as a litter box.

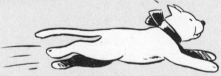

▷ **Mosquito repellents.** At your next barbecue, lay out the unwelcome mat for blood-thirsty skeeters by tossing a handful of **CITRUS** peels onto the coals. (Choose the kind that works best with whatever you're cooking.)

▷ **Seed-starter pots.** Hollow out half rinds of **LEMON, LIME, ORANGE,** or **GRAPEFRUIT,** and punch holes in the bottom using an awl or large nail. Fill the shells with starter mix, add your seeds, and set them in a tray. When your plants emerge, move them to the garden, "pots" and all.

▷ **Slug and snail traps.** Shortly before dark, set hollowed-out **ORANGE** or **GRAPEFRUIT** rinds among your plants. By morning, the skins will be filled with the slimy troublemakers. Pick up the traps and dump them—and the pesky pests—into a bucket of water with about a half cup of soap added to it. Then toss it on the compost pile. (If you don't have a compost pile, just bury it in your garden; the peels, soft bodies, and snail shells will all decompose and enrich the soil.)

▷ **Ultra-safe insecticide.** Put 1 cup of chopped **CITRUS** peels in a blender, and pour $1/4$ cup of boiling water over them. Liquefy, then let the mixture sit overnight at room temperature. Strain the slurry through cheesecloth or old pantyhose, pour the liquid into a hand-held spray bottle, and fill the balance of the bottle with water. Use it to polish off destructive caterpillars, or other soft-bodied insects, including whiteflies and aphids.

TIP **ROSEMARY,** like pennyroyal (see page 107), does a dandy job of keeping ticks and fleas away from you and your four-footed pals. It's an evergreen shrub with pale blue flowers and aromatic, grayish foliage. It's hardy only in Zones 8 to 10, but in colder territory, you can grow it in a pot outside, as Grandma Putt did, then bring it indoors at the first sign of frost. It'll sail right through the winter in a sunny window. To make your repellent powder, dry the leaves,

and grind them up in a blender. Then, rub the powder into your pets' fur, and sprinkle it around in their (and your) outdoor play areas.

TIP If you prefer a tick-and-flea repellent in liquid form, make a big batch of one of Grandma's favorites: **ROSEMARY** tea. Just boil 4 cups of spring water in a pan, and toss in 1 cup of rosemary leaves, either dried or fresh. Cover the pan, remove it from the heat, and let it cool. Strain the tea into another pan or jar, and let it sit while you give Rover a bath with a high-quality dog shampoo—*not* the flea and tick kind. (Use puppy shampoo if he's less than a year old—or 18 months for a giant breed like a Great Dane or Saint Bernard.) Rinse well to remove all traces of the shampoo, then pour the tea onto his coat, work it in well, and let it dry. Those blood-sucking bugs will dine elsewhere.

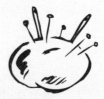

TIP If you're looking for a small gift for all the sewing buffs on your list, follow Grandma Putt's example, and make up a bunch of **ROSEMARY** pincushions. Just buy some small muslin bags at a craft shop (or, as Grandma did, make your own from scraps of pretty fabric and ribbon). Then pack the pouch as full

In Grandma's Day

When I was a small boy, Grandma Putt taught me how to grow an indoor "lawn," and it quickly became one of my favorite wintertime projects. Here's all there is to it: Find a natural sponge with large pores (not the synthetic kind), and soak it in water for a couple of minutes, until it's sopping wet. Squeeze it until it's about half dry, and sprinkle **GRASS SEED** into the openings on top. Then set the sponge on a plate in a sunny window, and sprinkle it lightly with water every day. Before you know it, you'll have a tiny patch of green to remind you that spring is just around the corner!

as you can with dried rosemary, and stitch it closed. Besides giving off a wonderful aroma, the rosemary will keep your sewing needles sharp and free of rust.

The great
OUTDOORS

TIP Grandma Putt loved her **BRUSSELS SPROUTS,** and she always grew plenty of them. But she never dreamed that they could help her fight weeds. Recently, though, scientists have discovered that these mini cabbages are jam-packed with thiocyanate, a chemical that's toxic to newly germinated seeds, especially small ones. And that makes them the perfect tool for attacking weeds that spring up in hard-to-reach places. Here's all you need to do: In early spring, blend 1 cup of Brussels sprouts in a blender or food processor, add enough water to make a thick mush, and whirl 'em for another few seconds. Add ½ teaspoon of dishwashing liquid, and pour the mixture into cracks in your sidewalk, driveway, or anyplace you want to stop weeds from germinating.

GRANDMA PUTT'S
Secret Formulas

FLOWERY BUG BUSTER

Whenever Grandma hand-watered her garden, she'd use this double-duty formula. It gave her plants a drink, and repelled all kinds of bad-guy bugs at the same time.

¼ **cup of marigold flower tops**
¼ **cup of geranium flower tops**
¼ **cup of garlic cloves**
5 gal. of water

Chop the flower tops and garlic (I use a food processor), and mix them in a bucket with the water. Let the mix sit overnight, and strain it into your watering can. Sprinkle your garden with this elixir, then scatter the solids on the ground to deliver even more bug-chasing power.

TIP Grandma had a simple way to trap slugs and snails in her garden: In the early evening, she'd set **CABBAGE** leaves among her troubled plants. By the morning, the leaves would be full of the slimy pests, and she'd just scoop the cabbage leaves up (bugs and all), and dump 'em into a bucket of soapy water (just a tablespoon or so of dishwashing liquid will do the trick). Then she'd toss it all onto the compost pile.

TIP If you'd rather not get close to touching slugs, bury some shallow cat food or tuna cans up to their rims. Then slice your **CABBAGE** leaves into thin strips, put them into the cans, and fill each one with salt water (about 1 teaspoon of salt per can of water). The slugs and snails will home in on the cabbage, fall into the drink, and drown.

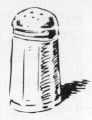

TIP If you grow "mildew magnets" like garden phlox, asters, and mums, it pays to have a prevention plan. One of the best I know of is this ultra-easy spray that Grandma would use to fend off both downy and powdery mildew. Here's all there is to it: Boil 10 cloves of **GARLIC** in 4 cups of water for half an hour. Strain, let the liquid cool to room temperature, and pour it into a hand-held spray bottle. When you get a spell of warm days and cool, humid nights—prime mildew weather—spray your trouble-prone plants every four or five days.

TIP Use the same **GARLIC** tea (see the tip above) to protect seedlings from damping-off fungus. Start mist-spraying your baby plants with the brew as soon as their little heads appear above the starter mix.

TIP This easy-to-make "condiment" is a must-have in your pest-control "pantry." Mince one whole bulb of **GARLIC,** mix it with 1 cup of vegetable oil, and put it in a glass jar with a tight lid. Set it in the refrigerator, and let it steep for a day or two. To test it for "doneness," remove the lid and take a sniff. If the aroma is so strong you want to drop the jar and run, you're good to go. If the scent isn't that strong, add half a minced garlic bulb, and wait another day. Then, strain out the solids, pour the oil into a fresh jar, and store it in the refrigerator.

TIP Turn your **GARLIC** oil (see the previous tip) into a potent pesticide by whirling 1 tablespoon of the oil in a blender with 4 cups of water and 3 drops of dishwashing liquid. Pour the mixture into a hand-held spray bottle, then take aim, and fire. The potion will deal a death blow to any soft-bodied insects, including aphids, whiteflies, and destructive caterpillars.

TIP There are jillions of mosquito repellents on the market these days, but for my money, none of them can beat the ones that Grandma grew in her **HERB** garden: lemon thyme *(Thymus* x *citriodorus),* lemon balm *(Melissa* *officinalis)*, and lemon basil *(Ocimum basilicum* 'Citriodorum'). To put them to work, all you have to do is crush the leaves to release their volatile oils, and rub them on your skin. You'll love the strong, citrusy scent—but skeeters will avoid you like the plague!

ONE MORE TIME

 When your **GARDEN HOSE** springs an irreparable leak or two, don't fret. As Grandma Putt would say, that little accident is a blessing in disguise, because holey hoses can perform a whole lot of useful chores around the yard. Here's a sampling.

▷ **Blade guards.** To protect the "business end" of a saw, ax, or knife, cut a piece of hose that's the same length as the blade. Then cut a slit down the middle of the hose, and slip it over the blade.

▷ **Design aid.** Keep your old, worn-out hose in one piece, and use it whenever you want to lay out new garden beds. Just lay it on the ground, and move it around until you get the shape you want. Use a spade to mark the outline in the ground, then stash the hose back in the tool-shed until you need it again.

▷ **Fake snake.** If birds are making off with your fruit, cut an old black or green hose into 4- or 5-foot lengths. Then wrap strips of red or yellow tape around the hose every few inches to look like stripes, and set the scary serpents around your trees or bushes. When the fine feathered felons start to fly in for breakfast, they'll take one look at that pretend predator and move their appetites elsewhere.

▷ **Soaker hose.** Just poke more holes all along the length, using an ice pick. Block one end with a wine cork or duct tape, and lay the hose in the bed you want to water. (If you want to keep it there permanently, cover it with compost or other mulch to make it blend in with the scenery.) Then attach the open end to an outdoor tap, or—depending on the distance involved—to a regular hose, and turn the faucet on gently.

▷ **Tree protector.** When you must stake a newly planted sapling, cover your ties with pieces of hose, so they don't damage the baby tree's tender bark.

ONE MORE TIME

Around our place, nothing was ever simply thrown away—not even **WEEDS.** That's because Grandma knew that most of these unwanted plants contained valuable nutrients that would make fine additions to her compost pile. Of course, she gave them a little pretreatment first. She either spread them out in the hot sun until they dried to a crisp, or dumped them in a bucket of water until they rotted. Then she tossed them on to the heap, secure in the knowledge that their reproductive days were a thing of the past.

TIP Is there a fungus among us? Nix that nastiness in a hurry by spraying your plagued plants with Grandma Putt's **HORSERADISH** tea. Just put 1 part horseradish leaves in a bucket, and pour 4 parts boiling water over them. Let the brew cool to room temperature, pour it into a hand-held spray bottle, and spritz your plants from top to bottom.

TIP Here's a first aid tip for all you hikers, backpackers, and trail riders: If you cut yourself when you're out in the middle of nowhere, with no antiseptic on hand, a **JUNIPER** tree can save the day. Just pluck a handful of berries, mash then up, and apply the glop to your wound. Cover the site with a clean, wet bandanna (or whatever cloth you have on hand). Then go to sleep. By morning, you'll be well on the mend.

TIP There is no cure for a plant virus, but a "vaccine" made from a green **PEPPER** plant may fend off attacks. In a blender or food processor, liquefy 2 cups of leaves from a healthy green pepper plant and 2 cups of water. Dilute the mixture with an equal amount of water, add ½ teaspoon of dishwashing liquid, and pour the solution into a hand-held spray bottle. Drench your plants from top to bottom.

TIP Whenever Grandma's **PINE** trees shed their needles, she'd scoop up the prickly things, and put them in a big bucket. Then, anytime she needed to fend off cutworms, slugs, or other soft-bodied crawlers, she'd scoop out some needles, and scatter them around the base of each vulnerable plant.

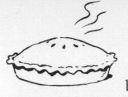

TIP Grandma told me that when she was a girl, folks swore by rotten **POTATOES** as a first-class dog repellent. They scattered them in new planting beds, around garbage cans, and anyplace else where they didn't want Rover to roam.

TIP **QUACKGRASS** may not be an attractive addition to your yard, but it's a very useful one if you're doing battle with slugs. That's because dried, dead quackgrass gives off a chemical that kills the slimy villains. So anytime you pull up a clump of the weeds, cut off the blades, and set them among the slugs' target plants. Leave the roots in the sun until they're good and dead, then toss 'em on the compost pile.

TIP This may seem like an odd thing to say, but I was always secretly overjoyed whenever aphids or whiteflies got out of hand in Grandma's garden. How come? Because I knew that she'd probably go at 'em with her **RHUBARB** spray. She'd pluck enough leaves to make about 1 pound, and boil them in 4 cups of water for about half an hour. She'd strain out the solids, and pour the liquid into a hand-held spray bottle. Then she'd mix in 2 teaspoons of dishwashing liquid, and spray those little bugs to

Kingdom Come. After that, she'd go back to the kitchen and use the stems to make my favorite strawberry-rhubarb pie! (Just one word of caution: Rhubarb leaves are highly poisonous, so don't even think of using this spray on edible plants.)

GRANDMA PUTT'S
Secret Formulas

FUNGUS-FIGHTER SOIL DRENCH

When a soilborne fungus strikes your flower or vegetable garden, fight back with this potent potion that Grandma swore by.

4 garlic bulbs, crushed
½ cup of baking soda
1 gal. of water

Combine these ingredients in a big pot, and bring the water to a boil. Then turn off the heat, and let the mixture cool to room temperature. Strain the liquid into a watering can, and soak the ground around your stricken (or fungus-prone) plants. Go very slowly, so the elixir goes deep into the soil. Then, dump the strained-out garlic pieces onto the soil, and work them in gently, so as not to disturb the plant roots.

Scat!

There's no doubt about it: Grandma Putt had some mighty power-ful pest-control potions (and you'll find a lot of them throughout this book). But she didn't have to reach for those weapons very often, because she knew an old-time secret that scientists have confirmed: The roots, leaves, and flowers of all plants send out chemicals, and some of these sub-stances repel particular insects and even bigger, four-legged critters. Here are some examples of how you can put 'em to work in your own yard.

To Keep These at Bay	Plant These Among Their Targets
Ants	Pennyroyal, southernwood, spearmint, tansy
Aphids	Chives, garlic, mint, nasturtiums, onions
Asparagus beetles	Basil, calendulas, nasturtiums, parsley, tomatoes*
Black vine weevils	Catnip
Borers	Garlic, onions, tansy
Cabbage loopers	Garlic, hot peppers, onions, rosemary, sage, tansy, thyme
Cabbage moths (the parents of cabbageworms)	Hyssop, mint, rosemary, sage, thyme
Cats	Rue
Colorado potato beetles	Catnip, horseradish, nasturtiums, tansy
Deer	Catnip, chives, garlic, lavender, onions, rosemary, scented geraniums, spearmint, thyme, yarrow
Flea beetles	Catnip, mint, wormwood
Fruit-tree moths	Southernwood
Gophers	Daffodils, squill
Japanese beetles	Garlic, larkspur, rue, tansy, white geraniums (*Pelargonium*)
Mexican bean beetles	Marigolds, nasturtiums, rosemary, savory
Mice	Mint
Moles	Mole plant (*Euphorbia lathyrus*), spurge (*E. cyparissias*), squill
Mosquitoes	Southernwood, wormwood

To Keep These at Bay	Plant These Among Their Targets
Plum curculios	Garlic
Rabbits	Dusty miller, garlic, Mexican marigolds (*Tagetes lucida*), onions, ornamental alliums
Root-knot nematodes	French marigolds (*Tagetes patula*)
Rose chafers	Geraniums (*Pelargonium*), onions, ornamental alliums, petunias
Slugs and snails	Prostrate rosemary, wormwood
Tomato hornworms	Borage, marigolds, opal basil

* Asparagus has a big appetite, and it suffers when any other roots share its food supply, so don't put these (or any other plants) directly into the soil of your asparagus bed. Instead, plant them in containers, and set them around the asparagus plants.

TIP Clubroot can cause big problems in cabbage-family plants (including broccoli, Brussels sprouts, and cauliflower). Fortunately, Grandma knew how to make sure that her brassica crops didn't join the club: She just buried stalks of **RHUBARB** in the planting beds. It worked like a charm—and it still does at my house!

TIP If roving cats are making mischief in your yard, here's a trick you can try the next time you prune your **ROSES.** Spread those thorny canes on freshly tilled soil to keep Fluffy from using it as a litter box. Or lay them on the ground under birdbaths, feeders, and nesting boxes to protect your fine feathered pals. (This same trick will keep raccoons out of your vegetable patch—or your garbage can.)

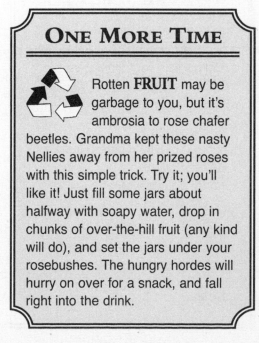

ONE MORE TIME

Rotten **FRUIT** may be garbage to you, but it's ambrosia to rose chafer beetles. Grandma kept these nasty Nellies away from her prized roses with this simple trick. Try it; you'll like it! Just fill some jars about halfway with soapy water, drop in chunks of over-the-hill fruit (any kind will do), and set the jars under your rosebushes. The hungry hordes will hurry on over for a snack, and fall right into the drink.

TIP Grandma always said that a patch of **STINGING NETTLES** is one of a gardener's best friends. Besides packing a load of nitrogen that's as potent as manure, they give off chemicals that repel all kinds of pesky pests. That's why, several times during the growing season, she brewed up a pot of nettle tea and served it to all of her plants. To make your own batch, just put 1 pound of stinging nettle leaves in a bucket, and pour in 1 gallon of water. Let the mix sit for at least a week, strain out the leaves, and give your plants a good drink.

TIP If you grow roses, you know what a pain in the grass black spot can be. Well, here's good news: If you reach the scene at the first sign of a breakout, a couple of garden vegetables can help you turn the tide. Just gather 15 **TOMATO** leaves and two small onions, chop them into fine pieces, and steep them in rubbing alcohol overnight. Strain out the solids, then use a small, sponge-type paintbrush to apply the liquid to both the tops and bottoms of any infected rose leaves.

TIP Grandma used **TOMATO** leaves in another fresh-from-the-garden potion to protect her flowers from flea beetles, whiteflies, and other pesky pests. To make your own supply, put 2 cups of chopped tomato leaves in a pan with 4 cups of water. Bring the water to a simmer (not a boil). Then turn off the heat, and let the mixture cool. Strain out the leaves, and add $\frac{1}{2}$ teaspoon of dishwashing liquid to the water. Pour the solution into a hand-held spray bottle, and spritz your plants from top to bottom. Tomato leaves are poisonous, so don't use this spray on any plants that you intend to eat.

GRANDMA PUTT'S
Secret Formulas

WILD MUSTARD TEA

Cabbage moths, cabbage loopers, and potato beetles all steered clear of Grandma's vegetable garden because she sprayed her plants with this tangy "beverage."

4 whole cloves
1 handful of wild mustard leaves
1 clove of garlic
1 cup of boiling water

Steep the cloves, mustard leaves, and garlic in the boiling water for 10 minutes. Strain out the solids, let the liquid cool, and pour it into a hand-held spray bottle. Then go get those bad bugs!

Avocados

Where we lived, in the snowy North, Grandma couldn't even dream of growing avocados. And in those days, before farmers started shipping their produce all over the country, she couldn't even buy them at her neighborhood grocery store. But if she could have, she'd have found plenty of great uses for these mellow, green fruits. Here's a rundown.

▶ *Bring dry, frizzy hair under control.* Peel and mash a ripe avocado, work it into your hair, and leave it on for 15 minutes. Rinse it out with cool water.

▶ *Deep-condition your hair.* (If your locks are showing the effects of heat and smog, this tip has your name on it.) Mash half of an avocado with 1/4 cup of mayonnaise (the real stuff, with eggs and oil in it). Massage the mixture into your scalp, and comb it out to the ends of your tresses. Cover your hair with a shower cap, and wrap a hot, wet towel around your head. Leave it on for at least 30 minutes, and then rinse.

▶ *Soften and invigorate normal to oily skin.* Mix 2 tablespoons of mashed avocado with 1 tablespoon of crushed almonds and 1/2 teaspoon of honey until the mixture is creamy. Smooth it onto your face with your hands, and leave on for 30 minutes or so. Rinse with lukewarm water, and pat dry.

▶ *Soothe, soften, and nourish dry skin.* Mix 1/2 mashed avocado with 1/2 mashed banana, and spread the "cream" on your face and neck. Wait 15 minutes, rinse with lukewarm water, and pat dry.

▶ *Soothe and soften some more.* This facial works wonders on any skin type. Mix 2 tablespoons of mashed avocado with 2 tablespoons of honey and 1 egg yolk. Spread the mixture over your face, leave it on for 30 minutes, rinse with warm water, and pat dry.

And About Those Covers...

Avocados got their nickname, alligator pears, from their tough, leathery—and hard-working—skins. Here's a sampling of what you can do with them.

▶ *Give yourself an ultra-easy facial.* Take an avocado peel with a thin layer of fruit left on it and rub the rind over your face. Its gritty texture will slough off dead skin, while the pulp that stays on your face moisturizes it. Wait 10 minutes, and rinse with cool water.

(continued)

(continued from page 119)

➧ *Say good-bye to rough skin.* Use plain old peels, minus the fruit, to soften the skin on your heels and elbows. Just sprinkle the inside of a peel with a few drops of lemon juice, and rub it across the rough body part. It'll feel a little strange at first, but your dry skin will love it— guaranteed!

➧ *Feed your flowers.* Bury avocado peels near your flowering plants (especially roses) to provide a potent dose of magnesium and potassium.

➧ *Trap slugs.* Just set avocado peels in your garden at night. Come morning, collect the slug-filled rinds, and drop them into a bucket of soapy water. Then dump it all on the compost pile.

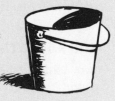

➧ *Start seeds.* Poke a few holes in the bottoms of avocado peels, and put them in a tray or shallow pan. Fill each "pot" with a commercial starter mix, and plant your seeds. When it's time to move the seedlings to the garden, plant 'em pot and all.

Don't Forget the Seeds

Talk about versatile fruit! Even the seeds (pits) of avocados do yeoman's work as beauty aids. Here's a duo of dandy ways to use them in your skin-care routine.

➧ *Give yourself a massage.* Rinse all of the fruit off an avocado pit, and rub the pit over your arms, legs, hips, and as much of your back as you can reach. It'll improve your circulation, and make you feel good all over. (Some folks also claim it helps conquer cellulite.)

➧ *Add punch to cleansing cream.* Remove the fruit from three or four avocado pits. Put the pits in a heavy-duty, zip-top plastic bag and smash them with a hammer until the pieces are about the size of peas. Then spread the little chunks on a baking sheet to dry for a few days. When they're completely dry, put them into a coffee grinder or food processor, and grind them into a powder (about the consistency of ground coffee). Again, spread them out to dry, and store them in an airtight container (a clamp-top canning jar is perfect). When you wash your face, add a teaspoon or so of the ground pits to your favorite liquid soap or cleansing potion.

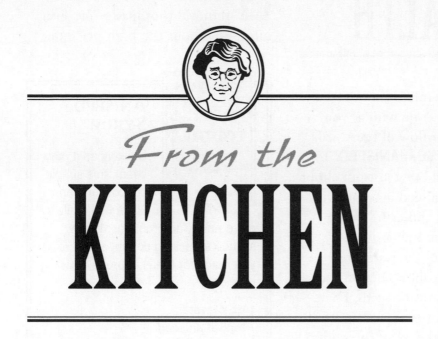

CHAPTER FOUR

From the

KITCHEN

121

Aluminum foil

Baking soda

Beer

Bread

Cayenne pepper

Coffee

Cola

Cornmeal

Eggs

Flour

Food coloring

Honey

Milk

Molasses

Mustard

Oatmeal

Olive oil

Salt

Sugar

Vegetable oil

Vinegar

Yogurt

and more...

To your HEALTH

flavored extract, like peppermint, vanilla, or cinnamon.

TIP For all the power of a stain-removal toothpaste—or even more—without the high price tag,

TIP If you're a nursing mother, or know someone who is, you can increase your flow of breast milk with a tea made from **ANISEED.** To make this helpful brew, just put about 7 teaspoons of aniseed in a pan with 1 quart of water, and bring it to a boil. Reduce the heat to low, simmer until the water has reduced to about 3 cups, and strain out the seeds. Then, once or twice a day, drink two cups of the potion, sweetened to taste with honey if you like. (This same tasty beverage also relieves indigestion and stomach upset.)

TIP Grandma Putt never bought a tube of toothpaste in her life. Instead, she kept her teeth and gums healthy by brushing twice a day with a little **BAKING SODA** on a wet toothbrush. If you don't care for the taste of plain soda, mix it with a few drops of your favorite

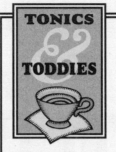

TONICS & TODDIES

ANISEED SYRUP

Unlikely as it may seem, this simple concoction can solve two of life's more annoying problems: It can silence a hacking cough, and (are you ready for this?) improve your memory.

1 qt. of water
7 tsp. of aniseed
4 tsp. of honey
4 tsp. of glycerin*

Bring the water to a boil, and add the aniseed. Reduce the heat to low, and simmer until the water is reduced to about 3 cups. Strain out the seeds, and while the brew is still warm, stir in the honey and glycerin. For cough relief, take 2 teaspoons of the syrup every few hours until your hacking stops. To give the old gray cells a boost, take 2 tablespoons three times a day as long as you feel the need.

* Available at drugstores

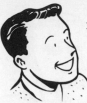 mash a ripe strawberry, and mix it with enough **BAKING SODA** to make a paste. Use it as you would any other toothpaste, and watch those pearly whites brighten up!

TIP Fight the bacteria that cause gum disease by brushing with a paste made of 3 parts **BAKING SODA** and 1 part hydrogen peroxide.

TIP Get rid of painful canker sores by rinsing your mouth with a solution of ½ teaspoon of **BAKING SODA** in half a glass of warm water. Repeat every few hours, as necessary, until the bothersome bumps are gone.

TIP Before commercial denture cleansers came along, folks cleaned their false teeth by soaking them in a bowl of water (2 cups or so) with 2 teaspoons of **BAKING SODA** added to it. And it still works just as well today!

TIP After a long day in the garden, Grandma Putt relaxed her tired, stiff muscles by soaking in a tub of warm water with ½ cup of **BAKING SODA** added to it. (This simple treatment will also make your skin feel softer and smoother.)

In Grandma's Day

When Grandma Putt was a youngster, folks couldn't run to the drugstore for antibiotic salves and ointments. Instead, they got their medicine wherever they could find it. And sometimes, they found it in the breadbox. For instance, this was a favorite treatment for infected cuts, and even dog bites: Soak a few slices of slightly moldy **BREAD** in condensed milk or half-and-half, apply the poultice to the wound, and fasten it on with a gauze bandage and adhesive tape. Change the dressing daily until the inflammation and redness are gone. (Grandma never had to use this on me, but she swore it acted almost overnight.)

TIP When you spend as much time outdoors as Grandma Putt and I did, you tend to get more than your share of bug bites. Fortunately, she knew a lot of ways to reduce the pain, itch, and swelling—including this tried-and-true routine. Dissolve 1 teaspoon of **BAKING SODA** in 1 cup of water. Then dip a clean, soft cloth into the solution, and hold it on the bite for 20 minutes or so.

TIP All kinds of things can make your skin break out in hives and rashes. But no matter what caused the itchy, red blotches, this old trick will send 'em packin' in no time. Just add 3 or 4 tablespoons of **BAKING SODA** to a tub of warm bathwater, and settle in for a long, soothing soak (cool drink, glowing candle, and nonserious reading matter optional).

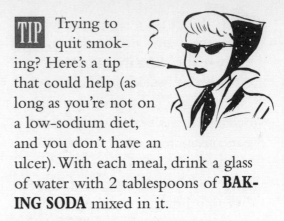

TIP Trying to quit smoking? Here's a tip that could help (as long as you're not on a low-sodium diet, and you don't have an ulcer). With each meal, drink a glass of water with 2 tablespoons of **BAKING SODA** mixed in it.

TIP Just like any other teenager, I was mortified when my face erupted in pimples. As always, though, Grandma rose to the occasion. She mixed equal parts of **BAKING SODA** and wheat germ with enough water to make a paste. Then she gave me the mixture, and told me to dab it onto the zits, wait about 10 minutes, rinse with warm water, and pat dry.

TIP Relieve heartburn the way Grandma did. Whenever you feel those annoying symptoms coming on, drink half a glass of water with $\frac{1}{2}$ teaspoon of **BAKING SODA** dissolved in it. Just one word of caution: If you're on a low-sodium diet, are over age 60, or are treating a child under age 5, consult your doctor before using this remedy.

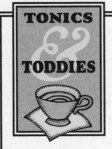

TONICS & TODDIES

SUPER-CHARGED CHICKEN SOUP

We all know that chicken soup is a powerful weapon in the fight against cold and flu germs. Well, here's a formula that will add even more *oomph* to your favorite recipe (or even instant chicken broth).

1 cup of chicken soup or broth
1 tbsp. of vinegar
1 garlic clove, crushed
Hot sauce

Heat the soup or broth, and stir in the vinegar, garlic, and hot sauce to taste. Then pour it into a bowl or mug, and sip yourself to health. Repeat as necessary until you're back in the pink again.

TIP When you feel yourself coming down with a cold, try this old-as-the-hills trick: Fill your bathtub with water that's as hot as you can stand it. While the tub is filling, pour a jigger of **BOURBON** into a glass of hot lemonade. Then settle into the tub, and sip your toddy. When you've finished, dry off and dive into bed. By morning, you'll be on top of the world again. (If you don't care for bourbon, or just don't have any on hand, substitute Irish whiskey, Scotch, or rum.)

TIP Grandma Putt had a remedy for boils that couldn't be beat—and it couldn't be simpler. Here's all there is to it: Soak a slice of **BREAD** in a bowl of milk until the bread is damp, but not sopping wet. Put the slice on top of the boil, fasten it on with a strip of cloth, and leave it there for 20 minutes or so. Repeat several times a day until the painful bump is history.

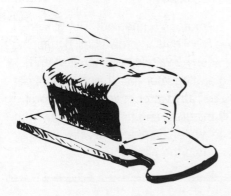

In Grandma's Day

The minute anyone in our house showed signs of a cold or flu, Grandma Putt (like mothers and grandmothers everywhere) put a big pot of **CHICKEN SOUP** on the stove, and served up bowl after bowl of the yummy stuff. But back in the Middle Ages, folks didn't think of chicken soup as a tasty germ fighter—they considered it an aphrodisiac!

TIP Once when my cousin Mary Ellen came to spend a few weeks at our place, she was struck with a nasty bout of menstrual cramps. But Grandma Putt cleared them up fast with this simple tea: Put 4 teaspoons of **CARAWAY SEEDS** on a cutting board or a sheet of wax paper, and flatten them slightly with the back of a spoon. Bring 2 cups of water to a boil, add the seeds, and simmer on low for five minutes. Remove the pan from the heat, and let the tea steep for another minute or two (but not enough to cool off). Sweeten with honey, if you like, and drink up. Just one cup should take care of the problem, but if not, sip a cup every hour or so until the pain vanishes.

TIP If you suffer from migraines, here's an old-time tip that could help end your agony: At the first sign of symptoms, dip a flat-ended toothpick into a jar of **CAYENNE PEPPER,** and sniff a tiny bit into each nostril. This remedy works for two reasons: Hot pepper contains both magnesium, which helps ward off migraines, and capsaicin, which blocks pain impulses from traveling to the brain. Just be sure you don't overdo it—a dash of pepper in the nose will deliver a HOT surprise!

TIP When you cut yourself in the kitchen, don't rush for the bathroom medicine chest. Instead, after washing the wound, sprinkle a pinch of **CAYENNE PEPPER** onto it. It'll stop the bleeding and help the wound close up fast.

TIP Nowadays, lots of people pay big bucks to have their teeth bleached. But I know an easier, cheaper—and much more enjoyable—way to keep your pearly whites white. What is it? Just say **CHEESE!** Eating that yummy treat

---

ONE MORE TIME

When Grandma ruled the kitchen, nothing went to waste—not even leftover **COOKING WATER.** Here are some of the ways she put that "experienced" liquid to use. (You might want to take special note of these tips if you live in a place where water shortages are becoming an all-too-frequent fact of life.)

▷ **Asparagus.** Clear up blackheads, pimples, and other facial sores by dabbing them with asparagus water twice a day.

▷ **Eggs.** Clean pewter by immersing the objects in egg water and letting

them sit for a few minutes. Then dip a soft cloth in the water, and rub your treasures clean. Rinse with clear water, and wipe dry.

▷ **Peas.** Relieve the itch of poison ivy and other rashes by sponging the skin with pea water. (Repeat as often as necessary.)

▷ **Potatoes** (unpeeled). Put glistening highlights in brown hair by dipping a pastry brush in potato water, and saturating your hair (being careful not to get any water in your eyes). Wait 30 minutes, and rinse thoroughly with cool water. Repeat every few weeks to retain the highlights.

(and other calcium-rich foods such as walnuts, almonds, rice, and oats) helps prevent your teeth from turning yellow.

TIP When you eat too much or too fast, and pay for it with heartburn, don't pop an antacid pill (unless your doctor has advised it, that is). Instead, grab a stick of **CHEWING GUM,** and chew it for half an hour or so. This will get your saliva flowing, so it can wash away the stomach acid that's leaking into your esophagus and causing the burning sensation.

TIP Need to calm a throbbing tooth? Do what Grandma did: Bite down gently on a whole **CLOVE** until you can get to the dentist's office. It will have a powerful taste, but it's also one of the best mouth-pain relievers around!

TIP Yikes! You were slicing a tomato for sandwiches, got distracted for a second, and sliced into your finger instead. Just reach for the powdered **CLOVES,** and pour a thin layer over your cut. It'll stop the pain and help prevent infection.

TIP Grandma Putt always kept a bottle of Coke syrup on hand, and used it to cure any kind of

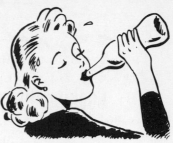

digestive trouble. Just a couple of teaspoons could cure anything from a tiny tummy ache to a full-blown case of vomiting. You may be able to get Coke syrup at your local drugstore. If not, just keep some **COLA** on hand (any brand will do). Then, when trouble strikes, open up the can or bottle, and let it go flat. Then sip your way back to comfort.

TIP When the bug bites or the bee stings, make a paste of **CORNSTARCH** and lemon juice, and apply it to the stricken spot. (Three parts cornstarch to 1 part lemon juice should be about right, but use more or less juice as needed.)

TIP As a boy, my hands were prone to blisters—and, of course, being a typical kid, I sure didn't want to wear gloves when I worked in the garden! As usual, Grandma had the answer to my problem: Before I headed out to do my chores, she'd have me rub a tablespoon or so of **CORNSTARCH** on my palms. The powdery stuff absorbed perspiration and prevented blisters from forming.

Cooking Oil Spray

Cooking oil in aerosol cans first hit supermarket shelves in the early 1960s, after Grandma Putt had departed from her earthly kitchen. But take my word for it: She'd have loved the convenience of spritzing her pots and pans—and dozens of other things, too. Here's a sampling of ways you can use this handy lubricant, indoors and out.

Indoors

▶ *Clean your grimy hands.* Coat them with cooking oil spray, rub it into your skin, then wash with soap and water. Dirt, grease, and latex paint will come right off.

▶ *Defrost your freezer easier.* The next time you do that messy chore, spray the bottom and sides of the compartment with cooking oil spray. The ice will be much easier to get off.

▶ *De-scum your shower door.* Spray a soft, cotton cloth with cooking oil spray, and wipe the gunk away.

▶ *Get a stuck ring off your finger.* Aim the nozzle at the spot between your skin and the metal intersect, and spray! Hold the digit up for a few seconds to let the oil penetrate, then slide the ring right off.

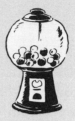

▶ *Get the gum out.* When a child gets chewing gum stuck in her hair, coat the lump with cooking oil spray (being careful not to get it in the youngster's eyes). Work the oil in with your fingers, then comb the sticky stuff out.

▶ *Keep plastic food containers stain- and odor-free.* Before you fill that holder with tomato sauce or any other colorful or aromatic food, spray the inside with cooking oil. This will help keep the contents from staining, or smelling up, the container.

▶ *Keep your dough together.* Spritz your table or work board with cooking oil spray before you roll out your dough. Your cookies or pie crust will peel right off, without leaving pieces stuck to the surface.

▶ *Loosen a screw.* Blast the stuck thing with cooking oil spray, and wait a few minutes to let it penetrate. That little piece of hardware should come right out.

▶ *Measure sticky stuff.* Before you pour honey, molasses, or other clingy fluids into a measuring cup, coat the surface with cooking oil spray. That way, the entire contents will flow out, and cleanup will be a breeze.

▶ *Prevent boilovers.* Spray the sides of a pot before you add water. That way, the liquid won't bubble up and over the sides when it's boiling.

▶ *Quiet squeaky hinges.* Spritz them with cooking oil spray, and they'll hush right up.

▶ *Remove labels and price tags.* Saturate the piece of paper (or the glue, if that's all that's left). Let it sit for five minutes or so, and slide it off with a plastic scraper or an old credit card.

▶ *Unstick a lock.* Give the lock and/or key a shot of cooking oil spray and say, "Open sesame!"

Outdoors

▶ *Clean your barbecue grill—fast.* Before you light the coals or turn on the gas, coat the grill with cooking oil spray. When the metal has cooled completely, just wipe it clean.

▶ *Cut it—smoothly.* Before you head out to prune plants or clip grass, "shoot" cooking oil spray into the working parts of your shears or clippers. They'll glide through their work, and your hands will say "Thank you!"

▶ *Dig it—easily.* Whether you're moving plants around your garden or digging new beds, spritz your shovel with cooking oil spray before you start, and every so often as the job progresses. It'll make digging in the dirt a snap!

▶ *Don't get frozen out.* Of your car, that is. Coat the door gaskets with cooking oil spray. It'll seal out water without harming the gaskets.

▶ *Lighten your snow load.* Coat your shovel with cooking oil spray. The white stuff will slide right off—making your job faster and easier.

▶ *Lubricate your bike chain.* Spritz it with cooking oil spray to keep it moving freely.

▶ *Protect your tools.* Lightly spritz the metal parts of all your tools to keep them free of rust and corrosion.

▶ *Say "No!" to grass.* Spray the blade, and the whole undercarriage of your lawn mower, with cooking oil spray before you start cutting the lawn. That way, the grass won't stick to the metal and gum up the works.

▶ *Speed across the snow.* Coat the bottom of a toboggan, snow tube, or saucer before you start down a snow-covered slope—if you want a *fast* ride, that is!

TIP When it came to treating minor burns, Grandma's kitchen was a gold mine of possibilities, and yours is, too. Like this one, for instance: Separate a raw **EGG** and gently apply the white part to the affected skin. It'll take the heat out fast!

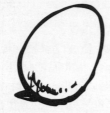

TIP To treat a sty or cyst on the eye, doctors often prescribe a hot compress, applied three or four times a day. And you'll find just what the doctor ordered in your refrigerator: an **EGG.** Pull one out, and hard-boil it. Wrap the hot egg (still in its shell) in a washcloth, and lay it against your sore eye for 10 minutes. When it's time for your next egg-laying session (sorry, I couldn't resist), put that same piece of "hen fruit" back in a pot of water, and reheat it.

TIP If you're a migraine sufferer, chances are you're always looking for new ways to conquer the pain and nausea those dreadful headaches bring on. Well, here's an old-time cure that folks still swear by: As soon as you feel the first hint of an attack, mix about ¼ teaspoon of ground **GINGER** in a glass of water, and drink up.

TIP When your stomach's doing flip-flops—whether the cause is the flu or a night on the town—reach for one of Grandma Putt's favorite tummy-tamers: **GINGER ALE.** Just pour yourself a big glass, and drink up. You'll be feeling ginger-peachy in no time!

TIP Once, Grandpa Putt got a cut on his heel that just wouldn't close up—until a retired doctor who lived down the street suggested a remedy that worked like a miracle. Here's all there is to it: Every night

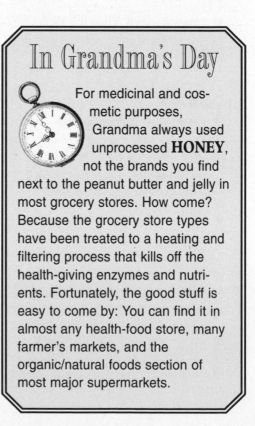

In Grandma's Day

For medicinal and cosmetic purposes, Grandma always used unprocessed **HONEY**, not the brands you find next to the peanut butter and jelly in most grocery stores. How come? Because the grocery store types have been treated to a heating and filtering process that kills off the health-giving enzymes and nutrients. Fortunately, the good stuff is easy to come by: You can find it in almost any health-food store, many farmer's markets, and the organic/natural foods section of most major supermarkets.

before bedtime, soak your foot for half an hour in a porcelain bowl (not metal) filled with enough Concord **GRAPE JUICE** to cover the sore. Gently pat the spot dry with a soft, cotton cloth, but don't rinse off the grape juice, and don't get the area wet when bathing. Healing time varies with the depth of the cut, but it should be gone after two to three weeks of nightly treatments.

TIP To heal stubborn sores elsewhere on your body, saturate a gauze pad in Concord **GRAPE JUICE**, apply it to the wound, and fasten it in place with adhesive tape. Replace the dressing every day, but don't wash the affected area. Before you know it, the nasty "owie" will be history.

TIP For simple sore-throat relief, you can't beat this trick: Just put a tablespoon or two of **HONEY** into a cup of hot water, stir in a teaspoon of lemon juice, and drink up. Repeat every few hours throughout the day. (But if your sore throat lasts longer than a couple of days, call your doctor.)

TIP To relieve a cough, mix a full cup of **HONEY** with 4 tablespoons of lemon juice and a half cup of olive oil. Heat the mixture for five minutes, then stir vigorously for two minutes. Take 1 teaspoon every two hours, and before you know it, your hacking will be history!

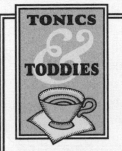

TONICS & TODDIES

RELIABLE MUSTARD RUB

This versatile formula clears up coughs and chest congestion, and delivers fast relief to sore muscles and stiff, achy joints. For best results, administer this treatment just before you go to bed.

2 tbsp. of olive oil
1 tsp. of dry mustard
1 tsp. of powdered ginger

Mix the ingredients together, and rub a tiny dab on your inner arm. Then wait 10 minutes. If the skin shows no sign of irritation, rub the rest of the mixture onto the troubled area until you feel a warm, tingling sensation. Depending on what body parts you've massaged with the oily mixture, either put on an old T-shirt, or cover the area with a soft, cotton cloth (thereby protecting your sheets). Then hop into bed and get a good night's rest. In the morning, wash off the residue with soap and water. Repeat as often as necessary.

Here's something that Grandma Putt knew: In addition to its many other virtues, **HONEY** is the only food on earth that never goes bad. In fact, archaeologists exploring the tombs of Egyptian pharaohs have found perfectly good honey that was thousands of years old!

TIP When acid indigestion strikes, strike back with **HONEY.** For immediate relief, take 1 to 3 teaspoons. To ease a chronic problem, take 1 tablespoon each night at bedtime, on an empty stomach, until you feel better. (Of course, if your discomfort continues for more than a few days, or if you experience other symptoms, call your doctor.)

TIP Like any other red-blooded American kid, I spent as much time as possible romping in the great outdoors—which meant that I got my full share of bug bites. But Grandma knew exactly how to eliminate the pain and itch: She just smoothed a dab of **HONEY** on each spot.

TIP I picked up a lot of cuts and scrapes in my day, and if Grandma happened to be in the kitchen when I came hollering for help, she'd wash the wound and spread **HONEY** over it. It dried to form a natural bandage and (as modern science has proven) hastened the healing process.

TIP To stop a migraine before it starts, take 1 teaspoon of **HONEY** the minute you feel the early warning signs.

TIP If you're too late to stop the pain, send a migraine packin' by taking 2 teaspoons of **HONEY** with each meal until your headache is history.

TIP Grandma Putt never had a weight problem, but whenever her friends wanted to shed a few pounds, they'd mix 2 teaspoons of **HONEY** in a glass of water, and drink it half an hour before each meal. It worked like a charm!

TIP It happens to most of us every now and then: We go to a party, imbibe a little too much, and wake up with the morning-after blahs. Well, don't take that hangover lying down. Instead, take 1 teaspoon of **HONEY** every hour until you feel better—which will be a lot sooner than you probably think possible.

TIP Got a stuffy nose? Grab a jar of prepared **HORSERADISH** from the refrigerator, and take a sniff. Repeat two or three times a day until you can breathe easier. (If the congestion lasts for more than a week, or if it's accompanied by green mucus, pain, or other symptoms, call your doctor pronto.)

TIP Looking for a *really* simple way to clobber cold symptoms? Just reach into the kitchen cupboard, grab a bottle of **HOT SAUCE,** and shake it well. Then put 10 to 20 drops of the fiery fluid into a glass of water, and drink it. Do this three times a day until you're all better.

TIP Do you keep **MEAT TENDER-IZER** in your kitchen? Well, Grandma did, and she probably used it more often to treat insect bites than she did to soften tough cuts of meat! It still works just as well as it did back then. All you have to do is mix it with a few drops of water, and spread it on the stricken site. The tenderizer will break down the protein in the poison, thereby nixing its pain-producing properties.

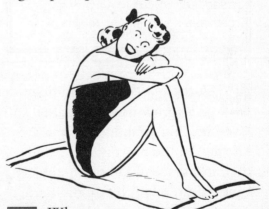

TIP When you head for the beach, tuck a shaker of **MEAT TENDERIZER** into your bag. It'll take the pain right out of a jellyfish sting. Just mix it with water, and apply it as you would for an insect bite.

ONE MORE TIME

A **LUNCH BOX** is just the right size for a first aid kit. So, if you've got a lunch box that's out of work, stock it with supplies, such as bandages, antibiotic ointment, and pain relievers, and stash it where you can grab it fast when you need it. (Of course, if it's a vintage collectible, decorated with pictures of, say, Davy Crockett or Zorro, keep it out in the open to be "wowed!" at.)

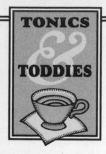

TONICS & TODDIES

GRANDMA'S BASIC BATH BLEND

Modern medical science has proven what Grandma always knew—that stress (or getting all hot and bothered, as she put it) is bad for your health. So do your body a favor, and keep a supply of this simple soother on hand.

2 cups of powdered milk
1 cup of cornstarch
Your favorite scented oil (optional)

Mix the ingredients together, and store the mixture in an airtight container. Then, whenever you feel the need, add ½ cup to a tub of hot bathwater, sink in, and relax.

TIP Although I never admitted this to my boyhood pals, I loved helping Grandma Putt in the kitchen. In the process (not being the most graceful kid on the block) I picked up more than a few burns on my hands and arms. And the minute I'd yelp in pain, Grandma would reach into the icebox, grab a bottle of **MILK,** and pour some into a bowl. Then she'd soak a soft cloth in it, and lay the compress on my burned skin. My job was to hold it there for 20 minutes or so, then rinse the milk off with cool water. She'd repeat the process every two to four hours, until the pain and redness went away. *Note:* If you try this trick at home, be sure to use whole milk or (better yet) half-and-half—it's the fat content that soothes the burn and helps it heal faster.

TIP That same whole **MILK** treatment works like magic on sunburn. If you don't believe me, just give it a try the next time you spend too much time in Ol' Sol's company.

TIP It's happened again. Modern science has confirmed two more of Grandma Putt's firmly held convictions: One, that the road to good health starts with a sound night's sleep, and two, that a glass of warm **MILK** at bedtime will help you drift off faster and snooze more restfully. Now, researchers at Cornell University have found that getting too little sleep may actually shorten your life span by as much as 8 to 10 years. As for the milk, well, it helps your brain produce a relaxing, sleep-inducing chemical called serotonin.

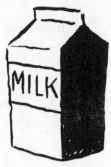

TIP Eczema has to be one of the most miserable afflictions on the planet. Fortunately, when a flare-up strikes, help is as close as your fridge. Just pull out a carton of whole **MILK,** mix some in a bowl with an equal amount of water, and saturate a gauze pad or soft, cotton cloth with the solution. Apply it to the affected area for about three minutes. Perform this maneuver two to four more times in quick succession. Repeat as needed throughout the day. Just be sure to rinse your skin with cool water after each treatment—otherwise, before you know it, you'll be smelling like sour milk!

TIP If the question on your mind is how to cure sore, swollen eyelids, my answer is "Moo"—moo juice, that is. Just soak a couple of cotton pads in ice-cold, whole **MILK,** lie down, put one over each eye, and rest for 5 to 10 minutes. Then, jeepers creepers, those peepers will be back to their old selves again!

TIP The next time you get a headache, try this trick of Grandma Putt's. Fill a basin with water that's as hot as you can tolerate, and mix 1 teaspoon of dry **MUSTARD** in it. Then, pull up a comfortable chair, put your feet in the water, and cover the basin with a towel. (This step is crucial, because you need to keep the heat in.) Sit back and soak your tootsies for about 15 minutes, keeping your eyes closed and your muscles as relaxed as possible. By the time the water cools down, your ol' noggin should be pain-free.

TIP Ease muscle aches and pains by soaking in a bathtub of hot water (as hot as you can stand it) with a handful each of dry **MUS-TARD** and sea salt mixed in it.

TIP Take the itch and pain out of hemorrhoids with this sweet and spicy remedy. Just mix equal parts of dry **MUSTARD** and honey to make a cream, and rub it (gently!) on the affected areas. Repeat as often as necessary to bring relief.

ONE MORE TIME

Don't cry over sour **MILK**—and don't dump it down the drain either. Instead, use it to clean your silver. Pour the milk into a basin, insert your pieces, and let them soak for half an hour to loosen the tarnish. Then wash them in soapy water. They'll sparkle like diamonds!

NUTCRACKER. It'll give you the torque you need to open that lid. Just don't squeeze too hard, or you'll crack the cap and it won't be usable.

TIP When you're constipated, get your innards back on track the way Grandma did. First thing in the morning, on an empty stomach, drink ½ cup of cool water with ½ teaspoon of dry **MUSTARD** mixed in it. Then follow up with your usual breakfast if you want to. Do the same thing the following day, and before you know it, things will be moving smoothly again.

TIP When the cap on the medicine bottle says, "Squeeze while turning," but your fingers refuse to cooperate, grip the cap with a

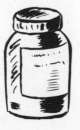

TIP It's all but impossible to get a good night's sleep when you're itchin' all over from allergies, eczema, insect bites, or poison ivy. Well, here's a bedtime routine that should let you get your 40 winks. Grind a cup of dry **OATMEAL** (not instant) into a powder using a blender, food processor, or coffee grinder. Stir the oat powder into a warm bath, and soak your discomfort away.

TIP Don't want to bother with the daily grind? Then just cut a leg off of an old pair of pantyhose, stuff the foot with **OATMEAL,** and tie the top to your bathtub spigot. Then turn on the water, and settle in for an oh-so-soothing soak.

TIP Grandma Putt knew a jillion ways to take the heat and pain out of sunburn. This was one of her favorites: Just wrap about 1 cup of dry **OATMEAL** in cheesecloth and run cool water through it. Wring out the excess H_2O, and apply the poultice to your burned skin for about 20 minutes every two hours. (You can use the same oatmeal

sachet over and over, but give it a cold shower before each treatment.)

TIP Whoops! That first jolt of hot java gave your throat a nasty burn! Put out the fire fast by drinking 2 teaspoons of **OLIVE OIL.**

TIP Nothing soothes an aching ear better than plain old heat. But what do you do when an earache strikes and you have no heating pad or hot water bottle on hand? It's simple: Just put a heatproof **PLATE** in the oven until it's toasty warm. Then wrap a towel around it, lie down, and rest your ear on the "package." Repeat as necessary—there's no chance of an overdose with this remedy!

TIP Need a temporary splint for an injured finger? Use a clean **POPSICLE® STICK!**

TIP Grandma did a whole lot of cooking in cast-iron **POTS,** pans, and skillets. And, although she didn't know it at the time, she was dishing up more than great food— she was also adding important iron to our diets. Scientists have found that foods cooked in that heavy gear actually absorb some of the iron.

What's more, highly acidic foods do the best job of picking up good old Fe. (*That* term should take you back to high school chemistry class!) So what are you waiting for? Haul out your favorite cauldron and whip up a big batch of marinara sauce!

TIP Boosting the humidity in the air can go a long way toward clearing up head congestion. But that doesn't mean you have to buy a humidifier. Instead, when a cold or flu clogs up your nasal passages, perch a big **POT** of water on a radiator, or simmer it on the stove.

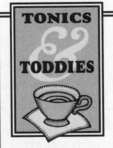

HYDRATION FORMULA

Even a brief bout of vomiting or diarrhea whisks crucial fluids and electrolytes right out of your body. But this simple beverage will put them back where they belong.

4 tsp. of sugar
1 tsp. of salt
1 qt. of water

Mix the ingredients together in a pitcher. Then drink 2 cups of the mixture every hour until you're in tiptop shape again.

TIP Headaches are an unfortunate fact of life—and that's why it pays to add this simple, Grandma-approved tool to your first aid kit. Mix about 1½ cups of uncooked **RICE** with five or six drops of lavender essential oil (available in herb, craft, and many health-food stores). Stuff the mixture into a soft, clean cotton sock and sew it closed. Then, whenever that old familiar throbbing starts, lie down and lay the fragrant sock over your eyes. The lavender scent will soothe you, while the weight of the rice will provide massage-like pressure against your eyes and forehead to help stop the pain.

TIP Grandma must have known a million drinkable, edible cures for sleeplessness. But here's one that relies on a simple kitchen utensil—a wooden **ROLLING PIN.** Just lay it on the floor in front of your favorite chair, sit back, and take off your shoes (you can remove your socks, too, if you like, but it's not necessary). Then put both feet on the pin, applying as much pressure as you can tolerate, and roll your tootsies back and forth for three minutes. Repeat this proce-

dure each evening, within an hour or two of bedtime, and within a week you should be getting a full eight hours of shut-eye every night.

TIP For hands-on relief of aches and pains, fill a new, clean **RUBBER GLOVE** with a half-and-half mixture of rubbing alcohol and water, and pop it into the freezer. Then, the next time a bruise, muscle strain, or other injury demands cold treatment, pull it out. Because alcohol doesn't freeze, you'll have a cold, but pliable, hand to drape over the trouble spot.

TIP Got a stuffy nose? Clean it out the way Grandma did, with a simple saline solution (just like the ones they sell in the drugstore). Dissolve ¼ teaspoon of **SALT** and ¼ teaspoon of baking soda in 1 cup of water. Use a medicine dropper to spritz the liquid into your nose whenever you need some air.

TIP Everybody on earth gets a sore throat now and then. Grandma Putt knew all sorts of remedies to nix that nastiness and get back to her song-singin' self, but this was the simplest: Just mix 1 teaspoon of **SALT** in about 2 cups of warm water. Then tip your head back and use it to gargle that sore throat pain away!

TIP The next time your head starts pounding, tell that ache to dry up. Here's how: Heat a few tablespoons of **SALT** in a dry pan until it's hot, but not too hot to touch. Pour the salt into a thin dish towel, and fold it up into a packet. Then hold it to the back of your head (yes, even though you feel the throbbing in the front), and gently rub. The dry heat should draw the pain right out.

TIP Good old NaCl is just about the best friend your mouth ever had. An 8-ounce glass of warm water with a teaspoon of **SALT** mixed in it can relieve tooth pain, reduce swelling in your gums, and even disinfect nasty abscesses. Just take a mouthful of salt water at a time, and swish it around for 10 to 30 seconds, directing it toward the painful area as much as possible. Proceed until you've drained the glass dry, and repeat as needed throughout the day. (*Note:* If you're on a low-sodium diet, use Epsom salts instead of table salt.)

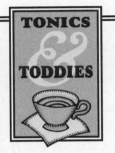

SPICY FLU FIGHTER

The next time you come down with a cold or flu, show those germs the door with this powerful (and pleasant) potion.

1 cinnamon stick
3 to 4 whole cloves
2 cups of water
1½ tbsp. of blackstrap molasses
2 shots of whiskey
2 tsp. of lemon juice

Put the cinnamon, cloves, and water in a pan, and bring the mix to a boil over medium heat. Let it boil for three minutes or so. Remove the pan from the stove, and mix in the molasses, whiskey, and lemon juice. Cover the pan, and let it sit for about 20 minutes. Drink ½ cup of the toddy every three to four hours, heating it up again before drinking. Before you know it, you'll be back in full swing!

TIP Cures for athlete's foot don't come any simpler than this one Grandpa used: Toss about ½ cup of **SALT** into a basin filled with warm water, and mix it well. Then soak your feet for 5 to 10 minutes. The briny solution will kill the trouble-causing fungus, and also soften your skin so that any antifungal medication you use can penetrate better. You say you don't have athlete's foot, but your dogs are dog-tired? Then treat yourself to that same salty bath, heated to the temperature of your choice. Sit back in a comfy chair, and soak your cares away.

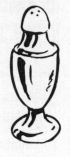

TIP Contrary to its name, ringworm is not a worm; it's a fungus that causes circular, scaly patches on the skin, and can spread like wildfire, even from one person to another. Fortunately, there's a simple way to douse the flames. First, soak a gauze pad in a solution made from 1 teaspoon of **SALT** dissolved in 2 cups of distilled water, and put it on the affected area for about half an hour. The next day, repeat the process using a gauze pad soaked in a solution made from 1 part vinegar mixed with 4 parts distilled water. Alter-

nate these compresses—salt one day, vinegar the next. In a week or so (depending on its severity), the foul fungus should be gone.

TIP When Ol' Sol really gets cookin', heat exhaustion can strike from out of nowhere. But this simple solution will put you back on your feet, fast. Just mix 1 teaspoon of **SALT** in a glass of water, and sip it slowly.

TIP I used to love Grandma Putt's homemade rye bread with **SESAME SEEDS.** But baking wasn't the only way she used those tasty tidbits. She also used them to make a first-class remedy for burns and bug bites. She mixed 3 to 4 tablespoons of ground sesame seeds with just

---

ONE MORE TIME

Whether you prefer loose **TEA** or bags for your daily "cuppa," don't throw away the leftover leaves! Instead, save them to make homemade scouring powder. Just mix 1 cup of black tea leaves with 1 teaspoon of baking soda and a few drops of dishwashing liquid, and use it as you would any commercial version.

enough water to make a coarse paste, then applied it to the scene of the "crime." In no time flat, it took away the pain and swelling. (You can either grind your seeds with a mortar and pestle, as Grandma did, or use a food processor or coffee grinder.)

TIP Here's a remedy for boils that'll suit you to a T. Rather, I should say **TEA.** Several times a day, hold a warm tea bag on the lump for about 15 minutes. Before you know it, the nasty thing will disappear. This same tea bag treatment will also help clear up painful cold sores.

TIP Even in these days of high-tech dentistry, having a tooth pulled is no picnic. And neither are the pain and swelling that often follow. Well, here's an old-time way to soothe your sore gums: Just put a warm, moist **TEA** bag against the affected area, and hold it there for 15 minutes. Repeat the procedure four times a day for three or four days, and your gums should be back to normal. (If they're not, call your dentist.)

TIP The next time a sleepless night or too many hours at the computer leave you with sore, puffy eyes, try

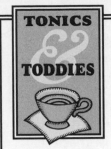

TONICS & TODDIES

SWEET-AND-SPICY SORE THROAT CURE

This double-dip gargle will send a sore throat packin', pronto!

⅛ tsp. of powdered cloves
⅛ tsp. of powdered ginger
⅛ tsp. of cayenne pepper
8 oz. of hot water
Ice-cold pineapple juice

Mix the spices in the water. Pour the juice into a glass, and set it aside. First, gargle with a swig of the spicy water mix. Then follow up by gargling with the pineapple juice. Switch back and forth between the hot and cold liquids one or two more times. Repeat the routine several times a day. The combination of hot and cold liquids will ease the burning sensation. And the dual action of the spices and bromelain (an enzyme in the pineapple) will loosen that irritating mucus in your throat.

this trick from *long* before computer days. Put a cold, wet **TEA** bag over each eye, and lie down for half an hour or so. (To keep the tea from staining your skin, you might want to wrap each bag in tissue first.)

TIP Soothe a sore throat with this tea-totaling toddy. Just mix 1 part hot **TEA** with 1 part warm lemon juice, add a generous amount of honey to taste (enough so that it coats your throat), and drink to your health!

TIP *Ouch!* You're sound asleep when, out of nowhere, a painful leg cramp jolts you wide awake. Well, don't just lie there losing shut-eye. Instead, hobble into the kitchen, pour an 8-ounce glass of **TONIC WATER,** and drink it down. The quinine in the fizzy mixer could be enough to uncramp your muscles. (If you don't care for the taste of plain tonic, jazz it up with a squirt of orange juice, a wedge of lime—or even a shot of gin!)

TIP Wax is in our ears for a purpose: to trap dirt and dust particles, and protect our ears from infections. But sometimes (especially as we get more, um, experienced) the wax can build up, become hardened, and even block the ear canal. Fortunately, there's a simple way to keep the stuff soft, so it can move right along: A couple of times each week, put a drop or two of warm **VEGETABLE OIL** into each ear. (Grandma used a medicine dropper, a.k.a. eyedropper, for this purpose.)

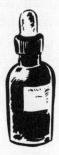

TIP To moisturize painful patches of eczema or psoriasis, gently wipe solid **VEGETABLE SHORTENING** onto the affected skin.

TIP I'm sure you know the classic way to soothe a black eye: Just slap a raw steak on it. It works, too. But it isn't the meat that does the trick; it's the cold temperature. So the next time you find yourself on the wrong side of a swinging door, save that T-bone for dinner. Instead, reach into the freezer, and grab a bag of frozen **VEGETABLES.** Wrap a soft cloth around it, lay it gently on your shiner, and leave it there until your face feels better. Then pop the bag back where you got it—or, better yet, cook the veggies and serve 'em up with that steak!

TIP If you suffer from arthritis pain, this simple remedy could give you relief. (It sure helped Grandpa Putt.) At each meal, drink 1 teaspoon of apple cider **VINEGAR** mixed in a glass of water. This remedy also works to loosen up leg cramps.

TIP One winter, I developed a bladder infection, and Grandma (with the doctor's okay) had me drink 2 teaspoons of apple cider **VINEGAR** in a glass of water three times a day. That solved the problem lickety-split.

TIP A dizzy spell can come on when you least expect it. When it does, drink a glass of water with about ½ teaspoon of apple cider **VINEGAR** mixed in it. Before you know it, you'll be steady on your feet again.

TIP When your problem is sinusitis or facial neuralgia, ease the pain by drinking ½ teaspoon of apple cider **VINEGAR** in

a glass of water once an hour for seven hours.

TIP Trying to lose weight? Here's a trick that may help: Before each meal, mix 1 teaspoon of apple cider **VINEGAR** in a glass of warm water (make sure it's warm!), and drink up. If you're like most folks, the elixir will decrease your appetite, so you'll just naturally want to eat less.

TIP To prevent indigestion, use the same procedure, but increase the **VINEGAR** to 2 teaspoons per glass of H_2O.

In Grandma's Day

Grandma Putt remained healthy, chipper, and sharp as a tack for her entire, long life. How did she do it? She always said it was because of one, unshakable habit: She ate three well-balanced meals a day, and with each one, she drank a glass of water with 1 teaspoon of **HONEY** and 1 teaspoon of apple cider **VINEGAR** mixed into it.

TIP By the time I came along, Grandma Putt's bouts of morning sickness were ancient history. But she always offered this tip to young women who were waiting for the stork: Every day, as soon as you get up, drink a glass of water with 1 teaspoon of apple cider **VINEGAR** mixed in it. It'll keep your stomach steady for the duration.

TIP Athlete's foot is no match for apple cider **VINEGAR.** Just wipe it on your afflicted tootsies several times a day, and kiss the itch good-bye!

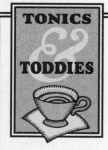

LEAPIN' LINIMENT!

A gentle rubdown with this vintage recipe will bring quick relief to arthritis pain and muscle aches.

2 egg whites
½ cup of apple cider vinegar
¼ cup of olive oil

Mix the ingredients together, and massage the lotion into your, or your patient's, painful body parts. (Be careful not to get any of the lotion on sheets or furniture!) Wipe off the excess with a soft, cotton cloth.

TIP Grandma Putt always kept a bottle of apple cider **VINEGAR** in the icebox. Then, whenever I got a sunburn, Grandma would pull out the bottle and pat my skin every 20 minutes with the cold liquid. It took the pain away fast and (because we didn't rinse it off), it prevented my burned skin from blistering and peeling.

TIP After a run-in with poison oak, poison ivy, or stinging nettles, mix equal parts of apple cider **VINEGAR** and water, and dab the solution onto your itchy skin.

TIP Grandpa Putt didn't like to wear gloves, even in the coldest weather. Well, one winter, he learned his lesson: He went out to split some firewood, 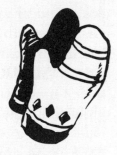 kept at it longer than he should have, and came back with his hands all chapped and sore. Grandma hit the ceiling. Then she mixed some of her favorite, rich hand cream with an equal amount of white **VINEGAR,** and told Grandpa to smooth it on his hands every time he washed them. Within days, his skin was back to normal.

ONE MORE TIME

After you've emptied a plastic **VINEGAR JUG,** use it to keep worms out of your apples—that is, once you've filled it with Grandma's "Worm-Free Fruit Tree Formula." You'll find the easy recipe on page 198.

TIP **VINEGAR** is also a handy thing to have on hand in the good old summertime. Whenever you spend too much time in Ol' Sol's company, just head for the bathroom, and pour 1 cup of white vinegar into a tub of warm water. Then ease on in, and heave a sigh of relief!

TIP Ease nasal congestion by boiling white **VINEGAR** in a pot, and inhaling the steam for a few minutes. Repeat several times a day until your sinus passages clear up. And be careful not to burn yourself!

TIP This corn-removing formula sounds too good to be true, but Grandma swore by it. At about your bedtime, put a slice of raw onion, a slice of white bread, and 1 cup of white **VINEGAR** in a bowl, and let it sit for 24 hours. The next night, put the bread on top of the corn, lay the onion on top, cover it with a bandage, and go to bed. There's a good chance the corn will fall off overnight. If it doesn't, repeat the procedure until the painful bump is history—it shouldn't take more than a couple of tries.

TIP When an insect sinks his choppers (or his rear end) into your skin, dab the site as soon as possible with apple cider **VINE-GAR.** If you've acted fast enough, it'll draw out the poison and swelling. Even if it's too late for that, the vinegar will still relieve the pain and itching.

TIP In the summers, I used to spend a *lot* of time at the old swimming hole. Grandma knew I was prone to "swimmer's ear," so before I headed out the door, she always had me rinse my ears with a half-and-half solution of rubbing alcohol and white **VINEGAR.** I still use it before I go swimming to prevent infections.

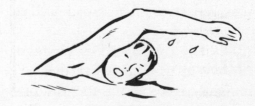

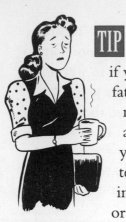

TIP We all get tired now and then. But if you feel constantly fatigued, the reason may be that lactic acid has built up in your system. (That tends to happen during periods of stress or strenuous exercise.) If that's the case, this simple trick may help: At bedtime each night, drink 3 teaspoons of apple cider **VINEGAR** mixed in ⅛ cup of honey. Continue the routine until your old vim and vigor return—but if that doesn't happen within a few weeks, call your doctor.

TIP Heal cold sores, and even soothe shingles, by dabbing the painful spots with apple cider **VINEGAR** on a cotton ball.

TIP Treat muscle strains and sprains the way Grandma did. Just mix a pinch of cayenne pepper in a cup or so of apple cider **VINEGAR,** dampen a cloth with the solution, put it on your sore body part, and leave it on for about five minutes. Repeat as often as you need to.

TIP If you're plagued by varicose veins, you know that their unsightly appearance is the least of the problem. They're also painful as the dickens—and even dangerous because they can trigger blood clots. Well, before you resort to drugs or surgery, try this old-time trick. Just soak a couple of cloths in apple cider **VINEGAR,** and wrap them around your legs. Then lie down with your feet propped up about 12 inches, and hold that pose for half an hour or so. Do this twice a day until those blue road maps hit the trail.

TIP Feeling down in the dumps? This old-time treatment often relieves mild depression: Drink about ½ cup of water with 1 teaspoon of apple cider **VINEGAR** mixed in it. Repeat once a day for a week or so, and your spirits should

In Grandma's Day

This was Grandma's surefire cure for a bloody nose: Soak a cotton ball in apple cider **VINEGAR,** and gently insert it into the dripping nostril. Then, holding your nose closed with your fingers, breathe through your mouth for about five minutes. Slowly remove the cotton. If the bleeding hasn't stopped, repeat the procedure.

perk up. (Of course, if you're struggling with serious depression, put down this book, and call your doctor *now*!)

TIP Grandma always stopped hiccups by mixing 1 teaspoon of apple cider **VINEGAR** in a glass of warm water. She'd sip it very *slowly* and bingo—no more hiccups!

TIP Annoying and unsightly warts will wander off into the sunset (so to speak) when you use this simple, old-time remedy. At bedtime, cover the bump with apple cider **VINEGAR**. (But *don't* rub it in! That could cause more warts to form.) Then, soak a gauze pad in apple cider vinegar, put it over the wart, and cover it with a bandage to hold in the moisture. Leave it on overnight. In the morning, remove the bandage, but don't rinse off the vinegar. Repeat each night until the lump is gone.

TIP If you're going through a period where bedtime is tossing-and-turning time, don't just lie there counting sheep—and don't rush off to the drugstore for sleeping pills. Instead, try this old

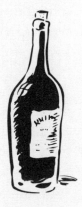

trick of Grandma's about an hour before you go to bed: Put 2 cups of white **WINE** in a pan, and heat it until it's *almost* boiling. (Don't let it boil!) Remove the pan from the heat, add 4 teaspoons of dill seeds, and let the mixture steep, covered, for half an hour. Drink it, lukewarm, 30 to 45 minutes before you hit the sack.

Your
GOOD LOOKS

TIP Hey, guys! If your facial skin is on the sensitive side, here's a little secret that you ought to know: **BAKING SODA** can end your razor burn once and for all. Mix 1 tablespoon of soda per cup of water, and splash the solution onto your face, either before or after you shave (or both, if you like).

TIP Hey, gals! Instead of coating your legs with shaving cream or soap before you shave them, use a solution of 1 tablespoon of **BAKING SODA** per cup of water. Your razor will glide right over your skin, leaving it satiny smooth.

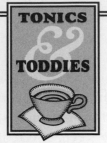

SWEET-AND-SOUR SCRUB

This simple, energizing rub will leave you rarin' to go—and make your skin feel squeaky clean and satiny soft all over.

½ cup of brown sugar
1 tsp. of honey
Juice of ½ small lemon

Mix all the ingredients together in a bowl. In the bath or shower, gently massage the mixture into your skin, and rinse it off. That's all there is to it!

TIP Take a tip from Grandma: Keep a jar of **BAKING SODA** by your bathroom sink, and use it to gently deep-clean your face. It'll lift out the traces of oil, dirt, and make-up that even the best cleansers leave behind. Here's the game plan: Wash your face with your regular soap or cleanser. Then, mix 3 parts baking soda with 1 part water, and gently massage the mixture into your damp skin. Rinse with clear, cool water, and pat dry.

TIP Fresh out of deodorant? Just dust a little **BAKING SODA** on your underarm skin. It'll absorb the perspiration (thereby eliminating odors), make you feel cooler and drier, and prevent stains on your clothes.

TIP Grandma Putt didn't need a fancy, high-priced mouthwash to keep her breath sweet and fresh, and neither do you. With her daily routine, you can neutralize odors in your mouth—not simply cover them up. Just mix a teaspoon or so of **BAKING SODA** in half a glass of water, swish it around in your mouth, and spit it out. Your breath will be kissin' sweet!

TIP In just a short time, styling gels, sprays, and even conditioners can build up in your hair and make those locks look dull and drab. But it's easy to keep the bright lights shining. At least once a week, pour about a teaspoon of **BAKING SODA** into your palm, and mix it with your regular shampoo. Then wash your hair as usual, and rinse thoroughly.

TIP When it comes to "hair pollution," styling products can't hold a candle to the high doses of chlorine and other chemicals used in public swimming pools. Get that stuff out with this intensive treatment. Mix 2 tablespoons of **BAKING SODA** with ¼ cup of fresh-squeezed lemon juice, and 1 teaspoon of mild shampoo. Wet your hair with water, and work the mixture thoroughly into your scalp and hair (clear down to the ends). Cover your locks with a shower cap or plastic bag, and go about your business for half an hour. Rinse well, and shampoo as usual. Repeat the process as necessary. (The frequency will depend on how often you swim, and how thoroughly you rinse your hair after each dip.)

Translation, Please!

Have you ever been stymied by the measurements in an old recipe, or in the instructions for some cosmetic or medicinal potion? Well, this chart will help you convert those terms to 21st-century lingo.

Old Recipe Calls For	Modern Measurement
1 jigger	1½ fluid oz. (a standard shot glass)
1 wineglass	¼ cup
1 gill	½ cup
1 teacup	A scant ¾ cup
1 coffee cup	A scant cup
1 tumbler	1 cup
A pinch or a dash	The amount you can pick up between your thumb and first two fingers (slightly less than ⅛ tsp.)
½ pinch	The amount you can pick up between your thumb and one finger
1 saltspoon	¼ tsp.
1 kitchen spoon	1 tsp.
1 dessert spoon	2 tsp.
1 spoonful	1 tbsp., give or take
1 saucer	1 heaping cup, give or take
Butter the size of an egg	¼ cup or half a stick
Butter the size of a walnut	1 tbsp.
Butter the size of a hazelnut	1 tsp.

TIP Grandma cleaned her hairbrushes and combs (and mine and Grandpa's, too) by soaking them overnight in a solution of 4 tablespoons of **BAKING SODA** per quart of water.

TIP The next time you're feeling so tense and stressed-out you could scream, relax with a **BEER.** Rather, make that beer*s*, plural. Pour three bottles of brew into a bathtub of warm water, lean back, and think lovely thoughts.

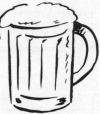

TIP Make your hair shiny and manageable the way Grandma did. Mix 3 cups of **BEER** with 1 cup of warm water, and use it as a final

---

ONE MORE TIME

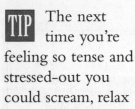
Are you concerned about cellulite on your hips and thighs? Well, wake up and smell the **COFFEE!** Then (after you've drunk a cup or two), let the grounds cool off, and rub them on the problem areas. They contain the same active ingredient—caffeine—as most cellulite creams.

---

rinse after your normal shampoo. (Don't worry—you won't smell like the corner bar. The aroma will disappear as your hair dries.)

TIP You could wait 'til the cows come home and not find a better facial cleanser than this one: Mix ¼ cup of **BUTTERMILK** with ¼ cup of whole, powdered milk (not nonfat) to form a paste. Spread it evenly over your face and neck, using a clean, new paintbrush or pastry brush. Let it dry for 15 to 20 minutes, and rinse with cool water. Store any leftovers in a covered container in the refrigerator.

TIP It never fails: You're rushing out the door to a meeting, and you realize that your breath smells, shall we say, less than soda-pop sweet. Quick—grab the jar of whole **CLOVES** from your kitchen spice rack, pop a few of the spicy things into your mouth, and chew them as you go on your way. You *and* your colleagues will be glad you did!

TIP Grandma Putt could never be bothered with coloring her hair, but she certainly knew how to go about it. If you ever told her you wanted to put red highlights in your curly locks, she'd have given you this advice: After shampooing in your

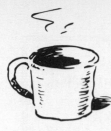

usual way, rinse with strong black **COFFEE** that's been cooled to room temperature. Give it 15 minutes or so to work its magic, then rinse thoroughly with cool water.

TIP Grandma Putt conditioned her hair with this old-time kitchen formula, and it still works as well as any product on the market—maybe even better. Beat the white of one **EGG** until it's foamy, then stir it into 5 tablespoons of plain, natural yogurt. Apply the mixture to one small section of your hair at a time. Leave it in for 15 minutes, then rinse.

TIP To reduce the appearance of large facial pores, beat one **EGG,** and mix it with about 1 tablespoon of honey. Spread the mixture onto your face, and leave it on for 20 minutes or so. Then rinse it off to reveal skin that's softer, firmer, and smoother than before.

TIP No matter what has caused the baggy pouches under your eyes, I'll tell you egg-zactly how to get rid of them: Separate a couple of **EGGS,** and apply the whites to your face with a clean, soft brush. (A new paint-, makeup, or basting brush will do fine.) Let the egg whites dry, and

In Grandma's Day

Every day, Grandma Putt drank a glass of water with unflavored **GELATIN** mixed into it. She was convinced that this simple trick made her hair thicker. At the time, of course, I thought that was just an old wives' tale. Then, not long ago, I read about a scientific study that proved Grandma was right. The folks in the study drank a daily ration of 7 teaspoons of gelatin dissolved in a glass of water, and after about two months, their individual hair strands had actually increased in diameter! (The only catch is that they had to keep it up; when they stopped drinking the potion, their hair returned to its normal size.)

rinse them off with cool water. Your facial skin will be tighter all over, including the under-eye zone.

TIP You say you've just been invited out, and there's not a dab of styling gel in the house? Well, if there's some unflavored **GELATIN** in the kitchen, you're in luck! Just mix the powder with half as much water as the instructions specify, and use it as you would hair gel—which you may never buy again!

TIP Here's a honey of a way to get rid of blackheads. Just heat about ⅛ cup of **HONEY,** and dab it onto the blemishes. Let it sit for a couple of minutes, wash it off with warm water, and rinse with cool water. Gently dry with a nice, soft towel.

TIP Been chopping onions or garlic? Get the odor off of your hands with dry **MUSTARD.** Just rub it in, and rinse it off.

TIP Banish blackheads the way Grandma did, by making a paste of roughly 3 parts **OATMEAL** to 1 part water, and rubbing it into the affected areas. Leave it on for about 10 minutes, rinse with warm water, and pat dry.

TIP Good old-fashioned **OAT-MEAL** is one of the best facial cleansers you can find anywhere. To use it, just grind about ¼ cup of oatmeal in a coffee grinder or food processor until it's the consistency of coarse flour. In a bowl, mix it with enough heavy cream to make a paste. (If you have oily skin, substitute skim milk.) Let the mixture thicken for a minute or two, then massage it into your face and throat. Rinse with cool water.

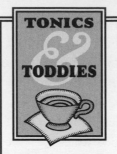

TONICS & TODDIES

DEEP-CLEANING FACIAL MASK

Women in Europe have been using this treatment for hundreds of years to get their skin deep-down clean. It still works like magic. Try it—you'll like it!

1 egg
¼ cup of nonfat dry milk
1 tbsp. of dark rum or brandy
Juice of 1 lemon

Combine the ingredients in a blender until the texture is creamy, and pour the mixture into a bowl or jar. Smooth it onto your face, and let it dry. There will be some cream remaining in the container; use this to remove the mask. Rinse well with warm water, and pat dry. Follow with your usual moisturizer.

TIP When Grandma Putt didn't have time to wash her hair, she gave herself a dry shampoo with **OATMEAL.** She'd put a handful on her head, work it through her hair with her fingers, and brush it out. That cereal removed all the oil, leaving Grandma's hair clean and shiny.

TIP If your hair is so dry that the ends are on the brink of splitting, head off trouble with this intensive conditioning treatment. Massage 1 cup of **OLIVE OIL** into your hair, and cover it with a plastic bag or shower cap. Cover that with a towel, secure it well with safety pins, and leave it on overnight. In the morning, wash your tresses with your regular shampoo, and rinse with a half-and-half solution of white vinegar and water.

TIP You'll never find a simpler—or more effective—moisturizer than this: Just rub **OLIVE OIL** onto your face, wait about 10 minutes, then rinse with warm water and pat dry.

ONE MORE TIME

Some **OLIVE OIL** comes in bottles that are almost works of art. So don't even think of sending the empties off in the recycling truck. Instead, wash them out well and use them as containers for your homemade cosmetic potions (with fresh corks, of course). Besides serving that practical purpose, they'll dress up your bathroom counter.

TIP Frequent dips in the ocean can make your skin silky soft. But even if you live hundreds of miles inland, you can still treat your skin to briny baths. Simply add ½ cup of **SALT** to a tub of warm water, and settle in for a good soak. When you get out, smooth on a good moisturizing body cream or lotion.

TIP One-half cup of **SALT** in a tub of warm water will nix the itch caused by poison ivy, insect bites, food-allergy rashes, or even post-sunburn peeling.

TIP You couldn't find an easier dandruff cure than the one Grandma used. Pour a tablespoon of **SALT** onto your head, rub it into your scalp, and shampoo as usual. Those white flakes will vanish like snow falling on warm ground!

TIP Here's a homemade bath mix that'll leave your skin feeling as soft and satiny smooth as the fanciest exfoliating cream. Mix about ¼ cup of sea **SALT** with 1 tablespoon of baking soda, and add enough almond oil to make a thick paste. In the bath or shower, rub the mixture all over your body, and rinse well.

TIP If you have oily skin, follow this routine to slough off dead cells and restore your skin's balance. First, cover your face with a hot, moist towel, and leave it in place for five minutes or so. Then mix 1 teaspoon of **SALT** with about 1 cup of water in a hand-held spray bottle, and spritz the solution onto your face. Then, without rinsing, blot your skin dry with a clean, soft towel. Your face will feel clean, healthy, and refreshed.

TIP Would you believe that you can find relief for puffy, swollen eyes in your cutlery drawer? It's true. Just pull out two metal **SPOONS** (either silver or stainless will do fine), and run cold water over them until they're good and chilly. Then lay one (curved side down) over each eye, and relax for a minute or two. Your peepers will feel—and look—a whole lot better!

TIP If your feet are a little, um, aromatic, get rid of the odor the way my Uncle Art did. Simply put a couple of **TEA** bags in a pan with 4 cups of water, and bring it to a boil. Remove it from the heat, and let it steep for 10 to 15 minutes. Pour the brew into a foot-size tub, add just enough cool water to bring the temperature down to your comfort level, and soak your feet in the brew for 30 minutes. Repeat the procedure once a day. After a week or so, your feet should smell as sweet as springtime. Well, *almost*.

In Grandma's Day

Grandma Putt always used to say that spilling **SALT** brings bad luck. Well, as with most superstitions, this one has some basis in fact: In ancient times, when this belief arose, salt was such a rare and valuable commodity, that losing even a little bit of it really *was* bad luck!

As for what you're supposed to do to stop the bad luck—toss a pinch of salt over your left shoulder—there's a reason for that, too. In most cultures, folks believed that good spirits followed you on your right side and evil spirits lurked behind you on the left. So, if you tossed some salt over your left shoulder, it would hit that bad guy square in the eye, and distract him from his dirty tricks.

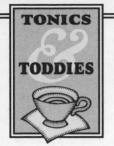

TONICS & TODDIES

SPICY BREATH SPRAY

This formula will kill odor-causing bacteria and keep your breath sweet and fresh.

¼ **cup of vodka**
5 drops of clove oil
5 drops of cinnamon oil
5 drops of orange oil
¼ **cup of water**

Mix all of the ingredients together, and pour the solution into a dark-colored glass bottle with a spray top. Shake well before using.

TIP Nowadays, you hear a lot about exfoliating creams and lotions, and you can pay big bucks for some of them. But you don't have to. This simple formula will get rid of layers of dead skin cells, and the ingredients are right in your kitchen. Just mix cold-pressed **VEGETABLE OIL** (like sunflower or safflower) with enough salt to make a gritty paste. Then add a few drops of your favorite essential oil. Rub this mixture over your wet skin—face, hands, elbows, and knees—and rinse well. You'll feel fresh, clean, and moisturized all over!

TIP Tired of paying an arm and a leg for fancy hand creams? Then stop buying them! Instead, do what Grandma did: Just pull out that can of **VEGETABLE SHORTENING** from your kitchen cupboard, and rub some into your hands. It'll soften those paws every bit as well as the priciest brand-name product.

TIP Hands that are really dry or chapped all but cry out for this super-softening routine: Just before you go to bed, rub **VEGETABLE SHORTENING** into your skin. Then put on a pair of old gloves, mittens, or even socks. Besides protecting your sheets, the covering will force the oil to penetrate deeper into your skin.

TIP Grandma Putt rarely wore eye makeup (or any other kind). But when she did brush on mascara for a *very* special occasion, like a wedding or christening, she took it off by dabbing a little **VEGETABLE SHORTENING** onto her eyelids, then gently wiping it over her lashes with a cotton pad.

For centuries before Grandma took her first breath, women have been using apple cider **VINEGAR** to shine and condition their hair. But with a few herbal additives, you can tailor the treatment to do more than that. All you do is add 1 cup of dried herbs to 1 quart of high-quality vinegar, let the mix steep for a few weeks, strain out the solids, and pour the liquid into a clean bottle. As for the type of herbs, that depends on the effect you're looking for. Here's the rundown:

- **Calendula** is a good, all-round conditioner.

- **Chamomile** puts highlights in blonde or light brown hair.

- **Lavender** and **lemon verbena** add enticing fragrance.

- **Nettles** control dandruff.

- **Parsley** and **rosemary** make dark hair come alive.

- **Sage** darkens graying hair.

Whichever combo suits your fancy, use the potion as a final rinse after shampooing, at a ratio of roughly 1 tablespoon of vinegar per gallon of warm water.

TIP Grandma never fussed with fancy astringents. After she washed her face, she just filled the bathroom sink about halfway with water, added a few tablespoons of apple cider **VINEGAR,** and splashed the solution onto her face. As they say on TV, try this trick at home for 30 days. If you're not satisfied that it closes your pores, restores the acid balance to your skin, and leaves your face feeling clean, soft, and refreshed, I'll...well, I'll be *very* surprised!

TIP Pimples—they're not just for teenagers anymore. And they never were. Why, even Grandma Putt got a few zits every now and again. They didn't last long, though, because she sent them packin' by dabbing them with a cotton ball dipped in white **WINE.** (Grandma had a fair complexion; if your skin is a little darker, use red instead.)

TIP Here's a terrific way to cleanse oily skin. Mix a tablespoon or so of brewer's **YEAST** with just enough warm water to make a paste. Rub it into your face, let it dry, and rinse with warm water. (You can find brewer's yeast at health-food stores or in the natural foods section of a drugstore or supermarket.)

TIP To cleanse and tone your skin at the same time, nothing beats plain, unflavored **YOGURT.** Just smooth it onto your face and throat, wait a minute or two, and rinse it off with warm water.

Around the
HOUSE

TIP When you serve bread, rolls, or muffins hot from the oven, keep them that way longer by putting a piece of **ALUMINUM FOIL** under the napkin in your bread basket. Besides keeping the goodies warm, the foil will protect the basket from grease stains.

TIP After a big family gathering, like Christmas dinner, when Grandma had a lot of silver cutlery to clean, she rinsed it all in cold water to get off any food residue. Then she launched into this routine: Cover the bottom of a large basin with **ALUMINUM FOIL,** lay the silverware on top, and cover it with boiling water. Add 3 tablespoons of baking soda, and wait 10

minutes. Then rinse the silver in clear water, and wipe it dry.

TIP In the summertime, **ALUMINUM FOIL** can help you keep your cool. Just tape or staple sheets of foil between the studs on the inside of your roof. They'll reflect the sun's rays outward—reducing the heat passing into your house by 20 percent or more.

ONE MORE TIME

 Those cardboard tubes from rolls of **ALUMINUM FOIL, WAX PAPER,** and **PLASTIC WRAP** must have a jillion-and-one uses. Two of my favorites are in the bedroom closet:

▷ **Boot trees.** For each one, tape three or four tubes together. Then slip one "tree" into each boot. To keep shorter boots shipshape, cut the tubes to the right length before you tape them together.

▷ **Pants hangers.** Cut the tube lengthwise, and pop it over the bottom of a wire coat hanger. Then fold your trousers over it. Because the roll is so stout, the legs won't get creases in the middle, the way they tend to do on plain hangers (even wooden ones).

TIP To make a radiator or base-board heater work more efficiently, wrap a piece of heavy-duty **ALUMINUM FOIL,** shiny side up, around a piece of cardboard or wood, and tuck it behind the unit. The foil will reflect heat into the room, so it won't be absorbed into the wall.

TIP Back when I got my first little apartment, it came equipped with a stove that was older than I was. It still worked fine, but the chrome trim had a lot of rusty patches on it. As always, Grandma knew exactly how to get them off. She told me to wrap a piece of **ALUMINUM FOIL** around my finger, shiny side out, rub the marks, then buff the chrome with a cotton cloth dipped in rubbing alcohol. When I was finished, that metal shone like a mirror!

TIP In one of my early attempts at cooking dinner in my first apartment, some food spilled onto a hot burner, and burst into flames. Fortunately, Grandma had taught me exactly what to do in that situation. I grabbed the **BAKING SODA,** and tossed it on the fire. It went out like a light!

TIP For routine cleaning, Grandma wiped her plastic laminate countertops with a paste made from 1 part **BAKING SODA** to 3 parts warm water. Then she rinsed the surface with cool water.

TIP To clean the grout between ceramic tiles, wet down the grout with a cloth or sponge, then dip a toothbrush in **BAKING SODA,** and scrub the dirt away.

GRANDMA PUTT'S
Secret Formulas

HOMEMADE SCOURING POWDER

This heavy-duty cleanser will get grease and grime off of pots and pans, appliances, tile floors, bathroom fixtures, and just about every other surface inside—and outside—your home, sweet home.

1 cup of baking soda
1 cup of salt
1 cup of borax

Combine these ingredients, and then store the mixture in a closed container. Use it as you would any powdered cleanser.

TIP If you have bathroom fixtures made of colored porcelain, you know how quickly stains and water marks can build up on those sinks and tubs. They stand out like sore thumbs—and they're the very dickens to get off without scratching the surface. Unless, that is, you tackle them with this simple, no-scratch cleanser: Mix 1 cup each of **BAKING SODA** and salt in a container with a tight lid, and keep it close at hand. Then, when the need arises, use it as you would any other scouring powder. This gentle powder also works wonders on kitchen counters and other easily scratched surfaces.

TIP Grandma cleaned painted-wood surfaces like floors, furniture, and woodwork with a solution of 1 teaspoon of **BAKING SODA** per gallon of hot water. She applied it with either a mop or a sponge, then wiped the surface dry with a soft cloth. (To dry a wooden floor, she wrapped the cloth around the business end of a dust mop.)

TIP Before you put on a pair of rubber gloves, sprinkle a teaspoon of **BAKING SODA** into each one, hold the top closed, and shake it to coat the inner surface. This will make the gloves slide on and off easily, instead of clinging to your skin.

GRANDMA PUTT'S
Secret Formulas

FLEA-FREE CARPET CLEANER

Here's an old-time, ultrasafe way to get rid of fleas that hitch a ride indoors with Fido—and keep your carpets clean and fresh-smelling at the same time.

½ cup of baking soda
½ cup of cornstarch
½ tsp. of rosemary, pennyroyal, or citronella oil*

Before you go to bed at night, mix the baking soda, cornstarch, and oil together. Spread the mixture evenly across your carpet, and scrub it into the fibers using a stiff brush or broom. Let it sit overnight, and vacuum it up in the morning.

* If fleas are not a problem and you simply want to clean your carpet, substitute any fragrant oil of your choice.

TIP To get rid of black scuff marks left by careless shoe-wearers on any kind of flooring, rub the spots with a paste made from 3 parts **BAKING SODA** to 1 part water.

TIP To freshen up a smelly drain, pour a cup of **BAKING SODA** into it, and flush with hot water.

Out, Darned Spot!

In the days before all those miracle sprays, gels, and sticks came on the scene, some of Grandma's most powerful laundry helpers came straight from the kitchen. These everyday products still do a first-class job of removing common household stains. Here's a rundown.

Stain	Material	How to Get It Out
Blood	Any fabric	Blot, then pour on cold **CLUB SODA.** Repeat if necessary.
Fruit or wine	Any washable fabric	Pour **SALT** on the spots, and soak the article in **MILK** until the marks are gone.
Grass	Any washable fabric	Rub the spots with **MOLASSES,** let the garments sit overnight, and wash them with mild soap (not detergent).
Grease or oil	Knit fabrics	Pour **CLUB SODA** (cold or room temperature) on the spot, and scrub gently.
Grease or oil	Any smooth fabric	Cover the spot with **CORNSTARCH,** wait 12 hours, and brush it off.
Ink (dry)	Any washable fabric	Dampen a sponge with **MILK,** and dab the stain until it's gone. (Be patient; it may take a while to get all of the ink out.) Then launder as usual.
Ink (still wet)	Any fabric	Pour **SALT** on the spot, and dab it gently (taking care not to spread the ink around). Let it sit for two to three minutes, and brush off the salt. Repeat if necessary.
Mildew	Any washable fabric	Moisten the spots with a half-and-half mixture of **SALT** and **LEMON JUICE,** then spread the item in the sun until the marks disappear.
Mustard	Any washable fabric	Soak the soiled area in a half-and-half solution of white **VINEGAR** and water until the spot disappears. Blot with a soft cloth, and launder as usual.

Stain	Material	How to Get It Out
Organic, protein-based substances (like milk, egg, and blood)	Any washable fabric	Make a paste of **MEAT TENDERIZER** mixed with a few drops of water, work it into the stain, and launder immediately.
Perspiration	Any washable fabric	Mix 4 tablespoons of **SALT** with 1 quart of water, and sponge the stains with the solution until they're gone. Launder as usual.
Rust	Any washable fabric	Mix equal parts of **SALT** and **VINEGAR.** Rub the paste into the stain, wait 30 minutes, and launder as usual.
Tar	Any fabric	Slather **MAYONNAISE** onto the spot, and let it soak into the fabric. Launder or dry-clean as usual.
Vomit	Any fabric	Remove the residue, using a plastic scraper or paper towels. Then cover the spot with **BAKING SODA,** let it dry, and brush it off. Launder as usual, or send the garment to the dry cleaner.
Wine (red or white)	Any fabric	Blot up any excess moisture, and saturate the stain with **CLUB SODA.** Rub lightly, and blot dry. Repeat if necessary. Then dry-clean or launder as usual.

TIP Over time, white cotton and linen can take on a dingy cast. Bring back the brightness by boiling the fabric for an hour in a solution made from ½ cup each of **BAKING SODA** and salt per gallon of water.

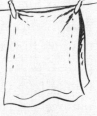

TIP Boxes of laundry detergent and cat litter can be all but impossible to open without breaking a fingernail. To avoid that frustration (and even pain), push the flap open with an old-fashioned **BOTTLE OPENER**—the kind we used to call a "church key."

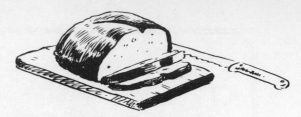

TIP Grandma's brown sugar always stayed soft and scoopable, because she put it in a glass jar along with a slice of **BREAD,** and stored it in the icebox.

TIP To freshen up a stale-smelling (or even foul-smelling) lunch box, soak a slice of **BREAD** in white vinegar for a minute or so. Then put it in the box, close the lid, and let it sit overnight. By morning, that food tote will be fresh as a daisy!

ONE MORE TIME

If you're remodeling your kitchen and decide to change the **CABINETS,** don't throw them away—put them to work someplace else in the house. If they're still in good shape, paint them and add new handles if you want to. Then use them to store (for instance) stationery supplies in your home office, towels and toiletries in a bathroom, soaps and cleaners in the laundry, or toys and books in a child's bedroom. Even if those cupboards are not much to look at, you can still haul them out to your shed or workshop, and fill 'em up with tools, hardware, or garden supplies.

TIP If you use your coffee grinder to pulverize spices, or even different flavors of coffee beans, you can wind up with a mighty strange aroma—not to mention foul-tasting coffee. To prevent that problem, after every use run a few chunks of **BREAD** through the grinder. Then your morning cup o' joe will always taste the way you expect!

TIP Are you spending an arm and a leg for bathroom deodorizers? Well, Grandma Putt would say, "Stop that right now!" Instead, when an, um, aromatic incident leaves the room smelling less than rosy, just light a **CANDLE.** Don't bother searching for a scented one. Any candle flame will burn away the foul-smelling gases.

TIP Unless you live in a very dry climate, wooden bookshelves tend to attract mildew—and, of course, pass it right along to the books. To protect your library, remove the volumes, sprinkle oil of **CLOVES** on the shelves, and rub it in well. Wait until the wood is dry, then replace the books.

In Grandma's Day

This piece of trivia falls squarely into the believe-it-or-not category—canned food was around for almost half a century before the **CAN OPENER** arrived on the scene. As a matter of fact, the opener that Grandma Putt was most familiar with didn't make an appearance until 1925! Here's the history lesson: A British merchant named Peter Durand invented what he called the "tin canister" in 1810, and used it to supply rations to the Royal Navy. But he neglected to develop a gadget to open the danged things. The sailors used pocket knives, chisels, bayonets—and sometimes even gunfire—to get to their vittles. Then in 1858, Ezra J. Warner of Waterbury, Connecticut, patented the first can opener. Unfortunately, it wasn't much of an improvement over guns and knives. It looked like a cross between a sickle and a bayonet, with a large, curved blade that had to be driven into the can's rim and then muscled around the perimeter.

But the story goes on. In 1870, an American inventor named William Lyman came up with a device that featured a cutting wheel that rolled around the can's rim. Then, finally, in 1925 the Star Can Opener Company of San Francisco modified Mr. Lyman's gadget by adding a serrated wheel that made the tin rotate against the cutting wheel. Bingo! The can opener as we know it was born! (The first electric model came on the market in December 1931.)

TIP When you need to wash greasy work clothes, add a can of regular **COLA** to the machine along with your detergent. It'll cut right through that nasty grime.

TIP Who says a **COOKIE JAR** is only good for storing cookies? A friend of mine uses her colorful collection of jars all over the house to hold toiletries in the bathroom, supplies in her home office, and odds and ends in her craft room.

TIP Anytime Grandma Putt needed a lid for a big pan that didn't have a topper, she used a **COOKIE SHEET** for the job.

TIP To keep damp books from getting mildewed, sprinkle **CORNSTARCH** throughout the pages. Wait several hours until all the moisture has been absorbed, and then brush out the starch. If any trace of dampness remains, repeat the process.

Coffee Filters

A German-born chemist named Peter Schlumbohm invented the paper coffee filter (along with the classy Chemex pot) in 1939. But it wasn't until the early 1970s, when electric coffeemakers took the United States by storm, that paper filters acquired the status of kitchen staples. That's too bad, because Grandma Putt would have found dozens of ways to use these sturdy, but porous marvels. You can, too. Here's a sample to-do list.

Fresh, Clean Filters

▶ *Blot a spill.* Accidents happen—even when you're fresh out of paper towels. So absorb the mess with a coffee filter (or two or three).

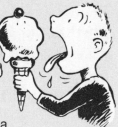

▶ *Catch drips.* Before you hand a young-ster (or even a grown-up) an ice pop or ice cream bar, poke a hole in a coffee filter, and insert the stick.

▶ *Clean glass.* Use coffee filters instead of paper towels to wash windows and mirrors. You can even use them to clean your eyeglasses—*if* the lenses are actually made of glass. Like any other paper product, coffee filters can leave tiny scratches on plastic.

▶ *Decork your vino.* When the cork crumbles and pieces wind up in the bottle, pour the wine through a coffee filter into a clean decanter.

▶ *Filter the air.* In a pinch, a coffee filter makes a fine stand-in for a dust mask. Just put it over your nose and mouth, and secure it with cord or a long rubber band.

▶ *Filter formulas, tonics, and tod-dies.* When you whip up one of Grandma's recipes that calls for straining out the solid ingredients, do the job with a coffee filter.

▶ *Freshen your fridge.* When you come home from vacation and discover a lot of, um, aromatic food that you forgot to pitch before you left, get rid of it *fast*. Then pull out six or eight coffee filters, and fill each one with $1/2$ cup of baking soda. Set them on the shelves and in the produce bins and other compartments. The filters will help the soda absorb the odors faster.

▶ *Hold that soil!* Line plant pots with coffee filters to keep the soil from seeping out through the drainage holes.

▶ *Make party favors.* Fill each one with candy, tiny toys, or other small goodies. Then gather up the sides to form a sack, and tie it closed with a colorful ribbon or length of raffia. If you like, tie a helium-filled balloon to each bundle, or (to make it double as a place card) add a name tag.

▶ *Make snowflakes.* Fold a filter in quarters, cut out shapes along the edges, then open it up. When you've made a full set of flurries, tape them onto a window, or hang them from the Christmas tree.

▶ *Nuke your food.* Use coffee filters to cover dishes when you put them in the microwave.

▶ *Pack your possessions.* Getting ready to move? Wrap your glassware and china in coffee filters. When you unpack, you can still use the filters to brew coffee.

▶ *Protect your china.* Separate stacked plates with coffee filters to keep the rough bottoms from scratching the smooth tops.

▶ *Recycle paint thinner.* After you clean your brushes, layer two filters over a clean jar, keeping them loose. Pour the old thinner through them into the jar, and cap it tightly (disposing of the filters). Save the thinner to clean your brushes again—but don't use it to thin paint or varnish, because there will be a little pigment left in it.

▶ *Save your skillets.* And other cast-iron pans, too. Put a coffee filter in the bottom of each one to absorb moisture and prevent rust from forming.

▶ *Serve hot dogs.* As the franks come off the grill, skip the paper plates. Instead, wrap each dog in a coffee filter. It's a holder and napkin in one convenient 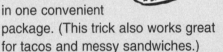 package. (This trick also works great for tacos and messy sandwiches.)

▶ *Shine your shoes.* Rub the polish on with a coffee filter instead of a cloth. Then throw it away when you're finished.

▶ *Start seeds.* If your future plants need chilly moisture to help them germinate, follow this routine: Put a coffee filter inside a small, zip-top plastic bag, pour 3 tablespoons of water on the filter, and space out your seeds. Then stash the bag in the fridge until the seeds sprout.

(continued)

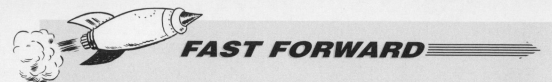

FAST FORWARD

(continued from page 165)

▶ *Weigh food.* Before you set chopped ingredients on a food scale, put the pieces in a coffee filter. They'll be less likely to spill, and the featherweight paper won't affect the numbers.

Used Filters, Grounds and All
▶ *Compost 'em.* Toss them onto the pile or into the bin. The paper will break down in no time, and the used java is a great source of high-nitrogen ingredients (a.k.a. greens). Just bear

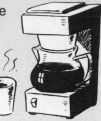

in mind that once the grounds have been composted, they'll no longer raise the acid level of your soil, because compost generally has a neutral pH.

▶ *Lower your pH.* Bury them in the ground near plants that prefer acidic surroundings (azaleas and rhododendrons, for instance). Besides increasing the acid level, the coffee will add valuable organic matter to the soil.

TIP Whoops! Your well-buttered toast fell off your plate, and landed butter-side-down on the carpet. Don't panic. Instead, pour **CORNSTARCH** on the stain to absorb the grease. Let it dry, and vacuum up the residue.

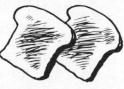

TIP When I inherited Grandma's books, some of them were sporting patches of mildew. (No matter how well you take care of your library, this nasty fungus can

creep in.) I didn't give it a thought, though. I just cleared it up the way she would have: I covered the spots with **CORNSTARCH** and let them sit for a few days. Then I brushed off the powder—outdoors, so the mildew spores couldn't latch on to anything else in the house. Those books, from Alcott to Twain, were (and still are) spotless.

TIP Get your carpet deep-down clean by sprinkling **CORNSTARCH** over the surface. Wait 30 minutes, and vacuum.

TIP Grandma had a super-simple way to make cut flowers last longer. She filled the vase with a solution of 2 tablespoons of clear **CORN SYRUP** per quart of water.

TIP Dang! You were writing out Christmas cards in bed, and your pen rolled out of your hand and onto your off-white carpet. Now what do you do? Sprinkle a teaspoon or so of **CREAM OF TARTAR** on the stain, and follow with a few drops of lemon juice. Rub the combo into the stain, and brush away the powder. Rinse immediately with warm water. Repeat as necessary until the ink has vanished.

TIP Keep a stone floor clean and sparkling by mopping it once a week with a solution made from a teaspoon or so of detergent-based **DISHWASHING LIQUID** per gallon of water. Rinse with clear water. (Don't use a soap-based product, because soap will leave a residue that will make the stone look dull.)

TIP There was nothing Grandpa Putt loved better than his favorite leather armchair. Grandma kept it looking as good as new by wiping it every couple of weeks with a soft, cotton cloth dipped in beaten **EGG** white. Then she buffed with a second cloth to give a sheen you could see yourself in!

TIP To make your refrigerator smell fresh and appetizing, dampen a cotton ball with the flavored **EXTRACT** of your choice, and tuck it onto a shelf.

GRANDMA PUTT'S
Secret Formulas

BRAVO BRASS CLEANER

Grandma cleaned all of the brass hardware in her house with this miraculous mixture. (It also works like a dream on copper cookware.)

1/2 cup of all-purpose flour
1/2 cup of salt
1/2 cup of dry laundry detergent (without bleach)
3/4 cup of white vinegar
1/4 cup of lemon juice (fresh or bottled)
1/2 cup of hot tap water

Mix the flour, salt, and detergent in a bowl. Add the remaining ingredients, and blend thoroughly. Dip a clean, soft, cotton cloth into the mixture, and rub it onto the brass, taking care to get it into all the nooks and crannies. Buff with a second, clean cloth. Store any leftover cleaner in a jar with a tight lid.

TIP In the wintertime, a closed-up house can develop a stale, unpleasant odor. But there's a simple way to make the air springtime fresh: Just apply a drop or two of lemon **EXTRACT** to the lightbulbs in lamps and ceiling fixtures, *before* you turn them on. (If lemon is not your favorite scent, substitute the extract of your choice, such as peppermint, almond, or vanilla.)

TIP For Christmas one year, I gave Grandma Putt a papier-mâché statue I'd made in art class—it was a life-size model of her dog, Charley. I was a little concerned about how she was going to keep the delicate surface clean, but as usual, she knew an old-time, fail-safe trick. First, she washed the whole thing with a sponge dipped in cold water (no soap). Then, while the surface was still damp, she dusted **FLOUR** all over it, and polished it with a cotton flannel cloth. This technique worked so well that I *still* have Charley's alter ego at my house! (P.S. You can use the same method to clean decorative plates, trays, or anything else made of papier-mâché.)

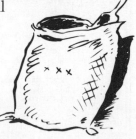

GRANDMA PUTT'S Secret Formulas

SCORCH-BE-GONE CARPET CLEANER

Whenever a light scorch mark appeared on her carpet—caused by, say, a fallen candle or a spark from the fireplace—Grandma cleaned it off with this easy-as-pie potion.

1 cup of white vinegar
1/2 cup of talcum powder (unscented)
2 medium onions, coarsely chopped

Put all of the ingredients in a pan, bring the vinegar to a boil, and continue to boil for about three minutes. Remove the pan from the heat, let the mixture cool, and spread it over the scorch mark. (Grandma used a soup ladle for this job.) Let it dry, then whisk it away with a stiff brush. Bye, bye, burn!

TIP Keep your stainless steel pans shiny-bright by rubbing them with **FLOUR** on a clean, soft, dry cloth. Then buff with a second cloth.

TIP To clean chrome faucets in your kitchen or bathroom, sprinkle a handful of **FLOUR** on them, rub with a clean, dry cloth, and polish with a second cloth.

TIP When you're using a dry material, like salt, cornmeal, or baking soda for cleaning purposes, sprinkling it evenly across a countertop, carpet, or other large surface can be tricky. So don't sprinkle. Instead, use a **FLOUR SIFTER** to spread your cleaner of choice over the surface.

TIP A leaking toilet tank can waste hundreds of gallons of water each day—without your even knowing about it. Fortunately, there's an easy way to find out if this is happening in *your* bathroom. Just drip a little **FOOD COLORING** into the tank. If the water in the toilet bowl turns color, call a plumber, who can dash right over and repair the seal.

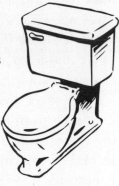

TIP Most of Grandma's home-made liquid cleaning formulas were colorless. Of course, she always labeled the bottles, but she also added a few drops of **FOOD COLORING** to each one. That way, she could tell her spot remover from her window cleaner at a glance.

TIP Your sheer curtains will always came out of the washer free of wrinkles if you use this trick: Just dissolve a package of unflavored **GELATIN** in 1 cup of boiling water, and add it to the final rinse.

TIP Have you ever found yourself with more fresh eggs than you could use before they went over the hill? Well, the next time that happens, do what Grandma's neighbor did when her chickens were extra generous. One by one, break each egg into a bowl, beat it lightly, and pour it into a compartment of a greased **ICE CUBE TRAY.** When the tray is full, pop it into the freezer. Once the contents are frozen, take them out, and store them in a freezer container or zip-top plastic freezer bag. Then, take out as many as you need for a recipe, let them thaw, and proceed as usual. They'll taste as fresh as they did the day you tucked them away.

TIP When it's time to move, wrap your dishes in your kitchen **LINENS.** You'll save space, because (of course) you have to pack your tablecloths, runners, placemats, and dish towels, anyway. What's more, the fabric won't leave smears, as newspaper would.

TIP Got a screw hole that's a tad too big for the screw? No problem! Just dip a wooden kitchen **MATCH** in some glue, stick it into the hole, and break it off flush with the surface. The screw should go in and stay put.

TIP Grandma often used pieces of oilcloth to cover tables, especially outdoors at picnic time. Like many of the things she took for granted, this vintage textile is back in vogue. If you have some at your house, keep it clean the way Grandma did: Wash it once a month with a solution made from equal parts of skim **MILK** and water. Then, once every three months or so, rub the surface with boiled linseed oil on a soft, cotton cloth, and polish it with a scrap of silk. (You can buy boiled linseed oil at your local hardware store. As for the silk, if you don't have a worn-out blouse or old silk tie on hand, you can use cotton instead—or check the rag-bag section of your favorite thrift store.)

TIP Don't cry over smeared ink—not even when it's leaked out of a ballpoint pen onto your favorite leather handbag or leather jacket. Instead, dip a soft, cotton cloth in **MILK,** and rub the marks away. Then wipe with a second cloth, dampened with clear, cool water.

TIP To declutter a desk drawer in a hurry, put a **MUFFIN TIN** inside it, and fill the compartments with all the small stuff, like push-pins, paper clips, stamps, and mini sticky-note pads.

TIP Remove odors from glass bottles or narrow-necked vases by soaking them overnight in a solution made from 1 teaspoon of dry **MUSTARD** per 4 cups of warm water. Rinse well, and let the pieces dry in the open before you put them away.

In Grandma's Day

Time for another trivia quiz! What classic American drink (and one of Grandma's favorites) made its debut at the 1904 World's Fair in St. Louis? The answer: **ICED TEA!** Ah, what would summertime be without it?

TIP No matter how careful you are, wooden tables tend to pick up water marks. Grandma removed them with this easy method: Put 4 tablespoons of virgin **OLIVE OIL** and 3 tablespoons of paraffin shavings in a double boiler, and heat until the wax has melted. Remove the pot from the heat, stir to mix the ingredients, and let cool. Then dip a clean, soft, cotton cloth in the paste, and rub it into the spotted area, using a circular motion. Then buff with a second cloth.

TIP When china plates sit stacked on a shelf, the bottom of one can scratch the surface of the plate below. To keep that from happening, put **PAPER PLATES** between them.

TIP There's nothing more annoying than cabinet and furniture drawers that constantly stick—and sometimes won't even budge. Fortunately, there's a simple solution to that problem. First, clean and sand all of the sticking surfaces of the drawer. Coat them with shellac, let it dry, and rub them with **PARAFFIN.** From then on, you'll have smooth sailin'!

TIP One day, Grandma Putt accidentally cracked her favorite ceramic vase. But she didn't get upset—in fact, she didn't bat an

eye. She just grabbed a block of **PARAFFIN** from her jelly-making cupboard, melted the wax, and poured the hot liquid into the vase. Then, she rotated the vase quickly so the wax covered the entire surface before it cooled off, and bingo! That old vase was as good as new. (This technique also makes porous surfaces waterproof—which means you can turn just about any container into a vase.)

GRANDMA PUTT'S
Secret Formulas

HOME-SAFE ANT BAIT

When ants are driving you bananas, indoors or out—and you have pets or young children on the scene—send the pests packin' with this formula. It's so safe kids and pets won't be harmed if they take a taste.

½ **cup of honey**
⅜ **cup of baker's yeast**
⅜ **cup of sugar**

Put the ingredients in a bowl, and mix thoroughly. Spread the mixture on bottle caps or pieces of plastic or cardboard, and set the traps in the ants' pathways. The tiny pests will flock to the sweet feast, and that'll be all she wrote.

Plastic Trash Bags

When Harry Wasylyk and Larry Hansen invented plastic garbage bags in 1950, they intended them for commercial use. (Their first customer was the Winnipeg, Manitoba, General Hospital.) It wasn't until the late '60s, when Union Carbide bought the rights to the idea, that GLAD® garbage bags became available to the home consumer. I've always been sad that GLAD didn't appear a couple of decades earlier, because Grandma Putt would have found countless uses for these weighty, waterproof wonders. Like these, perhaps:

▶ *"Babysit" your house-plants.* Before you take off on trip, line your bathtub with trash bags, and cover them with a big, wet towel. Set your plants on the towel, and just before you leave, water them thoroughly. Assuming the pots have drainage holes at the bottom, your green pals should stay in fine fettle for two weeks or so.

▶ *Change diapers on the go.* When you hit the road, or take to the air, with a tiny tot, pack a trash bag (or even three or four) to use as an emergency diaper-changing mat.

▶ *Chase birds from your vegetable garden.* Starting at the open end of a bag (the top), cut strips about an inch wide to within 3 inches or so of the bottom. Tape or staple the 3-inch band to your fence, or to posts that you've pounded into the ground. When a breeze comes up, the fringe will flap in the wind—making the startled birds scurry in a hurry!

▶ *Conquer clutter.* Tie the handles of drawstring trash bags to coat hangers, and hang one in each closet in the house. Then, each time you come across a gadget you haven't used in ages, a dress you wouldn't be caught dead in, or a toy the kids no longer play with, toss it into the bag. When the sack's filled up, take it to your local thrift store.

▶ *Foil raccoons.* Lay a 3-foot-wide strip of heavy-duty trash bags around your trash can, bird feeder, vegetable garden, or anything else you need to protect. Raccoons have hairless and very sensitive feet, and they don't like walking on slippery plastic. When they feel the slick surface, they'll clear out in a hurry.

▶ *Keep a cast or bandage dry.* Just cover it with a trash bag before you head for the showers—or out into a rainstorm.

▶ *Keep yourself dry.* Cut a head hole and armholes in a giant trash bag, and stash it in your car's glove compartment to use as an emergency rain slicker. Better yet, keep several of these slickers on hand so your passengers can stay dry, too!

▶ *Move your clothes.* When you're packing for a move, improvise a garment bag. Cut a small hole in the bottom of a large or giant-size trash bag. Then, gather a few hanging garments, and slip the sack over the hangers, so the hook sticks through. For extra protection, tape the bottom closed so nothing falls out in transit.

▶ *Paint at will!* Before you start to paint a room, cover light fixtures—and every other immovable object—with a trash bag (or two or three).

▶ *Protect your clothes.* Use a giant lawn-and-leaf bag as a waterproof smock for sloppy cleaning chores, indoors and out. Just cut a head-sized hole in the bottom and an armhole in each side, and slip the sack over your head.

▶ *Recycle cans and bottles.* Hang a drawstring trash bag on the inside of a closet or pantry door, and toss those empties into it. Then (depending on how your town handles these things), either take the containers back to the store and collect your deposit, pour them into your recycling bin on your regular pickup day, or haul them off to the recycling section of your local dump.

▶ *Sleep dry.* When your kids or grandkids have a campout, spread trash bags on the ground under their sleeping bags.

▶ *Waterproof a backpack.* Just put the pack in a trash bag, and cut slits for the straps to poke through.

▶ *Waterproof a mattress.* When a tyke in diapers (or an older person with an incontinence problem) comes to spend the night, cut open a giant trash bag and spread it out under the sheet.

▶ *Winterize your windshield.* If your car has to stay outdoors overnight in cold weather, cover the windshield with a trash bag or two to keep the glass free of frost, ice, and snow. Anchor the plastic under the wipers.

TIP When you need to move or store fragile knickknacks, or any small, breakable objects, reach into your kitchen cupboard and pull out some **PLASTIC FOOD CONTAINERS.** Then wrap your little treasures in bubble wrap or soft, thick fabric, tuck them inside the containers, and snap on the lids.

TIP Catalogs, bills, and other mail can pile up fast in an entryway or home office. But an old-fashioned kitchen gadget can stop postal clutter in its tracks. Just find or buy a wooden **POT-LID RACK,** paint or stain it if you like, and put it on a desk or hall table. Then put all your mail in the slots, with cards and letters in front, and catalogs, magazines, and large envelopes toward the back.

TIP I'll never forget the day I found Grandpa Putt's old guitar in the attic. When he said it was all mine, I jumped for joy. (In my 10-year-old head, I was thinking, "Move over, Roy Rogers—here I come!") As you might expect, there was a whole lot of dust inside the instrument, but Grandma knew how to fix that. She just poured a handful of uncooked **RICE** into the center hole, shook the guitar gently, and poured the rice out, dirt and all. Then, to make sure the inside was clean as a whistle, she reprised the performance a few times (as they say in the music biz). This same trick works just as well with violins, mandolins, and any other stringed instrument.

TIP If you use your coffee grinder to grind spices and citrus peels as well as java, here's a simple way to keep all those odors from mixing and mingling: Just put a teaspoon or two of uncooked **RICE** in the reservoir, grind it up, and toss it out. Presto—odor-free blades!

TIP Dang! As you were putting an egg into a pan of water, you accidentally cracked the shell. Don't fret. Just do what Grandma always did when that happened: Bring the water to a boil, add 1 teaspoon of **SALT,** and then put in the egg. The salt will make the egg white set quickly, so it won't ooze out through the crack.

TIP Whenever one of Grandma's glass decanters or vases started looking dull, she'd put a handful of **SALT** and 2 teaspoons of white vinegar in it, and give it a few good shakes. Then she'd rinse it with clear water. That thing would sparkle!

TIP As you know if you're a coffee or tea drinker, these beverages tend to leave ugly brown stains on ceramic cups, mugs, and teapots. But there's an easy way to get rid of those "souvenirs." Just mix equal parts of **SALT** and white vinegar, and scrub the marks away.

TIP A wooden cutting board will last for years—and stay free of nasty bacteria—if you follow Grandma's maintenance plan. Every two or three weeks, cover the board's surface with a layer of coarse **SALT** (either kosher or sea salt), then rub it thoroughly with the cut side of a lemon half. When you're finished, rinse the board with hot water, dry it, and rub on a light coat of vegetable or mineral oil.

TIP Coarse **SALT** will keep cast-iron pans clean and rust-free. Just sprinkle the salt over the inside, and scrub the bottom and sides with a soft, slightly damp sponge. Then rinse with clear water, and dry the pan thoroughly.

TIP When wine spills on your carpet, immediately give it a shake—of **SALT.** Sprinkle the NaCl lightly over the spot, and blot it up. If any liquid remains, add more salt, let it sit until it's absorbed all of the wine, then vacuum.

ONE MORE TIME

When you empty a sturdy, round **SALT CONTAINER,** don't throw it away. Cut the top off, and use the container to hold (for instance) wooden spoons in your kitchen, knitting needles and scissors in your craft room, or screwdrivers and chisels in the workshop.

Grandma's Substitutions

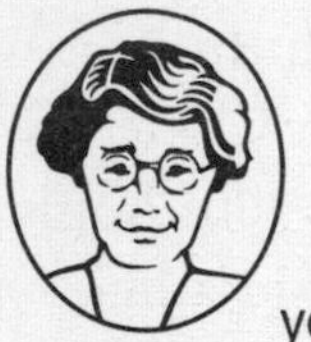

It happens to all of us now and then: You're cooking dinner or whipping up a special treat for the kids, and you discover that you're fresh out of a crucial ingredient. What a pain! Well, for Grandma Putt and her cohorts, who had to feed their families during the Great Depression and World War II, lacking a specific product was often business as usual. Did they complain? No sir! They simply found stand-ins that worked just as well as the originals. And you can, too. Here's how.

If You Lack This	Use This Instead
1 tsp. of baking powder	½ tsp. of cream of tarter + ¼ tsp. of baking soda
1 cup of buttermilk	1 tsp. of vinegar or lemon juice + enough milk to measure 1 cup
1 cup of cake flour	⅞ cup of all-purpose flour
1 tbsp. of cornstarch	2 tbsp. of all-purpose flour
¾ cup of cracker crumbs	1 cup of bread crumbs
1 cup of dark corn syrup	¾ cup of light corn syrup + ¼ cup of molasses
1 garlic clove, minced	⅛ tsp. of garlic powder
1 tsp. of garlic salt	⅛ tsp. of garlic powder + ⅞ tsp. of salt
1 cup of half-and-half	1 tbsp. of melted butter + enough whole milk to measure 1 cup
1 cup of honey	1¼ cups of sugar + ¼ cup of liquid *
1 tsp. of lemon juice	¼ tsp. of apple cider vinegar
1 tsp. of lemon peel	½ tsp. of lemon extract
1 cup of light corn syrup	1 cup of sugar + 1 cup of liquid *
1 cup of molasses	1 cup of honey
1 small onion, chopped	1 tsp. of onion powder, 1 tbsp. of dried, minced onions, or 2 tbsp. of frozen, diced onions
1 tbsp. of prepared mustard	½ tsp. of powdered mustard + 2 tsp. of vinegar
1 square of semisweet chocolate (1 oz.)	3 tbsp. of semisweet chocolate chips or 1 square of unsweetened chocolate (1 oz.) + 1 tbsp. of sugar
1 cup of sour cream	1 cup of plain yogurt

If You Lack This	Use This Instead
2 tsp. of tapioca	1 tbsp. of all-purpose flour
1 cup of tomato sauce	$^3/_4$ cup of tomato paste + 1 cup of water
1 cup of white sugar	1 cup of packed brown sugar or 2 cups of confectioners' sugar, sifted
1 cup of whole milk	$^1/_2$ cup of evaporated milk + 1 cup of water

* May be water or whatever other liquid your recipe calls for, such as milk, cream, or fruit juice.

TIP If you have a marble-topped table or two, you know that this soft stone is a magnet for liquid-based stains. Fortunately, there's a simple trick for removing them. Just cover the stain with **SALT,** wait a few minutes, then brush it off. Repeat until the salt has absorbed the "trespassing" fluid.

TIP For extra-stubborn stains on marble, try this: Cover the marks with **SALT**, pour sour milk over it, and leave it for three or four days. Then wipe it off with a soft, damp (not wet) cotton cloth.

TIP Grandma had a simple method for getting white water rings off of wooden tabletops. She used a pinch of **SALT** and a drop of water, rubbing it into the wood with a soft cloth until the stain disappeared. Then she followed up with her regular furniture polish.

TIP Even if you have a self-cleaning oven, this old-time trick is worth having in your repertoire. (After all, your next rental cabin or beach house might not have all the latest, greatest appliances.) The minute you discover something bubbling over in the oven, cover the spatters with **SALT.** That way, the food won't adhere to the surface, and when the oven has cooled down, you can just wipe the spill away with paper towels.

TIP Tackle stove-top spills in a similar way. Sprinkle **SALT** on the spots while the burners are still hot. When they're cool enough to touch, clean them off with a cloth, sponge, or nylon scouring pad.

TIP As Grandma always said, a new broom sweeps clean. And it'll sweep cleaner, longer if you soak it in a bucket of hot water with 1 cup of **SALT** added to it *before* you use it for the first time. Half an hour should do the trick. *Note:* This works only with natural-bristle brooms (and brushes, too), not the synthetic kinds.

GRANDMA PUTT'S
Secret Formulas

OLD-TIME ALUMINUM CLEANER

Grandma Putt kept her aluminum pots and pans looking brand-spanking new with this simple, homemade cleanser. (It'll also work its magic on your aluminum outdoor furniture!)

½ **cup of cream of tartar**
½ **cup of baking soda**
½ **cup of white vinegar**
¼ **cup of soap flakes (such as Ivory Snow®)**

Combine the cream of tartar and baking soda in a bowl. Add the vinegar and mix to form a paste. Stir in the soap flakes, transfer the mixture to a glass jar with a tight lid, and label it. Apply the paste with a plain steel wool pad, and rinse with clear water.

TIP To get tarnish off of brass or copper, mix **SALT** with just enough lemon juice to make a paste, and rub the spots away. Then rinse the piece in cool water, and wipe dry.

TIP Folks who live in the cold, cold North have all sorts of ways to keep water pipes from freezing in the winter. Grandma's favorite method was to toss a handful of **SALT** down each drain just before she went to bed at night.

TIP Before you wear new pantyhose for the first time, soak them for three hours in a solution made from 2 cups of **SALT** per gallon of water. Then rinse them in cold water and drip dry. This treatment will help prevent runs, and make your hose last a whole lot longer.

TIP I don't know about you, but I spend most of my weekends (and a lot of weekdays) in blue jeans. And believe me, I want those pants to be soft and comfortable from day one! So before I wear a new pair for the first time, I add ½ cup of **SALT** to the water in my washing machine. Then I toss in the detergent, and press the "On" button. Those pants come out so soft, I could swear I'd worn them for years.

TIP Like most housewives of her day, Grandma made a *lot* of gelatin salads. And whenever she was in a hurry to get one chilled and set, she sped up the process by filling a big bowl with ice cubes, and sprinkling **SALT** over them. Then she put the salad (in its container of course!) on top. In no time flat, that colorful, wiggly treat was ready to serve.

TIP Does your septic system seem a little sluggish? Chances are that's because the underground breakdown squad (a.k.a. anaerobic bacteria) needs an energy boost. So serve up this power-packed snack: Mix 1 pound of brown **SUGAR** and 1 package of baker's yeast in 1 quart of warm water, and pour the mixture into the toilet bowl. Let it sit for 10 minutes, then flush. Before you know it, things will be flowing free and easy again.

TIP Grandma Putt was a live-and-let-live kind of person, even where bugs were concerned. But one fall, when ants began making first-class nuisances of themselves in her

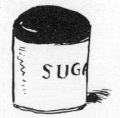

kitchen, she fought back hard. And you can, too. Just mix 2 tablespoons of **SUGAR** and 1 tablespoon of baker's yeast in 1 pint of warm water. Then spread the mixture on pieces of cardboard, and set them in the problem areas. The ants' antics will be ending in a flash.

TIP Grandma had a sterling silver coffee-and-tea set that she'd gotten as a wedding present and used only when company came to call. Between visits, she stored the pieces (coffeepot, teapot, sugar bowl, and creamer) with their lids off, and tucked a couple of white **SUGAR** cubes inside each one. That kept them from developing a stale, musty smell.

FABULOUS FURNITURE POLISH

When it comes to making fine furniture look its elegant best, this easy-to-make polish gets the Grandma Putt Seal of Approval!

$\frac{1}{4}$ **cup of linseed oil**
$\frac{1}{8}$ **cup of vinegar**
$\frac{1}{8}$ **cup of whiskey**

Mix the ingredients in a glass jar with a lid, and wipe the mixture onto your wooden furniture with a clean, soft, cotton cloth. Then buff with a second cloth. Cap any leftovers tightly, and store at room temperature.

TIP After you've cleaned your good jewelry, put it in a **TEA STRAINER** to rinse it. That way, there's no risk of having any tiny treasures tumble down the drain.

TIP To keep a covered pot from boiling over on the stove, insert a **TOOTHPICK** between the lid and the top edge of the pot. This will make an opening that's just big enough to let the steam escape.

TIP Besides our regular, big Christmas tree, Grandma Putt always kept a small one on a table in the entryway. And when it came time to squirt water into its tiny stand, she did the job with a **TURKEY BASTER.**

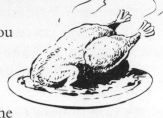

TIP When you put too much water into a big, heavy pot on the stove and it starts to run over the top, don't manhandle the thing over to the sink. Just use a **TURKEY BASTER** to siphon off the excess H_2O.

TIP We had a big bronze bust of Mozart that sat on the piano. It had been in the family for so long that Grandma didn't even know where it came from, but she sure treasured that sculpture! She kept it spotless and gleaming by wiping it every week or so with a few dabs of **VEGETABLE OIL** on a soft cloth.

TIP Why bother buying furniture polish, when it's so easy to make your own better "brand"? Just mix 1 cup of **VEGETABLE OIL** with $\frac{1}{2}$ cup of lemon juice, and rub it into your wooden pieces every time you dust them. Then buff them with a soft cloth until the wood shines—and will it ever!

TIP Clean and protect wood floors by rubbing them with a half-and-half mixture of **VEGETABLE OIL** and white vinegar.

TIP Get a ceramic-tile floor squeaky clean by mopping it with ¼ cup of white **VINEGAR** mixed in a bucket of warm water.

TIP Whenever Grandma found burn marks on her brick hearth, she'd sponge them off with white **VINEGAR,** and rinse with clear water. For routine cleaning of brick or stone, she used 1 cup of white vinegar in a bucket of warm water.

TIP The scaly crust that builds up at the base of faucets can be the very dickens to get rid of—and, there's no way to give it a full-immersion treatment as you can with a spigot (see page 182). But the crud will float right off it if you go at it Grandma's way. Just soak paper towels in white **VINEGAR,** and lay them over the faucets. Wait an hour or so, then scrub the gunk away with a toothbrush, and rinse with fresh water.

TIP Keep the bottom of your steam iron clean by wiping it every now and then with a soft, cotton cloth moistened with white **VINEGAR.** (Just be sure the iron is unplugged and cool!)

TIP To keep deposits from building up on the inside of your iron, periodically fill the water holder with white **VINEGAR,** set the dial on high steam, and go about your business while the appliance cleans itself. When the reservoir is dry, flush it with clear water. (How often you need to perform this maneuver depends on how much ironing you do; let your eyes be your guide.)

TIP When water leaves lines on your favorite vase, do what Grandma did: Saturate a towel or washcloth (depending on the size of the container) with white **VINEGAR,** and 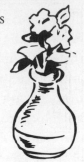 stuff it in so it has contact with the sides. Let it sit overnight, and by morning those unsightly marks will wash right off.

TIP Over time, soap residue tends to build up on baked enamel surfaces, like the outsides of your stove and other kitchen appliances. Eventually, it dulls the finish, but it's a cinch to restore the shine. Just mix equal parts of white **VINEGAR** and water, dip a sponge in the solution, and wipe the film away.

TIP Keep your good crystal—and even those vintage Howdy Doody jelly glasses—shiny bright by following the same routine Grandma used on her glassware: After every washing, rinse them in a solution made from ½ cup of white **VINEGAR** per gallon of water.

TIP Clear the openings of a clogged showerhead by soaking it in a bowl of warm, undiluted white **VINEGAR** until the scale deposits loosen up and float away. If some holes remain blocked, clear them out with a toothbrush, toothpick, or darning needle.

TIP To remove scale from a sink spigot, fill a strong plastic bag about halfway with white **VINEGAR,** and tie the bag over the spigot so it's

GRANDMA PUTT'S
Secret Formulas

SAFE-AND-SOUND BATHROOM DRAIN CLEANER

Soap scum and hair can make a yucky mess in tub and sink drains. But you don't need toxic chemicals to clean the stuff out. This gentle formula will have those pipes flowing freely again in no time.

1 cup of baking soda
1 cup of salt
½ cup of white vinegar
2 qt. of boiling water
Hot tap water

Mix the soda, salt, and vinegar together, and pour the mixture down the drain. Wait 15 minutes, then follow with the boiling water. Turn on the hot water, and let it run into the drain for one minute. For really stubborn clogs, repeat as necessary.

submerged in the vinegar. Leave it until the crud has dissolved, then rinse with clear water.

TIP Almost nothing in the bathroom gets grimy faster than the track for a sliding shower door (at least it seems that way). But I know an easy way to clean it. Just pour white **VINEGAR** into the channel, wait two or three minutes, and rinse. Presto—gunk leavin' on Track Number One!

TIP Call me old-fashioned, but I love writing with a genuine fountain pen. (In fact, I still have the one Grandma Putt gave me when I graduated from high school.) To keep that, and my newer models, clean and free-flowing, I take them apart every so often and soak the pieces in white **VINEGAR.** I leave them there for an hour or so, then rinse them in warm water, and lay them on a paper towel to dry.

TIP Even your washing machine needs a good washing every now and then. To get rid of built-up soap scum, hair, lint, and heaven knows what else, pour 1 gallon of white **VINEGAR** into the drum, and run the washer through a regular large-load cycle.

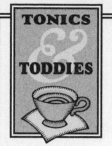

TONICS & TODDIES

GRANDMA'S HOMEMADE VINEGAR

Grandma Putt used to make her own apple cider vinegar, and you can, too. The process takes time, but the recipe couldn't be simpler. Here it is.

12 ripe apples, unpeeled and diced
1 package of baker's yeast
Pure spring water

Put the apples (cores and all) in a stoneware crock, or a deep glass or ceramic bowl. Add the yeast, and pour in enough spring water to cover the apples. (It will probably take about a quart.) Cover the bowl with a piece of cheesecloth, and fasten it on with a rubber band. Put the container in a warm place (ideally where the temperature will stay at roughly 80°F), and let it sit for three to four months, or until the natural sugars have been converted to alcohol. (You'll know by the taste that you now have hard cider.) Strain out the apples, and pour the liquid into a fresh crock or bowl. Set it back in its warm place, uncovered, and leave it for another three to four months. Then pour the vinegar into a glass bottle or jar, and store it at room temperature.

TIP For my money, nothing gets the day off to a rip-roaring start like a good, fresh cup of coffee—and you can't get one from a coffeemaker that's built up a supply of mineral deposits. To keep your machine clean, fill the water reservoir with equal parts of white **VINEGAR** and water, put the pot in place, and turn on the switch so the vinegar cycles through the machine. Then dump out the resulting "brew," and follow with a pot of clear water. How often you need to perform this maneuver depends on how much coffee you make, so let your nose and your taste buds be your guide!

TIP Although new wallpaper is a cinch to strip off, the ones applied in Grandma's time are something else again. To loosen that glue, you need to use a potent stripper—like the one you can make by mixing about $\frac{1}{2}$ cup of white **VINEGAR** in a bucket of hot water. Then, just paint the solution onto the wall, let it soak in, and scrape the paper right off. (If the paper is especially stubborn, add more vinegar to the water.)

TIP There was nothing Grandma loved for breakfast more than

ONE MORE TIME

Even the tidiest, most efficient people I know have trouble keeping their home offices neat and well organized. Here's a Baker's dozen **KITCHEN CONTRAPTIONS** that can help you corral the clutter that's clogging up your desk, work-tables, and supply cupboards:

▷ **Baking pans**

▷ **Berry baskets**

▷ **Breadboxes**

▷ **Canisters**

▷ **Cutlery organizers**

▷ **Dish drainers**

▷ **Glasses**

▷ **Mugs**

▷ **Napkin holders**

▷ **Pot-lid racks**

▷ **Spice racks**

▷ **Utensil crocks**

▷ **Wire-mesh produce baskets**

poached eggs. And to make sure they kept their shape in the pan, she always added a few drops of **VINEGAR** to the cooking water. (Either white or apple cider vinegar will do the job.)

TIP When you need to get the smoky smell out of a room, fill a glass jar with **VINEGAR** (any kind will do), and sink a large oil-lamp wick into it. The wick will absorb the noxious odors, and the vinegar will kill them dead.

TIP Like a lot of the things Grandma had in her house, linoleum floors have staged a big-time comeback. If you have this classic covering underfoot in your kitchen (or any other room), keep it fresh and clean by mopping the floor once a month with a solution made from ½ cup of apple cider **VINEGAR** per gallon of warm water. This stuff will cut right through grease and dirt—and leave the air smelling sweet, too.

TIP You've found a terrific table for peanuts at a flea market. There's just one problem: There's a thick buildup of polish on the wood. How do you get the stuff off? Simple: Wipe it with a half-and-half solution of white **VINEGAR** and

water, and rub it off immediately. Repeat if you need to (but you probably won't).

TIP Anytime Grandma Putt got a new wooden spoon, she soaked it in apple cider **VINEGAR** overnight, and dried it off with a towel the next morning. This treatment kept the wood from absorbing food odors, so Grandma didn't have to worry about having her chocolate chip cookies come out of the oven smelling faintly of spaghetti sauce!

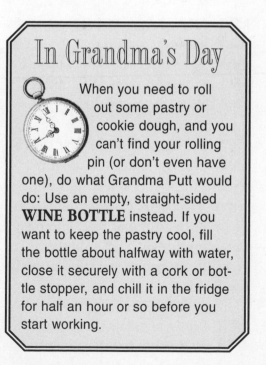

In Grandma's Day

When you need to roll out some pastry or cookie dough, and you can't find your rolling pin (or don't even have one), do what Grandma Putt would do: Use an empty, straight-sided **WINE BOTTLE** instead. If you want to keep the pastry cool, fill the bottle about halfway with water, close it securely with a cork or bottle stopper, and chill it in the fridge for half an hour or so before you start working.

TIP To clean plastic piano keys (which are found on all the instruments made in the last 30 years or so), wipe them with a chamois dampened with a solution of warm water and white **VINEGAR.** About 1 tablespoon per quart of H_2O should do the trick.

TIP **VINEGAR** can also keep odors from seeping into your skin. So the next time you have to handle aromatic food, like onions, garlic, or fish, pour a few drops of apple cider vinegar into one palm, and rub your hands together *before* you touch the smelly stuff.

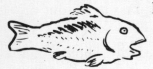

TIP Over time, metal curtain rings tend to pick up rust spots. Get the things bright and shiny again by boiling them in white **VINEGAR** until the marks disappear.

TIP For the softest, fluffiest towels this side of a five-star hotel, try this trick: Just add 2 cups of white **VINEGAR** to the rinse water in your washing machine. The next time you dry off after a shower, you'll think you've died and gone to the Ritz!

TIP Nowadays, fabrics tend to be a lot more colorfast than they

ONE MORE TIME

There's nothing like a wooden knife block for keeping those kitchen cutting tools sharp and free of nicks. But if you need to store your knives in a drawer with other cutlery, here's the next-best way to avoid damage: Cushion the point of each knife by sticking it into a used **WINE CORK.**

were in Grandma's time. Still, unless you're sure the dye will stay put, it doesn't pay to take chances. Before you wash a new, bright-colored garment for the first time, soak it for about 15 minutes in a solution made from 2/3 cup of white **VINEGAR** per gallon of cold water. Then wash and dry the article according to the guidelines on its care tag.

TIP In a pinch, shine your shoes with **WAX PAPER.** Just rub it across the leather, and buff with a soft cloth.

TIP When company's coming, and you want to give your tile floor an instant shine, wrap a sheet of **WAX PAPER** around your mop, and scoot it over the floor.

TIP Grandma had a special way of making Grandpa's trousers look neat and crisp—and stay that way longer. Before she ironed each leg, she folded a sheet of **WAX PAPER** over it, and ironed across the paper. A little bit of the wax seeped into the fabric, making the crease hold better.

TIP If you have an old piano, you know that those ivory keys can turn yellow faster than you can say "rose of Texas"—much less play it. Well, keep them shiny-bright by cleaning them with a dab of plain **YOGURT** on a soft, cotton cloth.

Family and
FRIENDS

TIP Keep Fido off of the couch by laying strips of **ALUMINUM FOIL** on the seat cushions. When he jumps up, the crackly sound will startle him, and he'll jump right back off. (At least most dogs will.)

TIP Fight diaper rash the way Grandma did: by wiping baby's bottom with a solution of 4 tablespoons of **BAKING SODA** per quart of warm water.

TIP Clean a toddler's white shoes by sprinkling **BAKING SODA** onto the leather and wiping with a damp cloth.

TIP When my buddies and I were going through a "let's be spies" phase, Grandma showed us how to write invisible messages. You just mix 1 teaspoon of **BAKING SODA** with 2 teaspoons of water, dip a fountain pen into the solution, and scrawl your crucial note on a piece of paper (in code, of course). When the "ink" has dried, hold the paper near a lightbulb. Bingo—brown writing will materialize. Then all you have to do is remember how to decode your message....

TIP What do you do when a child's—or dog's—favorite stuffed critter gets dirty, and it happens to be unwashable? Simple: Just fill a bag with **BAKING SODA,** pop the toy inside, and shake the sack until the fabric is covered. Wait 15 minutes or so, to let the soda absorb the dirt and oils. Then remove the toy, and shake or vacuum off the excess white stuff.

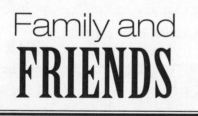

ONE MORE TIME

Here's a brainteaser for you: What do you get after you remove the cutting strip from a box that once held **ALUMINUM FOIL?** The answer: a playing-card holder for young children, or anyone else who has trouble grasping a full hand of cards. You just close the lid, and slip the cards into the slot between the flap and the side of the box. (Of course, this trick works just as well with plastic wrap and wax paper boxes.)

TIP When you play as many card games as we did at Grandma's house, the cards can get dirty and greasy mighty fast. Grandma kept ours clean by rubbing them frequently with a slice of white **BREAD.**

TIP Is there a teething puppy in the house? Then safeguard your furniture, woodwork, and heaven knows what else, by giving young Rover a steady supply of big, cold **CARROTS** to chew on. The cool temperature will soothe his sore gums, and he'll love the satisfying crunch. (Just don't tell him that these tasty treats are good for him!)

TIP Want to know a spicy secret for keeping cats and dogs away from your houseplants? Just shove a few **CINNAMON** sticks into the soil in each pot. Felines and canines both seem to dislike the aroma.

TIP When you're entertaining a crowd of youngsters for a Christmas or birthday party, use **COOKIE CUTTERS** to make sandwiches in festive shapes—for instance, Santas, stars, animals, or cowboy boots.

TIP **COOKIE CUTTERS** also make great stencils. Just trace around them to make patterns for wall decor, homemade wrapping paper, hand-painted fabric, or a jillion-and-one other craft projects.

TIP When Christmastime rolls around, make one-of-a-kind tree ornaments using cookie cutters and the Play Clay recipe on page 193—or encourage the kids to do it. And, to make sure the cutters cut cleanly, spritz them with **COOKING OIL SPRAY** before pushing them into the clay.

TIP Like any other self-respecting feline, Grandma Putt's cat, Eleanor, flatly refused to go near any body of water that was bigger than her drinking bowl. So, whenever Her Ladyship needed a bath, Grandma would rub **CORNMEAL** into her fur, and brush it out. Presto: a squeaky clean kitty with no hissy fits!

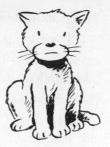

TIP Nowadays, there are special foods designed to prevent hairballs in cats, but they weren't around when Grandma's Eleanor needed them. So once a week, Grandma added a teaspoon of **CORN OIL** to Eleanor's dinner. That did the trick!

TIP No matter how careful you are when you're clipping a cat's or dog's toenails, it's easy to cut them a little too short. When that happens, dab the bleeding end with a pinch of **CORNSTARCH.** It'll speed up the clotting process and (more important to Fluffy and Fido), help ease the pain.

TIP Fresh out of baby powder? No problem! Just use **CORN-STARCH** instead. It'll keep the little tyke dry, comfortable, and free from heat rash—even in the hottest weather.

TIP When Halloween rolls around, whip up some makeup for your young clown, monster, or movie star—or even for your own costume. Just mix 2 tablespoons of **CORNSTARCH** with 1 tablespoon of solid shortening, then stir in the food coloring of your (or the trick-or-treater's) choice.

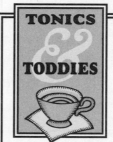

TONICS & TODDIES

BABY BATH FORMULA

Whenever one of her young friends had a baby, Grandma gave her a jar or two of this extra-gentle bath mixture.

¼ cup of nonfat dry milk
¼ cup of whole, dry buttermilk
1 tbsp. of cornstarch

Mix all of the ingredients together, and put the mixture in a covered glass jar. When baby's bath time rolls around, pour 1 tablespoon of the powder into a baby bathtub, or ¼ cup into a full-size tub.

TIP For every holiday, Grandma pulled out all the stops. She even served up food in the appropriate, festive shades—with the aid of **FOOD COLORING.** For instance, at her annual Fourth of July picnic, dessert was always a three-layer, red, white, and blue cake. And on Christmas, she made red and green pancakes for breakfast (in separate batches, of course).

TIP If your kids or grandkids love Dr. Seuss as much as mine do, surprise them one morning with *real* green eggs and ham. And how, you may ask, do you produce green eggs? Simple: Add a few drops of *blue* **FOOD COLORING** to the eggs before you scramble them.

TIP Add a **GARLIC PRESS** to your young artists' supply kit. It's just the ticket for producing "hair" to use on clay or dough creations. Just put a lump of the material in the bowl of the press, squeeze the handles, and out come the makings of, say, Santa's beard or a lion's mane.

TIP To stop a case of the runs in a child, mix a 3-ounce package of fruit-flavored **GELATIN** with 1 cup of cold water, and have the youngster drink it down. If that doesn't halt the flow, or if other symptoms are present, call your doctor pronto.

ONE MORE TIME

To you, extra pieces of **KITCHEN GEAR** may just add up to clutter, but to a small child, those gadgets and gizmos can mean hours of good old-fashioned fun. Here are a dozen dandy castoffs you might donate to a collection of bathtub, sandbox, or wading-pool toys. (And you can probably think of a lot more.)

▷ **Colanders**

▷ **Funnels**

▷ **Ice cream scoops**

▷ **Measuring cups**

▷ **Measuring spoons**

▷ **Mixing spoons**

▷ **Plastic ice cube trays**

▷ **Plastic food-storage containers**

▷ **Pots and pans**

▷ **Soup ladles**

▷ **Strainers**

▷ **Turkey basters**

TIP On more than one occasion I "caught" a fly ball square in the eye. And Grandma always had the perfect cure for my shiner. She pulled an **ICE CREAM BAR** out of the deep-freeze, wrapped a clean dish towel around it, and had me hold it over my sore eye. After the pain eased up, I got to eat the compress (minus the wrapper and towel, of course)!

TIP Summers always flew by when I was a boy, and my pals and I never wanted to waste a minute of our outdoor playtime. We didn't even like to go inside for lunch! Fortunately, Grandma Putt understood exactly how we felt (after all, she'd been a child once herself). So she found a clever way to bring lunch to us: She served it up in flat-bottomed **ICE CREAM CONES.**

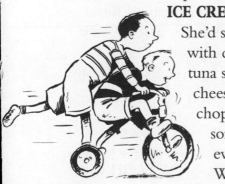

She'd stuff them with chicken or tuna salad, cottage cheese with chopped fruit, or sometimes even hot dogs. We loved it!

TIP Looking for a clever gift for a child? How about a **LOLLY-POP** "plant"? Just get a clay flowerpot in the color of your choice, and a Styrofoam® ball that's a little bigger

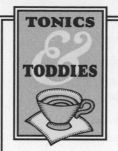

TONICS & TODDIES

SKUNK-AWAY PET BATH

Nothing can ruin your day—or your good night's sleep—like discovering that your dog has gotten up close and personal with a skunk. Fortunately, you can rely on this super-duper deskunking solution to get Rover smelling sweet as a rose again. Well, almost. (This formula also works on skunked humans.)

1 qt. of hydrogen peroxide
1 cup of baking soda
2 tbsp. of dog or puppy shampoo*

Mix the ingredients in a bucket or basin and, using a washcloth or sponge, apply the solution to your dog's coat (but don't get it on his head or near his eyes or ears). Rub it in thoroughly, then rinse with clear water.

* In a pinch, substitute liquid soap or mild, soap-based dishwashing liquid.

than the top of the pot. Glue the ball to the rim, then insert colorful lollypops into the foam (stick first, of course!) until you've covered the globe. Tie a ribbon around the pot, add a whimsical gift card, and present it to the youngster.

In Grandma's Day

If your children or grand-children love **POPSICLES**® (and Grandma's sure did!), here's a tale they should hear: That tasty—and fortune-making—treat was invented, quite by accident, in 1905 by an 11-year-old boy named Frank Epperson. It seems that one day, Frank mixed up a jar of powdered soda pop mix and water, and set it on his back porch, where he could sip from it as he played in the yard. Then, as kids will, he forgot to take it with him when he went back inside. The next morning he found it, frozen stiff, with the stirring stick standing straight up. When he pulled on the stick, out came the frozen pop. Frank knew at glance, and a lick, that he had stumbled onto something pretty darn good.

The following summer, he made what he called "Epperson Icicles" (soon changed to "Epsicles") in the family icebox, and sold them around the neighborhood for five cents each. Later, he changed the name to "Popsicle" because he'd made his prototype (so to speak) with soda pop. And the rest, as they say, is history.

TIP Get chewing gum out of a child's hair by rubbing **PEANUT BUTTER** into the lump. Massage it in with your fingers, then comb the gum and peanut butter out, and follow with the youngster's usual shampoo.

TIP The next time you send a fragile present through the mail, forget about filling the box with foam packing "peanuts." Use real **PEANUTS** instead. They'll cushion the contents as well as the fake type—and the recipient can eat them!

TIP Need a trunk for a young child who's headed off to camp? Use a **PICNIC COOLER.** Put clothes in the bottom, and toiletries and other small necessities in the top tray. The handles make it easy to carry, and it can double as a bench in the youngster's bunkhouse or cabin.

TIP As a little tyke, I was convinced that my Uncle Art was a genuine magician. He could even make the flames in our fireplace turn from their normal orangey red to bright yellow! Later, I found out that he performed this feat by tossing a handful of **SALT** into the fire. Now I do this same magic trick for all my grandchildren (until they get old enough to catch on, that is).

TIP For a baby, a stuffy nose is pure misery. But you can unclog that tiny schnozolla the way Grandma did. Just dissolve ¼ teaspoon of **SALT** in 8 ounces of water, and insert two drops of the solution into each nostril, using a medicine dropper. Then use a suction bulb to draw out the saline mixture and mucus. Just one word of caution: Don't use this treatment more than six times a day.

TIP To keep a toddler from sliding off of a chair, put a rubber **SINK MAT** on the seat.

TIP Every youngster needs a magic carpet ride now and then. Luckily for me, anytime I was itchin' for a flight, Grandma provided my "transportation," in the form of a colorful, fringed **TABLECLOTH.**

TIP It's easy for us grown-ups to forget how scary it can be to lose your first baby tooth and see the blood come flowing out of your mouth. But you can stop the flow and set the youngster's mind at ease the way Grandma always did. Just roll a moist **TEA** bag into a tight cylinder, and hold it on the spot where the tooth used to be.

GRANDMA PUTT'S
Secret Formulas

PLAY CLAY

Your young sculptor can turn out creations galore with this kitchen-counter modeling medium.

2 cups of baking soda
1 cup of cornstarch
1½ cups of water
Food coloring (optional)

Mix the ingredients together in a pan, and cook over medium heat, stirring continuously, until thickened. Spread the mixture on a plate or cutting board, cover it with a damp cloth, and let it sit until it's cool enough to handle. Knead the dough until it's smooth, adding food coloring if you'd like. (Use as much as it takes to reach the shade you want.) Store the clay in an airtight container in the refrigerator.

You have two drying options for the finished products: Let them sit, uncovered, for a few days, or bake them in the oven on the lowest setting for half an hour or so, checking every few minutes to make sure they don't "overcook." (With either method, drying time will vary, depending on the thickness of the objects.) When they're good and dry, the artist can display them unadorned, or paint them with acrylic paint.

TIP Use a **TURKEY BASTER** to top off your bird's water dish—just shove it through the bars of the cage, take aim, and squirt. (Of course, at least once a day, you'll still want to pull out the dish, clean it, and add fresh water.)

TIP The next time your dog or cat has a run-in with a bush full of burrs and prickles, pour a few drops of **VEGETABLE OIL** on the stickers, then gently comb your pet. The stick-ups should glide right out; if they don't, just add a little more oil, and comb again.

TIP Before you 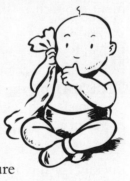 put a fresh diaper on a baby, wipe a light coat of **VEGETABLE SHORTENING** onto his bottom. It'll form a moisture barrier and help prevent diaper rash.

TIP When I was a boy, I kept a few white mice as pets. They were great little pals, but there was one problem: No matter how clean I kept their cage, the little rodents always gave off a distinctive odor. To absorb the aroma, Grandma had me put a bowl of **VINEGAR** next to the cage (but not *in* it). I replaced it with a fresh supply every few days, and my room always smelled as fresh as a daisy.

In Grandma's Day

Grandma knew that even the best-trained dog or cat has an accident once in a while. Of course, she wasn't overjoyed when it happened on her carpet—and she didn't have the fancy enzyme cleaners that can whisk the odor right out. But fortunately, she had products that worked just as well, and they'll work for you, too. Here's the routine: First, blot up as much of the urine as you can with paper towels or old rags. (If the deed has just been done, this step alone will take care of 90 percent of the problem.) Then flush the spot with **CLUB SODA,** let it sit for a minute or two, and blot again. Follow up by mixing equal parts of white vinegar and cool water, and scrubbing the solution into the rug with a stiff brush. Blot up the excess liquid, rinse with cool water, and let the spot dry. If a stain remains, reapply the vinegar and water solution, wait 15 minutes, then rinse and blot again.

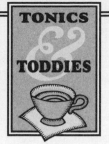
FROZEN BIRD TREATS

Want to give your pet bird a cool and healthy treat? Whip up a batch of these goodies.

1 qt. of vanilla yogurt
1 cup of mashed fruit*
2 tbsp. of peanut butter
2 tbsp. of honey

Puree the ingredients in a blender or food processor, and freeze the mixture in ice cube trays or, for larger birds, 3-ounce plastic cups. Then, when Polly wants a snack, pop one into the microwave, nuke it for a few seconds, and serve it up. Or, if you're partial to Grandma's slower, easier ways, pop the frozen treat into a heat-proof dish, and set it into a 350°F oven for about 20 minutes.

* Don't use avocados—they're poisonous to birds!

TIP Although I loved to play outdoors, I never minded rainy days because Grandma knew lots of ways to help the time fly inside. One of my favorites was a science experiment we called "bubble-blowing seashells." Just fill a glass or bowl one-quarter of the way with **VINEGAR** (any kind will do). Then gently drop in two or three seashells, and watch the bubbles rise to the surface. Grandma explained that this happens because the acetic acid in the vinegar reacts with the limestone in the shells to form carbon dioxide—the same stuff that gives soda pop its fizz.

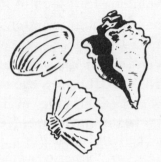

TIP To help keep her dog free of fleas and ticks, Grandma always added 1 teaspoon of apple cider **VINEGAR** to each quart of water in his drinking bowl.

TIP Do you have kids or grandkids who collect stickers? If so, the next time they get a new set, give them a sheet of **WAX PAPER** to try out their designs. They can move the stickers around on the slick surface time after time while they decide on a permanent arrangement for their scrapbook pages.

The great
OUTDOORS

TIP Grandma Putt used to root a lot of cuttings in water, and she had her own special system. She always stretched a piece of **ALUMINUM FOIL** across the top of the glass and poked holes in it. Then she inserted the cuttings through the holes. The foil held the stems securely in place, and kept the water from evaporating as quickly as it would have in an uncovered container.

TIP When Grandma brought her herbs and geraniums indoors for the winter, she always set the pots on windowsills that she'd lined with **ALUMINUM FOIL,** shiny side up. It reflected light onto the plants and kept them going strong all winter long.

TIP After your next barbecue, lay a sheet of **ALU-MINUM FOIL** on the hot grill. Then, when it's cooled down,

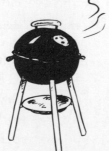

peel off the foil, crinkle it into a ball, and rub the grill clean. All those burned-on burgers will be gone faster than you can say, "Make mine medium rare."

TIP Heading off on a camping trip? Brighten up your camp-site by giving your lanterns a reflective backdrop. Just wrap pieces of wood or cardboard in **ALUMINUM FOIL,** shiny side up, and set one behind each light.

TIP For my money, there's nothing more relaxing than sitting back in the shade of a tree and sipping a nice, cool drink. And there's nothing more annoying than batting at a bunch of bugs who want to share that drink. To stop 'em from diving in, cover the top of your glass with **ALUMINUM FOIL,** poke a hole in it, and push a straw through the hole. Then sip to your heart's content—and the bugs' frustration.

TIP Need a one-time funnel for a really grimy job, like pouring oil in your lawn mower? Double over a piece of **ALUMINUM FOIL** and roll it into the shape of a cone.

TIP Clean a fiberglass boat hull by scrubbing it with a damp sponge sprinkled with **BAKING**

SODA. Then rinse with clear water and dry with a soft, cotton cloth. For extra-tough stains, leave the baking soda on until it dries, then wipe it away with a damp cloth or sponge.

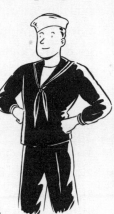

TIP If you're a sailor, you know how quickly verdigris—that unsightly green tarnish—can build up on a boat's brass fittings. Well, you can get that nautical hardware shipshape in a flash. Just mix **BAKING SODA** with enough lemon juice to make a paste, rub it onto the metal, and leave it for three to five minutes. Then rinse with clear water. If any green stuff remains, apply more paste, and scrub the crud away.

TIP Even before I learned how to drive, Grandma taught me how to put out small gas, oil, or engine fires: Stand at a safe distance away and throw **BAKING SODA** at the flames. I always keep a big box of soda in my garage, the trunk of my car, and my boat just in case—and you should, too!

TIP When corrosion builds up on your car's battery, clean the posts and cable connectors by scrub-

---

ONE MORE TIME

 When it was seed-starting time at Grandma's house, she couldn't just run down to the local garden center and pick up a lot of fancy containers, because those things didn't exist back then. She had to make her own starter flats and pots, using things she had around the kitchen, or waiting to go out with the trash. I still start my seeds in **KITCHEN CASTOFFS.** Here are some of the containers I like to use (after I've washed them thoroughly and poked holes in the bottoms, of course):

▷ **Cracked china cups and mugs**

▷ **Margarine, cottage cheese, and yogurt containers**

▷ **Milk cartons**

▷ **Muffin tins**

▷ **Paper, plastic, and foam drinking cups**

▷ **Pie and cake tins**

▷ **Plastic and foam take-out containers from restaurants and delis**

---

bing them with a paste made of 3 parts **BAKING SODA** to 1 part water. Then dry the cleaned parts with a soft cloth, and coat them lightly with petroleum jelly.

WORM-FREE FRUIT TREE FORMULA

You won't wind up with wormy fruit when you trap the egg-laying moths with this simple recipe.

½ **cup of apple cider vinegar**
½ **cup of sugar**
1 tbsp. of molasses

Mix the ingredients together, and pour the mixture into a clean plastic jug or (for smaller plants) yogurt containers with a hole punched in each side of the rim. Hang two or three traps in each tree or bush.

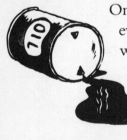

TIP Grandpa Putt loved to putter with his car, and he was mighty careful about keeping oil from spilling onto the garage floor. Once in a while, though, even he would end up with messy splotches on the concrete. He cleaned them by covering the spills with equal parts of **BAKING SODA** and cornmeal. He'd wait until the oil had been absorbed, and then he'd sweep up the residue. If any stains still showed, he'd wet the floor with clear water, and scrub the spots with baking soda on a stiff brush, then rinse.

TIP Towels you use at the beach or swimming pool tend to pick up more than their share of odors. So, when you wash them, give your detergent a freshening boost by adding ½ cup of **BAKING SODA** to the final rinse cycle.

TIP To remove greasy stains from your car's cloth floor mats or cloth upholstery, cover them with equal parts of **BAKING SODA** and salt. Brush lightly, so the powder penetrates into the fibers, leave it for a few hours, then vacuum.

TIP Grandma Putt had the biggest, showiest hydrangeas in our neighborhood. She swore they bloomed like gangbusters because she gave them an occasional drink of **BAKING SODA** dissolved in water. She never measured, but I'd say 2 teaspoons of soda per gallon of H_2O would do the job. And, by the way, begonias, geraniums (*Pelargonium*), and any other flowers that prefer alkaline soil enjoy this treatment, too.

TIP Before I head outdoors to do my winter chores, I put on a pair of thin socks. Then I grab a thicker, warmer pair, and shake about

½ teaspoon of **CAYENNE PEPPER** into each sock. I slip these over the thinner ones, and I'm good to go. My feet stay toasty warm, even when everyone else has *foot*sicles!

TIP Calling all gardeners, car mechanics, and boat buffs! Get your grimy paws clean by mixing **CORNMEAL** with enough apple cider vinegar to make a paste. Scrub your hands thoroughly, working the mixture into all the joints and crevices. Then rinse well, and dry off. If dirt still lingers, repeat the procedure. (Unlike chemical cleaners, this stuff won't harm your skin—in fact, it'll make it softer and smoother.)

TIP The dirtiest car windows in town will turn crystal clear—with almost no elbow grease—when you wash them with Grandma's favorite formula: Mix a pinch or two of **CORNSTARCH** and a cup of ammonia in a bucket of water, and wipe the solution onto the glass with paper towels. Rinse with clear water.

TIP The day I got my first car, Grandma showed me how to make this super-easy (and super-cheap) cleaner. Just pour ½ cup of **DISHWASHING LIQUID** and ¼ cup of baking soda into 1 gallon of cool water in a bucket, and stir it *very* slowly (to keep suds to a minimum). Pour 1 cup of that formula into a bucket of warm water, mix well, and bathe that old jalopy! Keep the "starter formula" close at hand because you'll probably need to mix up several buckets of cleaner as you go along.

TIP Back when Grandma Putt was fighting mosquitoes in her yard, they were garden-variety nuisances—not the vile disease carriers they are today. But although the stakes may be higher now, Grandma's battle plan works as well as ever to keep the population down. Set some old pans around your lawn, fill them with water, and add a few squirts of **DISHWASHING LIQUID** to each one. When the mama skeeters set down to lay their eggs, they won't be able to get up again. Better yet, when the eggs hatch, the larvae will drown!

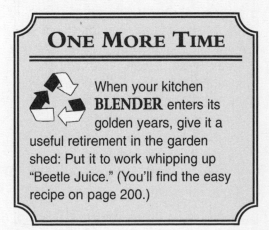

ONE MORE TIME

When your kitchen **BLENDER** enters its golden years, give it a useful retirement in the garden shed: Put it to work whipping up "Beetle Juice." (You'll find the easy recipe on page 200.)

BEETLE JUICE

When beetles, weevils, or any other bugs are driving you to drink (or just increasing your consumption), haul out your retired kitchen blender. Then round up a bunch of the troublemakers, and whip 'em up into this potent potion.

½ **cup of trouble-causing bugs (adults, larvae, or both, either dead or alive)**
2 **cups of water**
1 **tsp. of dishwashing liquid**

Whirl the bugs and water in an old blender (one you'll *never* use again for the preparation of human food, pet food, or cosmetic treatments). Strain the goop through cheesecloth, and mix in the dishwashing liquid. Pour ¼ cup of the strained, soapy mixture into a 1 gallon hand-held sprayer, and fill the rest of the jar with water. Spritz your plants from top to bottom, and make sure you coat both sides of the leaves. *Note:* You can also use the juice to kill hibernating adults and larvae in the ground (generally in fall or early spring). Pour the liquid into a 2-gallon bucket, fill it the rest of the way with water, and drench the soil around the plant.

TIP Grandma Putt marked off straight-edged planting beds with stakes and string, but when she wanted fancy shapes like circles or crescents, she "drew" the outlines on the ground with all-purpose **FLOUR.** If she didn't like the result, she just brushed the white stuff away and tried again.

TIP Mice can make mischief around your yard, all right, but their big cousins are downright dangerous. If rats are starting to show up at your place, don't pull any punches. Hit 'em hard with this homemade poison. Mix equal parts of **FLOUR** and powdered cement, and put it in a shallow container, like a big jar lid or disposable pie pan. Set it next to a pan of water in a place where the rats will find it, but children and pets can't get at it. The wretched rodents will eat the powder, then take a drink. The cement will harden inside their bellies, and that'll be all she wrote!

TIP **FOOD COLORING** makes a great stain for wooden planters, birdhouses, or anything made from unfinished wood (white pine absorbs the color best). Mix 1 part food coloring with 5 or 6 parts water. Saturate the wood surface, wait about five minutes, and wipe with a soft cloth. Let the piece dry overnight, then wipe again.

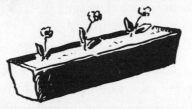

TIP Here's one of the easiest ways I know of to trap Japanese beetles. Just set a pan of soapy water on the ground about 25 feet from a plant you want to protect. In the center of the pan, stand an opened can of **GRAPE JUICE** with a piece of window screening over the top. The beetles will make a beeline for the juice (they can't resist the sweet, purple stuff!) and fall into the water. Then the story ends happily—for *you*, that is!

TIP Keep your outdoor ferns lush and lovely by feeding them two or three times during the summer with ½ cup of **MILK** and 1 tablespoon of Epsom salts per gallon of water.

TIP Grandma Putt saved the seeds from most of her vegetables and annual flowers. To keep them fresh until planting time, she

ONE MORE TIME

Don't send that old **DISH DRAINER** off with the trash! Take it out to your garden shed. It's just the ticket for rinsing off vegetables before you bring them into the house. Just put the veggies in the rack, give 'em a gentle shower from the hose, and let the water and dirt run right off.

stored them in powdered **MILK.** She put 1 part seeds to 1 part milk in a glass jar with a tight-fitting lid, and stashed it in the icebox (*not* the freezer).

TIP Plain old **MOLASSES** makes a great, all-purpose fertilizer. Apply it to any of your plants at a rate of 4 or 5 tablespoons per gallon of water.

TIP One summer, hordes of grasshoppers descended on our garden from out of nowhere. Grandma spoiled their fun by sinking jars up to their rims in the soil, and filling each one with a mixture of equal parts **MOLASSES** and water. The 'hoppers dove right into the drink—and stayed there!

TIP Before I left on a camping trip with my Boy Scout troop, Grandma always made me a supply of waterproof, wooden matches. It was simple, too. She'd just melt some **PARAFFIN,** and dip the tip of each match into it. When the wax dried, she'd put the matches in a small tin, which I tucked into my knapsack. (If you don't have a tin on hand, you can use a small plastic box or a zip-top plastic bag.)

GRANDMA PUTT'S
Secret Formulas

BYE-BYE BLACK SPOT SPRAY

If you love roses as much as Grandma Putt did, this kitchen-counter helper belongs in your garden recipe book. It works like a charm to head off the dreaded black spot fungus.

1 tbsp. of baking soda
1 tsp. of dishwashing liquid
1 gal. of water

Mix the ingredients together, pour the solution into a hand-held spray bottle, and spray your roses every three days during the growing season. Then, there'll be no more singin' the black spot blues!

TIP **SALT** is a fail-safe slug killer. But never simply pour the stuff on the slimers—if your aim is off, you could do more damage to your plants than the slugs could! Instead, pour a quarter inch or so of salt into a paper bag or coffee can. Then pick up the slugs (I use old tongs for this job), drop them into the salt, and shake the container.

TIP Here's a sweet way to stop nasty nematodes in their tracks. Just dig **SUGAR** into the soil at a rate of 5 pounds per 50 square feet of planting area. The tiny little worms will gobble the stuff up—and it'll choke them to death! One word of caution, though: Don't use this trick more than once on the same piece of land, because sugar will also kill beneficial organisms in the soil, and then you'll *really* be in trouble.

TIP Earwigs rarely cause real trouble in a garden. Sometimes, though, the chomping bugs can get out of hand. If that happens at your place, pour equal parts of **VEG-ETABLE OIL** and soy sauce in empty cat food or tuna fish cans. Set out the traps at night, and toss them (and their contents) out early in the

In Grandma's Day

If your squash, peppers, tomatoes, and annual flowers aren't producing as well as they used to, there could be a four-letter reason: b-e-e-s. Or, rather, the lack of them. If the little buzzers aren't showing up in big enough numbers, the pollination rate—and therefore, your yield—will suffer. But don't worry. Grandma Putt knew of a sweet way to lure bees to her plants, and it'll work for you, too. Put 2 cups of water in a pan, add ½ cup of **SUGAR,** and boil, stirring until the sugar is completely dissolved. Let the mixture cool, dilute it with 1 gallon of water, and pour the solution into a hand-held spray bottle. Then spritz your bloomin' plants. Before you know it, willing winged workers will fly to your rescue!

morning before butterflies or good-guy bugs flit in for a drink.

TIP When you're faced with a gang of hungry slugs, you couldn't find a more potent weapon than white **VINEGAR.** Just pour some into a hand-held spray bottle, take aim, and fire. The slimy pests will die instantly.

TIP You say a skunk came to visit and left a fragrant calling card behind? Don't fret. Just mix 1 cup of white **VINEGAR** and 1 tablespoon of dishwashing liquid with 2½ gallons of water. Then thoroughly saturate walls, stairs, outdoor furniture, or any other nonliving thing that reeks of eau de skunk. (If you, your dog, or your kids have been the recipient of Pepé Le Pew's favors, use the Skunk-Away Pet Bath formula on page 191.)

TIP Azaleas, rhododendrons, camellias, and other acid–soil lovers will bloom to beat the band if you water them every few weeks with a solution of 2 tablespoons of **VINEGAR** per quart of water.

TIP To make new terra-cotta pots look as though Grandma herself had used them, just paint them with plain **YOGURT** and set them outdoors in a shady spot. As the yogurt dries, moss and lichen will grow on the clay surface. Keep an eye on the containers, and when they've aged enough to suit you, hose them off with clear water. It generally takes a week or so to produce an authentic-looking "antique."

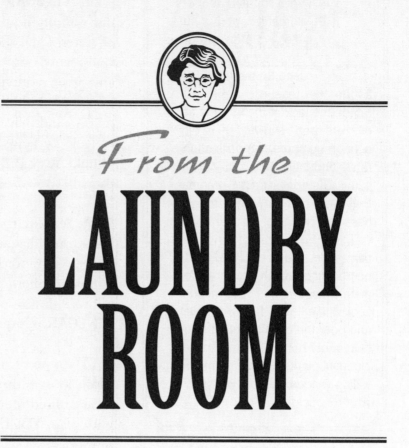

CHAPTER FIVE

From the
LAUNDRY ROOM

To your HEALTH

TIP The next time a mosquito sticks her blood-sucking snout into your skin, nix the itch and swelling by dabbing the spot with a few drops of **AMMONIA.** Act fast, though, *before* you start scratching. If you apply ammonia to broken skin, the sting will feel a whole lot worse than the skeeter's bite!

TIP Relieve the itch of poison ivy by patting the nasty red blotches with a solution of a teaspoon or so of household **BLEACH** per quart of water.

TIP **BLEACH** is also just the ticket for clearing out the fungus that causes athlete's foot—as my Uncle Art knew well.  Soak your feet twice a day in a solution of ½ cup of bleach per gallon of water. Before you know it, the burning and itching will be history. (*Caution:* If you have diabetes, check with your doctor before you soak your feet in *anything*.)

In Grandma's Day

Soaps, detergents, and bleaches earn their keep in the laundry by actually removing dirt and stains. But Grandma Putt's favorite wash-day whitener, **BLUING,** works its magic by optical illusion. I know that sounds strange, so let me explain.

Of the 300-odd shades of white that exist in the world, the brightest ones have a slight bluish tinge. But undyed cotton and wool are yellowish in tone, linen has a distinct hint of brown, and most synthetic fibers rank somewhere on the gray scale. In order to get the snowy look that we think of as "pure" white, manufacturers bleach their material, then treat it with bluing. This substance is actually a very fine iron powder that adds microscopic blue particles to the fabric, thereby making it look whiter. Over time, the bleach and bluing wash out, and the fabric regains its natural "dingy" appearance. When that happened at Grandma's house, she knew just what to do. She added about ¼ teaspoon of bluing to a gallon of cold water, poured it into the washing machine at the start of the wash cycle, and bingo—those whites came out as snowy as Frosty's belly!

TIP Hey, you folks in the Sunbelt! This tip has your name on it: You can douse the flames of a fire ant's bite by dabbing the area with a half-and-half solution of **BLEACH** and water. If it's applied within 15 minutes of the bite, it'll ease the pain and swelling. (But if you've been bitten multiple times or the pain is severe or spreads beyond the bitten spot, hightail it to the closest doctor.)

TIP When you spend as much time in a flower garden as Grandma Putt did, you're bound to find yourself on the wrong end of a bee now and then. And if you're smart (and was she ever!), you've got more than a few tricks up your sleeve for easing the pain and swelling. Well, one of Grandma's favorite bee-sting remedies came straight from her laundry room. After scraping out the stinger, she'd dab a few drops of **BLUING** onto the spot for instant relief!

TIP You say a rash has you scratchin' up a storm? Then step into the laundry room, grab a can of spray **STARCH,** and spritz that itch good-bye!

Your GOOD LOOKS

TIP Take it from me: The last thing Grandma Putt wanted to do to her clean, fresh hair was run a dirty comb through it. My guess is that you feel exactly the same way. So keep your combs spotless by washing them every week or so in 2 cups of cold water with a few drops of **AMMONIA** added to it.

TIP Ladies, if you're troubled by dark hair on your upper lip, this old-time tip is for you. Mix 1 teaspoon of **AMMONIA** with ¼ cup of hydrogen peroxide (6 percent), and dab the solution onto the offending hair with a cotton ball. Let it sit for 30 minutes, then rinse it off with cool water.

TIP Grandma Putt never dyed her hair, but when the gold had turned to silver (as the old song goes), she did have a little trick for keeping those tresses sparkling white: After she washed her hair, she added a few drops of **BLUING** to a quart of water, and used this as a final rinse. Some folks use this treatment after every shampoo, but Grandma only took the time for it when she felt she needed a whitening boost.

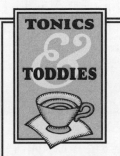 **TIP** To clean your hairbrushes, fill the bathroom sink with warm water and stir in ½ cup of **BORAX** and 1 tablespoon of laundry detergent (either liquid or dry). Swish the brushes around in the water a few times, then rinse them in clear water, and let them dry.

TIP It's no secret that good old **BORAX** can clean just about anything in your house. But here's something you may not know: This natural, slightly alkaline substance also makes a gentle, nondrying cleanser for your skin. You have your choice of methods: Either "power up" your favorite cleanser by adding about ½ teaspoon of borax to it when you wash your face, or use the borax straight from the box, with enough water mixed in to make a paste. Wash your face as usual, and rinse with clear, lukewarm water.

TIP **FABRIC SOFTENER** makes a fine stand-in for hair spray. Mix 1 part softener to 2 or 3 parts water (depending on how much hold you want) in a spray bottle, and spritz it onto your styled hair. It'll keep those locks in place, and make them shine like the sun!

TONICS & TODDIES

FABULOUS FACE FRESHENER

Dab this lotion onto your face after exercising, or anytime you feel like you need a pick-me-up. It also makes a great after-cleansing astringent to remove all traces of soap or cleansing cream.

½ **tsp. of borax**
¾ **cup of distilled water***
2 **tbsp. of vodka**

Mix the borax in the water until the powder is thoroughly dissolved. Add the vodka and stir well. Store the potion in a glass bottle with a tight lid to prevent the alcohol from evaporating. Then, when you feel the need for facial refreshment, apply the solution to your skin with a cotton ball or pad.

* If you prefer a scented lotion, use 6 tablespoons of distilled water and 6 tablespoons of your favorite flower water, such as orange, rose, or lavender.

TIP Fresh out of hair conditioner? No problem! Just mosey into the laundry room, and pick up the liquid **FABRIC SOFTENER.** Use it as you would your normal conditioner, pouring a similar-size dollop of the liquid into your hand, and working it through your hair. Wait two or three minutes, and rinse. (*Note:* Be sure you use a quality product for this job. The lower-priced brands don't seem to work as well—or so I'm told by my lady friends, who have a lot more hair than I have!)

Around the
HOUSE

TIP Self-cleaning ovens didn't exist when Grandma Putt was cookin' up a storm. But she knew a trick that was the next best thing for cleaning her oven walls. She mixed 1/4 cup of **AMMONIA** and 2 cups of warm water in a glass baking dish, put it in the oven, shut the oven door, and let it sit overnight. The next morning, she just wiped the grime away with a damp sponge— no elbow grease necessary!

GRANDMA PUTT'S
Secret Formulas

HEAVY-DUTY WALL CLEANER

When dirty walls have you climbing the walls, this potent potion can save the day. It works like magic on any kind of paint—oil-based or latex.

1/2 cup of ammonia
1/4 cup of washing soda*
1/4 cup of white vinegar
1 gal. of warm water

Mix all the ingredients in a bucket, and scrub your cares away. Store any leftover formula in a sealed container in a cool, dry spot.

* Available in hardware stores and the laundry section of your supermarket.

TIP A few scratches on a glass Christmas tree ornament can add character (and maybe bring back fond memories of Christmases past). But if the paint is peeling off in big patches, that's another story. You can still save those decorations, though. Just strip off the old paint with a half-and-half solution of **AMMONIA** and water. Then rinse with clear water. When the baubles are completely dry, paint them with glossy enamel (brush or spray it on; it's your call), and hang them on the tree. *Note:* Be sure to wear gloves for the stripping phase of this project—and any other time you're working with ammonia.

TIP Back in the 1950s—the heyday of live television—Grandma Putt had one of the first TV sets in her neighborhood. And, believe you me, she kept that screen spotless. (After all, any time Perry Como crooned or President Ike gave a speech, Grandma wanted a crystal-clear view!) Her simple formula: She made a solution from ¼ cup of **AMMONIA** and 2 quarts of warm water, and wiped it on sparingly with a soft, cotton cloth. Then she dried it with a second cloth.

TIP Some people like a little verdigris on their brass and copper pieces. But if you're not one of those folks—or if the metal has simply turned too green for your taste—bring back the original luster by rubbing the surface with a half-and-half solution of **AMMONIA** and salt, and rinse with clear water.

TIP To polish pewter, wipe it with a soft, cotton cloth dipped in a solution of 2 tablespoons of **AMMONIA** in 1 quart of hot, soapy water.

TIP Attention, chocoholics! The next time you wind up wearing some of your favorite food, don't despair. Just scrub the brown stains with full-strength **AMMONIA,** then wash the garment as usual. Your chocolate-spotted clothes will come out their normal shade of vanilla (or maybe strawberry or grape...).

In Grandma's Day

People have been using **AMMONIA** for thousands of years (the ancient Egyptians actually burned camel dung to produce it). But it wasn't until 1918 that a German chemist named Fritz Haber figured out how to make it in a laboratory. And Grandma Putt was in her middle years when the smelly, but useful, stuff became commonplace in laundry rooms around the world. We owe that advancement to another German chemist, Carl Bosh, who refined Haber's formula so that ammonia could be made commercially. Incidentally, both chaps won the Nobel Prize for their efforts.

TIP Back before polyurethane and other durable finishes came along, Grandma—and just about everybody else—protected their fine wooden tables by covering the surface with a sheet of glass. Grandma cleaned her glass-topped tables by spraying them with a solution of 2 tablespoons of **AMMONIA** per quart of water, and drying with a soft, cotton cloth. (One word of caution, though: If the glass you're cleaning is surrounded by wood, spray the solution in the center of the glass and work slowly toward the edges, being careful not to get any of the cleaner on the wood surfaces.) And since you're already cleaning, you can use this same solution to get your grimy windows sparkling again.

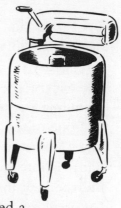

TIP Dang! You popped a load of clothes into the washer, then went about your business and forgot all about them. By the time you remembered to toss them in the dryer, they'd developed a sour smell. Don't worry. Just put those duds through the wash again, but this time with a tablespoon or so of **AMMONIA**—no detergent. They'll come out as fresh as a field of daisies!

GRANDMA PUTT'S
Secret Formulas

GREAT GROUT CLEANER

Even the grimiest grout will come clean as a whistle with this home-made "miracle" spray.

3 cups of rubbing alcohol
2 cups of bleach
1/2 cup of liquid floor cleaner
1 qt. of water

Mix the ingredients together in a bucket. Then pour the solution into a hand-held spray bottle, and use it as you would any spray cleaner. Store the leftover mix in a tightly sealed container, well out of reach of children and pets.

TIP Clean your jewelry by soaking the pieces for a few minutes in a half-and-half solution of sudsy **AMMONIA** and water. Use a soft toothbrush to get built-up dirt out of cracks, crevices, and intricate design work. Then rinse with clear water, and dry with a soft cloth. *Caution:* Don't use this technique on gold plate, or on anything that contains soft stones, such as opals, pearls, or jade.

TIP If you believe the magazine and television ads, you might think you can't possibly get along without those expensive spot-remover sprays. Don't you believe it! You can make your own "miracle" stain remover by filling a clean spray bottle with 2 parts water and 1 part **AMMONIA.** Spritz it on any stain (test for colorfastness first!), and most will wash right out.

TIP Whoops! Your dish of ice cream just toppled onto the sofa. Now what do you do? What Grandma did when I dropped an ice cream cone, that's what!

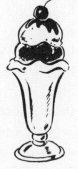

First, scrub the area gently with a mixture of a teaspoon or so of dishwashing liquid per cup of warm water. Follow up with a solution of 1 tablespoon of **AMMONIA** in 2 cups of water. Wash the spot again with dishwashing liquid and water. Finally, saturate a clean, cotton cloth with warm water, wring it out, and scrub gently. Then let the fabric dry naturally.

TIP There are lots of good ways to remove fresh blood stains, and you'll find some dandy ones in Chapter 4. Once those spots have dried, getting them out is trickier, but Grandma had great success with this routine: Soak the stained fabric in a solution of 2 tablespoons of **AMMONIA** per gallon of cold water until the spots have faded. Then, instead of using your regular laundry detergent, wash the piece in cold water and dishwashing liquid. (It'll do a better job of getting out the last traces of the stain.)

TIP To loosen a rusted screw or bolt, spray it with **AMMONIA.** Give the liquid a few minutes to penetrate, and that stubborn piece of hardware should screw right out.

TIP Grandma Putt cleaned her porcelain kitchen sink every few days by filling it with hot water and adding a few drops of household **BLEACH.** Then (wearing rubber gloves), she reached in and positioned the drain cover so that the water drained out very slowly—thereby giving the whole surface a thorough cleaning with no work on her part!

TIP Keep cut flowers fresh longer by filling their vases with a solution made from ⅛ teaspoon of **BLEACH** and 1 teaspoon of sugar per quart of water.

TIP Here's a super-simple way to clean a porcelain sink—even if the dirt has been building up for way too long. Cover the surface with a thick layer of paper towels, and saturate them with a half-and-half solution of **BLEACH** and water. Wait about five minutes, then remove the towels (wearing rubber gloves), and rinse with clear water.

TIP **BLEACH** is also just the ticket for getting tea stains off of china cups and teapots. Just fill the vessel with lukewarm water, add a few drops of bleach, and let it sit for

a minute or two. Then wipe the marks away, and follow with your usual dishwashing method. Just one word of caution: Don't use this trick on plastic dishes—it can damage the finish. (See the tip at right for a safer way to clean plastic.)

TIP Although Grandma Putt had a clothes dryer toward the end of her life, she always dried most of her laundry the old-fashioned way: by hanging it outdoors on a laundry line, using wooden clothespins. So it should come as no surprise that she kept those little clipping devices as clean as the clothes she used them on. How? Every couple of weeks, she soaked the pins for about 10 minutes in a bucket of warm water with half a cup of **BLEACH** and a tablespoon of laundry detergent added to it. Then she clipped them on the line to dry in the sun. Even if you use your wooden clothespins for nonlaundry jobs (like the ones you'll find in this chapter), this trick is still a great way to fend off both dirt and mildew.

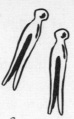

TIP To remove stains from wooden cutting boards or butcher block countertops, soak a white dishcloth in undiluted **BLEACH,** and lay it over the marks. Let the cloth sit for 10 to 15 minutes, then rinse the area with clear water.

TIP Don't bother with fancy (and expensive) bathroom cleansers. Plain old **BLEACH** works every bit as well for cleaning tubs and sinks, ceramic tile, shower curtains, and even grungy glass shower doors and stalls. Just pour the bleach into a spray bottle, spritz the dirty surface, and wipe it clean. For stubborn stains, wait a few minutes before scrubbing. (Wear rubber gloves anytime you work with bleach, and make sure to keep a door or window open for ventilation.)

TIP Plastic food containers come in mighty handy, all right, but sometimes they develop a sort of greasy feeling. Fortunately, you can put an end to that, fast. Anytime you wash those containers, or any other plasticware, add a capful of **BLEACH** to your dishwater, along with your regular dishwashing liquid.

TIP Want to make your silverware (and glassware) sparkle? Add a capful of **BLEACH** to a sink full of water and your regular dishwashing liquid, and that'll do the trick!

ONE MORE TIME

Let me take a stab in the dark and guess that dusting does not rank among your favorite pastimes. Well, I know a tool that just might make that chore a little easier, and maybe even fun (well, sorta). What is it? An empty, trigger-type spray **BOTTLE,** like the ones liquid cleaners and some laundry spot removers come in. Just wash the bottle and let it dry thoroughly. Then take aim, pull the "trigger," and blow the dust out of hard-to-get-at places, like the nooks and crannies in figurines, fancy picture frames, and carved furniture.

TIP Going out of town for a few days? If so, congratulations—you have a chance to avoid what is probably one of your least-favorite cleaning chores! Just before you head out the door, pour ¼ cup of **BLEACH** into your toilet bowl. When you get home, that porcelain will be as clean as a whistle—all you have to do is flush. (If any critters will be in the house during your absence, make sure you close the bathroom door before you leave.)

TIP Grandma Putt had a crystal chandelier that her grandma had left her. She loved that sparkly treasure—but cleaning all those little crystals was not exactly her favorite way to spend an afternoon, to put it mildly. Fortunately, she didn't have to do that chore too often, because she had a labor-saving trick up her sleeve: Each time she washed them, she added a few drops of **BLUING** to the rinse water. Somehow, the bluing repelled dust particles, which kept the glass cleaner, longer.

TIP If you think water may be leaking from your toilet's flush tank into the bowl, and wasting a whole lot of H_2O in the process, try this simple experiment: Pour a tablespoon or so of **BLUING** into the tank. If the water in the bowl takes on a sky-toned tint, you've got a leak to mend!

TIP Turn white flowers blue by adding ¼ cup or so of **BLU-ING** to the water in the vase. The color will travel up through the

GRANDMA PUTT'S
Secret Formulas

COCKROACH ELIMINATOR

Contrary to what some folks think, cockroaches can invade even the cleanest of houses. If they've moved into your domain, get 'em outta there with this simple formula.

4 tbsp. of borax
2 tbsp. of flour
1 tbsp. of cocoa powder

Mix the ingredients together, and put the mixture into jar lids. Set them in your kitchen cupboards, behind the refrigerator, and any-place else where the roaches are roaming—but be sure that you put 'em in places where children or pets can't get to the yummy powder.

stems and into the petals. (Of course, the more bluing you use, the darker the shade will be.)

TIP Each time you clean and refill your humidifier, add a tablespoon of **BLUING** to the water. This will prevent algae from building up and causing a yucky mess in the reservoir.

TIP Like any other red-blooded American kid, I managed to get my clothes splotched with a lot of brown mud. Fortunately, Grandma knew just how to get those stains out. After brushing off as much dirt as she could, she rubbed the spots with a solution of 1 tablespoon of **BORAX** in 1 cup of water. Then she tossed those duds in with the rest of the wash, and they always came out clean as a whistle.

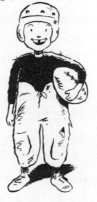

TIP If your tap water is on the hard side, you know how quickly the unsightly deposits can build up in a toilet bowl. But there's a simple way to send 'em packin'. Just make a paste of roughly 3 parts **BORAX** to 1 part white vinegar, slather it on the marks, and leave it

ONE MORE TIME

If you use a laundry spot remover that comes in a plastic squeeze **BOTTLE,** you've got a great addition to your, or your youngsters', craft-supply closet. Just rinse the bottle thoroughly, and use it to hold homemade paint (see the simple recipe on page 223). When the creative urge strikes, either pour the paint into a small dish, or use the bottle as a "brush," squirting your design right onto the paper.

for three or four hours. Then rinse with clear water.

TIP Stains from wine and other alcoholic beverages can be the very dickens to get out of a carpet—but not if you go at it Grandma's way. First, mix ½ cup of **BORAX** in 2 cups of water. Sponge the solution into the soiled area, wait 30 minutes, and follow with your regular carpet shampoo. Let the spot dry, and vacuum. Repeat the process if you need to. And remember: The sooner you attack any tough carpet stains, the better chance you'll have of getting out every trace of the marks.

HOMEMADE FABRIC FRESHENER

If you like the idea of using a fabric deodorizer, but you don't care for the heavy scent of the commercial products (or maybe the high price tag), try this easy alternative.

2 cups of unsigned, liquid fabric softener
2 cups of baking soda
4 cups of warm water
Essential oil of your choice

Mix the fabric softener and baking soda in the water, and add a few drops of your favorite essential oil, such as lemon, orange, or almond (let your nose be your guide as to quantity). Pour the mixture into a hand-held spray bottle, and use it on upholstered furniture, draperies, carpets, or any other fabric that's smelling less than springtime fresh.

TIP Back when Grandma Putt was brewing her breakfast coffee, electric drip coffeemakers did not exist. She, and just about everybody else, used a percolator. Well, like a lot of other good

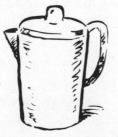

things from Grandma's era, these metal marvels are staging a comeback. If you've got one at your house, here's a simple way to keep it clean (and your coffee fresh-tasting). Just fill the pot with water, and add 1 teaspoon each of **BORAX** and powdered laundry detergent. Bring the water to a boil, and let it percolate for a few minutes. Then pour out the solution, and rinse thoroughly with clear water.

TIP No matter how well you wash a teapot after each use, those brown tannin stains still build up over time. But you can remove them by filling the pot with boiling water, tossing in a handful of **BORAX** (roughly ½ cup), and letting it sit overnight. Then give the pot a good washing before making your next cuppa.

TIP Are you looking for a simple (and economical) way to disinfect and deodorize the surfaces in your kitchen, bathroom, or baby's room? Well, look no further! Mix ½ cup of **BORAX** in 1 gallon of hot water, and go to town. You can either pour the solution into a hand-held spray bottle, or dip a sponge into the bucket and wipe dirt and germs away—it's your call.

ONE MORE TIME

 Those big, sturdy, colorful caps on **FABRIC SOFTENER** and **LAUNDRY DETERGENT** bottles are as versatile as the bottles themselves. On page 232, you'll find a whole lot of dandy uses for the empty jugs. And here's a rundown of helpful jobs for the caps. (Of course, you'll want to rinse them out thoroughly before you put them to work.)

▷ **Bathroom organizers.** Line up caps on the shelves of your medicine chest, and fill 'em up with lipstick tubes, tweezers, makeup brushes, cotton swabs, and all those other little things that can add up to big clutter.

▷ **Container-plant sticky traps.** When bad-guy bugs are munching on your potted plants, indoors or out, coat caps with corn syrup, petroleum jelly, or spray adhesive, and set them on the soil in the pot, or (depending on the size of the plant), nestle them among the branches. One cap will be large enough to debug a small- to medium-size plant; use two or three traps for larger ones. Choose your cap color by consulting "Color Them Gone" on page 231.

▷ **Mini paint buckets.** Pour in just as much paint as you need for a small craft project or touch-up job.

▷ **Pest-control helpers.** To keep rabbits, groundhogs, and chipmunks out of your flower beds, sink caps into the soil among your plants, and fill them with a mixture of 1 part bloodmeal to 2 parts water. This way, the bloodmeal won't vanish into the soil when it rains, thereby giving your plants an overdose of nitrogen.

▷ **Seed-starting pots.** Collect as many caps as you'll need, punch or drill drainage holes in the bottom of each one, and set them in a tray or shallow pan. Then fill each "pot" with starter mix to within about 1/2 inch of the top, and plant your seeds.

▷ **Soap dishes.** Keep a cap by the kitchen sink to hold scraps of soap and a small, soft sponge. Then, when you have a tiny cleaning job to do, soap up a corner of the sponge, and get to work.

▷ **Wading pool, sandbox, or bathtub toys.** Give a few caps to anyone between the ages of about two and six, and watch the fun begin!

▷ **Workbench sorters.** When it's finally time to sift through your homogenized stash of small hardware, line up a bunch of caps. Then toss each size screw (for example) into a separate cap.

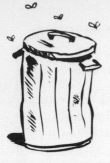

TIP Nobody expects a garbage can to smell like a bed of roses, but you don't want it to smell like, well, garbage. And it won't, if you sprinkle a tablespoon or so of **BORAX** in the bottom of the can before you put in the plastic liner. Then, when it's time to wash the container, just pour in a little water, and use that same borax as a scouring powder.

TIP Clean canvas shoes by scrubbing them with a toothbrush dipped in **CARPET SHAMPOO.** Rub the fabric until the shampoo foams up, then rinse with clear water.

TIP After you wash wool gloves, make sure they keep their shape by shoving a wooden **CLOTHESPIN** (either clip- or prong-type) into each finger.

TIP Clip-type **CLOTHESPINS** make perfect clamps to use when you're repairing broken china, or gluing small pieces of wood together.

TIP The next time you're tempted to buy some of those special clips to reseal food packages, or hold phone messages and office papers together, ask yourself, "Would Grandma do this?" You bet your life she wouldn't—because clip-type **CLOTHESPINS** will do the job every bit as well for a fraction of the price!

TIP It's frustrating, all right: You've just finished washing your windows, but your hard water has left spots behind. Fortunately, this

---

ONE MORE TIME

 The boxes that dry **LAUNDRY DETERGENT** comes in are some of the sturdiest cartons you can find. In fact, they're just about as strong as those upright file boxes designed to store catalogs and magazines—and they're absolutely free. To make your own publication holders, just cut the top off of an empty box, and clean out all the detergent residue. Then slice a diagonal piece all the way around the box, from the upper right corner to about 8 inches from the bottom (use a commercial magazine file, or a picture of one, as a guide if you need to). Add your choice of decorative coverings, such as fabric, wallpaper, or adhesive plastic, and stick on a label to show the contents.

problem has a simple solution. Just wipe **FABRIC SOFTENER** onto the marks, wait about 10 minutes, and wipe again with a damp cloth (no need to dry). Presto—spotless glass!

TIP Grandma Putt had a no-muss, no-fuss way to get baked-on food off a baking pan. She poured a teaspoon or two of **FABRIC SOFT-ENER** into it, filled the balance of the dish with water, and let it sit overnight. The next morning, she wiped the crusty spots away.

TIP Tired of getting static shock from your carpet? Then try this simple trick: Mix a capful of **FABRIC SOFTENER** with 2 cups of water in a spray bottle, and lightly spritz the rug.

TIP Clean paint-covered brushes the fast, easy way, by soaking them for 10 seconds in a mixture of ½ cup of **FABRIC SOFTENER** per gallon of water. They'll come out as soft and spotless as new. *Note:* This method only works on water-based paints, not oil-based products.

TIP If you're giving an old piece of furniture a fresh coat of paint, and want a finish that's out of the ordinary, use a **FEATHER DUSTER** instead of a paintbrush.

In Grandma's Day

Ready for another trivia quiz? Well, ready or not, here it comes: Where did the term *soap opera* originate? The answer: From Grandma Putt's favorite radio serial, *Ma Perkins*, which went on the air in 1933, sponsored by Procter & Gamble's Oxydol® **SOAP POWDER.** The show was such a hit with listeners that P&G began underwriting a slew of similar programs—and selling a whole lot of soap to faithful listeners. It wasn't long before the genre and the sponsor's products became entwined in people's minds, and a new phrase entered the American vocabulary.

TIP If you sew clothes (your own or anybody else's), you know that getting all of the pattern pieces back into the envelope they came in can be as hard as—if not harder than—folding a road map into its original configuration. Well, here's a simple solution to that frustrating dilemma: Set the smaller pieces on top of the larger ones, and press them lightly with a warm **IRON.** Then fold them to the right size, and slide them into the packet.

In Grandma's Day

No one knows exactly who invented the **WASHING MACHINE,** or when. The basic concept goes back centuries, to the days when sailors on long sea voyages would stuff their soiled clothes into canvas sacks, tie them to ropes, toss them overboard, and let the ocean waves tumble them clean. One thing we do know is that as early as the 1700s, women in western Europe were doing the family laundry by putting it into a wooden box, which they filled with soap and water, and tumbling the clothes by hand with a crank.

The first electric clothes washers appeared in England and the United States in 1915, and featured a motor that rotated a metal drum pierced with holes. These pioneer machines were a step in the right direction, but still demanded a fair amount of hard labor, including hauling wet laundry out of the tub and running it through a wringer. Then in 1939, the first truly automatic washers came on the market, complete with preset water levels, variable sturdiness cycles, and timing controls. And believe you me, Grandma and her fellow housewives stood up and cheered!

TIP To get grease marks off of wallpaper, use Grandma's simple method: Put a piece of brown paper over the spot, and hold a dry, warm (not hot) **IRON** on it for a minute or so. Then shift the paper, so that a clean portion covers the stain, and press it again. Keep repeating the process until all of the grease has been absorbed.

TIP Contrary to their name, clothes moths don't confine their egg-laying activity to clothing. Any natural-fiber object in your house—including your carpet—can be a moth maternity ward. If you suspect that larvae may be lingering in your floor covering, saturate a bath towel with water, wring it out, and spread it over the rug. Then grab your **IRON,** set it on high, and press the towel until it's dry. You don't need to push down hard; it's the steamy heat that kills the pesky little pests.

TIP Grandma had a no-fuss way to clean a grimy broiler pan. While it was still hot, she covered the surface with a thick layer of dry **LAUNDRY DETERGENT,** and topped that with a dampened paper towel. She let it sit for 20 minutes or so, and wiped it clean.

TIP Dry **LAUNDRY DETERGENT** makes a fine scouring powder for kitchen and bathroom sinks, tubs, and other ceramic or porcelain surfaces.

TIP Tuck some **LAUNDRY DETERGENT** bottle caps into your supply cupboard or desk drawer, and use them to corral pushpins, paper clips, and other tiny odds and ends.

TIP Grandma Putt cleaned unpolished marble by wiping it with a solution of ¼ cup of **SOAP FLAKES** per gallon of water. Then she rinsed it with clear water, and dried the clean surface with an old towel. (For best results on polished surfaces, use a commercial product that's specially made for cleaning marble.)

TIP When your vellum lampshades start looking dingy, clean them with this old-time routine: First, wipe them with a soft cloth that's been dipped in a solution of 1 part **SOAP FLAKES,** 1 part warm water, and 1 part denatured alcohol. Rinse with a second cloth 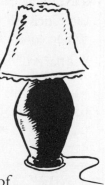 dipped in straight denatured alcohol, then rub the surface with a dab of furniture polish on yet another soft cloth.

TIP If you like to use single-knit, T-shirt-type fabric for sewing projects, you know the material has a frustrating tendency to curl up on the edges as you're trying to stitch into it. You can solve that problem in a hurry by lightly spritzing those edges with spray **STARCH,** and letting them dry before you start to work. The starch will sufficiently stiffen the fabric to curb its urge to roll, yet leave it pliable enough for your needle to penetrate easily.

TIP Patchwork quilts are as popular now as they were when Grandma Putt was making them for our beds at home. If you've just invested in a new one, or stitched one yourself, use this trick to lock the colors in: Soak it for two hours or so in a bathtub of cold water with 3 to 4 cups of **WASHING SODA** mixed into it. Then rinse the quilt thoroughly in cold water. To dry your creation, spread it out flat in a well-ventilated area away from direct sun. (Of course, this tip applies only to cotton quilts, not to those made from silk and velvet.)

Family and
FRIENDS

TIP Give a budding sailor a bath-time treat by adding a table-spoon or two of **BLUING** to his bathwater. Then he can sail his toy boats across his own mini ocean!

TIP Do you have a white dog, or maybe a horse with a white mane and tail? If the answer is yes, then this tip's for you. To make that coat sparkle like new–fallen snow, all you need is a bottle of good old-fashioned **BLUING.** Wash and rinse your pal as usual, then add two or three drops of bluing to a quart of water, and comb the solution through his coat as a final rinse. Say, I wonder if this is how Roy kept Trigger's mane so snowy white?

TIP Remove the scent of pet urine the same way Grandma did before those special enzyme cleaners came on the market. If the spot is still wet, blot up as much moisture as you can with paper towels or old rags. Then dampen the spot with water, and pour a gener-

GRANDMA PUTT'S
Secret Formulas

DRYER LINT MODELING CLAY

Young (and even not-so-young) craft artists can have a ball with this trash-to-treasure art medium.

1½ cups of dryer lint
1 cup of water
½ cup of all-purpose flour
Food coloring (optional)

Put the lint in a saucepan, cover it with the water, and let it sit until the lint is saturated. Add the flour, and stir until the mixture is smooth. Add 2 to 3 drops of food coloring, if you like. Cook the mixture over low heat, stirring constantly until it holds together, and you can form peaks with the spoon. Pour it onto a cutting board, aluminum foil, or newspaper, and let the clay sit until it has cooled. Then let your creative juices flow. When you've finished your masterpiece, let it dry for three to five days. After that, you can leave it unembellished, paint it, or deck it out in the trimmings of your choice.

ous layer of **BORAX** on top. Wait until it has dried completely, then vacuum the area. That should do the trick, but if the odor lingers, repeat the treatment a time or two.

TIP Whenever Grandma lit the candles on my (or anybody else's) birthday cake, she held the match in a clip-type **CLOTHESPIN.** That way, she knew she wouldn't wind up with singed fingertips.

TIP Make a family message center by gluing clip-type **CLOTHES-PINS** to a strip of wood, and attaching it to the wall by your telephone or in your entryway. If you want, you can add labels above the pins. For example, you could assign one to each member of the family, or identify the clips by category, such as "phone messages," "shopping list," and "weekend chores."

TIP Do you remember when you were so little that you had to reach up to dry your hands on a bathroom towel? Well, I don't, but I *do* remember when my children and grandchildren were tiny tykes—and how often the towel ended up on the floor because they had to tug at it. We solved that problem by draping the top quarter of each towel over the rod, and

pinning it at both sides, just under the rod, with clip-type **CLOTHES-PINS.** The youngsters got their hands dry with no trouble, and the towel stayed put.

TIP If your cat's gunnin' for your houseplants, protect that greenery the way Grandma did: Saturate a cotton ball with lemon oil **FURNITURE POLISH,** and set it on the soil in the pot. Fluffy will keep her distance.

TIP It's a dilemma, all right: You need to take your cat to the vet, but you don't have a pet carrier, and there's no time to get one from a pet shop. Not to worry! Just put Fluffy inside a plastic **LAUNDRY BASKET,** invert another one of the same size over it, and tie the edges together. Then get on the road! (This trick works just as well for bunnies, tiny dogs, and any other small critters.)

ONE MORE TIME

When you clean your dryer's lint filter, do you just toss those fabric leavings in the trash? You do? Well, stop that right now! That fluffy **LINT** has plenty of life left in it. Here's some for-instances:

▷ **Bird nest furnishings.** Fill mesh bags or cage-type suet feeders with 100 percent cotton lint, and hang the packages from tree branches in very early spring. Or simply shove wads of lint into holes in trees. Nest-making birds will pull out the downy, soft fibers and use them to line their nests. (*Caution:* Don't use lint from a wash load that's been treated with fabric softener, which can be harmful to birds.)

▷ **Compost makings.** Toss 100 percent cotton lint onto the pile or into the bin. Or if you have no place to "cook" compost, simply bury the lint among your plants. It'll break down in a flash, adding valuable organic matter to the soil.

▷ **Deer-tick eliminators.** Soak the lint in a pet shampoo that contains a flea and tick killer called permethrin. Then pull off a small wad, and push it into an empty toilet-paper tube. When you've filled a half dozen tubes or so, set them out in brushy areas or other sheltered spots where deer mice (carriers of deer ticks) are likely to find them. The mice will take the fuzzy stuff home to line their nests, and the disease-spreading ticks will be history.

▷ **Fire-starter nuggets.** First, cut a cardboard egg carton into 12 sections, and fill each one with dryer lint (but *only* from 100 percent cotton fabric). Then melt down old candle stubs or paraffin sealers from home-made jelly, and pour a layer of melted wax on top of the lint. When it's time to light your fireplace or charcoal grill, set one of your nuggets in the kindling or briquettes, and hold a match to the cardboard edge. You'll have a roaring fire in no time.

The great
OUTDOORS

TIP Grandma kept rascally raccoons out of her trash cans by saturating an old rag with **AMMONIA,** and tying it to the can lid. This trick also works (most of the time) to fend off dogs and skunks.

TIP If the 'coons are gunnin' for your corn crop in addition to your garbage, fill old margarine tubs or other small containers with **AMMONIA,** and set them among your plants. The masked gluttons will dine elsewhere.

TIP Gophers can eat their way through a garden in no time flat, but Grandma had a fragrant way to send 'em packin'. She soaked rags in **AMMONIA,** and stuffed one into each tunnel entrance. The hungry rascals beat a fast track to another dining establishment!

TIP For my money, the most effective way to deal with slugs, snails, beetles,

---

ONE MORE TIME

When you're decluttering your cleaning cupboard, and realize that it's time to toss out a few old **BROOMS** and **MOPS,** hang on to the handles. Those sturdy posts make first-class tomato stakes.

---

destructive caterpillars, and just about any other kind of large insect pests is to grab a pair of old tongs, pick the villains off your plants, and drop them in a bucket of water laced with a cup or so of a lethal ingredient—like good old-fashioned **AMMONIA.**

TIP If you'd rather shoot insect culprits than pick 'em off your plants, send 'em to you-know-where by spraying them with a half-and-half solution of **AMMONIA** and water. *Caution:* In order for this potion to be effective, it needs to make direct contact with the bugs, so whatever you do, don't spray the entire plant, hoping for long-term effectiveness. (Besides being counterproductive from a bug-elimination standpoint, it could do major damage to the plant.)

FAIRY RING FIGHTER TONIC

Fairy ring is a fungal disease that leaves your lawn littered with unsightly circles of mushrooms or puffballs. Fortunately, the cure is as close as your laundry room.

Dry, mild laundry soap (1 cup for every 2,500 sq. ft. of affected lawn area)*
1 cup of ammonia
1 cup of baby shampoo
1 cup of antiseptic mouthwash

First, pour the dry laundry soap into a hand-held spreader, and spread it lightly over the affected area. Then mix the remaining ingredients in a 20 gallon hose-end sprayer and apply to the point of run-off. Those 'shrooms will be history!

* Be sure to use soap, not detergent (Ivory Snow® is a good choice). And whatever you do, don't use more than the recipe calls for—more is *not* better! That goes for all of my tonics, and Grandma's too.

TIP Every year in early spring, when Grandma's forsythias were just starting to show buds, she clipped off armloads of branches, brought them inside, and put them in buckets of warm water. She dropped a cotton ball saturated with **AMMONIA** into each pail. Then she put the branch-filled container into a plastic dry-cleaning bag (you could also use a giant-size trash bag), and tied it tightly with twine. In what seemed like the blink of an eye, the ammonia fumes made those baby buds burst into bloom. (*Note:* This trick works just as well on lilacs, pussy willows, crab apples, and any other flowering trees or shrubs.)

TIP Oh, boy! You were changing the oil in your car, and somehow the stuff found its way onto your concrete driveway. Now what do you do? Exactly what Grandpa Putt did when this mishap occurred: Mix a cup of **AMMONIA** in a bucket with a gallon of warm water, and brush that petropuddle away. Then rinse with clear water. (And next time, be more careful!)

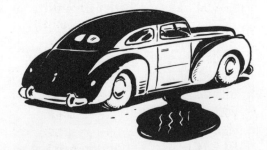

TIP As far as I'm concerned, a backyard barbecue is just about the most fun you can have in the summertime. That is, until it comes time to clean the greasy grill. I don't know anything that can make the chore enjoyable, but it *is* as easy as pie when you use this formula: After the rack has cooled, put it in a black plastic garbage bag. (The color is crucial, because only a black bag will draw enough intense heat from the sun.) Lay the bag on the ground, pour in enough **AMMONIA** to cover the rack, and close the bag tightly with a twist tie. Leave it lying in the sun for two or three hours, then turn it over and leave it for another two or three hours. When you open the bag (carefully, so you don't splash ammonia on yourself), that rack will be clean as a whistle. Just rinse it with clear water, and dry it off. Then call up the gang and invite them over for another barbecue!

TIP Clean golf balls by soaking them in a solution of ¼ cup of **AMMONIA** and 1 cup of water. Then rinse the balls in clear water, and dry them with a soft cloth.

TIP When mildew builds up on plastic-mesh lawn furniture, send it packing by scrubbing the fabric with a solution of 1 cup of **BLEACH** per gallon of water. (But first, test for colorfastness by wiping it onto an inconspicuous spot.) Then rinse well with clear water, and make sure the mesh is completely dry before you put the furniture away indoors.

TIP Before you set a plant in a pot that's been used before, disinfect the container the way Grandma Putt did: Soak it for 15 minutes or so in a solution of 1 part **BLEACH** to 8 parts water.

TIP To get rid of moss that's growing on brick, stone, or concrete, spray the patches with a half-and-half mixture of **BLEACH** and water, and wipe clean with a damp cloth.

In Grandma's Day

Anytime a plant disease reared its ugly head in Grandma's garden, she took precautions to make sure she didn't spread the germs around, and you should, too. After you've worked with diseased plants—and before you go near healthy ones—clean your tools with a solution of 1 part **BLEACH** to 3 parts water. And for good measure, dunk your gardening gloves in this bath, too.

TIP To keep moss from growing on roof or siding shingles, use a solution of 2 capfuls of household **BLEACH** per gallon of water. Sponge on the solution, and don't rinse. How often you need to repeat this procedure depends on the location of your house. In a damp, shady spot, it's a good idea to use this treatment at least once every two years.

TIP Would you like to find a way to turn the water in your swimming pool an enticing shade of Pacific Ocean blue? Then take a tip from pool dealers and hotel pool-keepers from coast to coast: Add **BLUING** to the water. To color a 20- by 40-foot pool, pour in one or two 8-ounce bottles at the point where the water flows in from the filter. Wait a couple of hours to let it circulate thoroughly, and dive right in. Over time, the sun will fade the color. When you

Bring on the Boron

Boron is what gardeners call a micronutrient, but when some vegetables don't get enough of it, they suffer from macrotrouble. Fortunately, a deficiency is simple to fix: All you need to do is sprinkle a tablespoon or so of **BORAX** around each plant. Then, at the end of your growing season, have your soil tested, and add whatever amount of borax the results call for. But how do you know when your veggies are crying out for the big B? It's simple—just keep watch for these symptoms.

Vegetable	Signs of Boron Deficiency
Beets	The inside of the root turns brown and corky.
Cabbage	The whole head turns brown.
Celery	Margins of leaves show brownish mottling; horizontal cracks later appear on the stems.
Corn	New leaves develop elongated, watery, or transparent stripes; ears (if they appear at all) have corky, brown bands at the base.
Rutabagas	The inside of the root turns brown and corky.
Swiss chard	Horizontal cracks appear on the stems.
Turnips	The inside of the root turns brown and corky.

notice that starting to happen, simply pour in another bottle of bluing. Just a few words of caution: Take care not to splash the bluing on your pool's walls or coping, and don't use in aerated models like whirlpool baths or hot tubs. Although this stuff won't hurt a single living thing, in undiluted form, it may leave spots on some hard surfaces.

TIP A few drops of **BLUING** added to the water in a birdbath will reduce the growth of algae—without harming so much as a feather on your flying friends.

TIP Creeping Charlie and other spreading, broadleaf weeds can be a real pain in the grass. But you can nix their rampage by dosing your lawn with a mixture of 5 tablespoons of **BORAX** per gallon of water early in the spring and again in the fall.

TIP Every autumn, Grandma Putt dried flowers and leaves from her garden to use in wreaths, potpourri, and other craft projects that she gave as Christmas gifts. Her method was simple: First, find a cardboard box that has a lid and is big enough to hold your plant parts. Next, mix 1 part **BORAX** and 2 parts cornmeal, and pour a 1-inch layer of the mixture into the box. Lay your

plant material on top, then very gently cover it with more of the mix, leaving no air space around the flowers. (If you're working with many-petaled posies, such as roses or carnations, sprinkle some of the mixture directly into each bloom before you place it in the box.) Tape the carton closed, and store it in a dry place at room temperature for 7 to 10 days. At the end of the waiting time, pour or gently brush away the covering, and carefully lift out your treasures.

TIP When lime and hard water leave unsightly deposits on flowerpots, stone or concrete patios, water spigots, or any other hard surface, get rid of them with this simple routine: Dissolve ½ cup of **BORAX** in 1 cup of warm water, and stir in ½ cup of white vinegar. Sponge the mixture onto the spots, let it sit for 10 minutes or so (longer for really stubborn stains), and wipe clean.

TIP When you're cutting roses to take inside, protect your fingers by holding each thorny stem with a clip-type **CLOTHESPIN.**

TIP It used to be that whenever I was playing golf, I had a dickens of a time hanging on to my scorecard—I'd always lay it down somewhere to make my shot, then stroll off down the fairway, leaving the card behind. But that was before I discovered this nifty trick: I clip the card to my golf bag with a clip-type **CLOTHESPIN.** That way, I always know what my score is (even when I'd rather not!).

In Grandma's Day

Grandma Putt was a great believer in an old-time method of gardening called electroculture. Practitioners of this system did everything they could to draw static electricity to their crops. For instance, they used only metal poles for staking tomatoes, and they grew vine crops like beans and peas on metal trellises. So what does this have to do with laundry products? Just this: When a lightning bolt cracks through the air, the electrical energy makes the resident nitrogen and hydrogen combine to form **AMMONIA.** The ammonia, in turn, combines with rainwater and falls on plants in the form of dilute nitric acid—exactly the form of nitrogen plants need for good growth. And that explains why your grass, and every other plant in your yard, turns greener after a thunderstorm.

TIP You say when your big spring bulb display bursts into bloom, there are some noticeable patches of bare ground? Don't fret. Just stick **CLOTHESPINS** into the places where there should be tulips, daffodils (or whatever). That way, you'll know exactly where to plant more bulbs in the fall.

TIP Once, when I was headed off on a camping trip with my Boy Scout troop, I couldn't find hide nor hair of my tent pegs. There was no time to buy new ones, but Grandma knew just what to do: She gave me a bunch of wooden **CLOTHESPINS** to use instead. They worked just fine. In fact, I still keep some on hand for just that purpose.

TIP I have Grandpa Putt's old scythe hanging in my tool-shed, and believe me, it still comes in mighty handy for cutting down vegetable plants at the end of the harvest season—not to mention weeds that have gotten out of hand. (And unlike a newfangled string trimmer, it's as quiet as a lamb, and doesn't demand constant supplies of string and gasoline.) That blade does require a little TLC, though. I keep it free of nicks, and safely stored, the way Grandpa did: After each use, I wrap the blade in a heavy-duty **LAUNDRY BAG,** and tie the bag's drawstring tightly around the scythe's handle.

Color Them Gone

Plastic bottles that once held liquid **LAUNDRY PRODUCTS** make terrific traps for all kinds of pesky pests. Not only are these jugs sturdy and waterproof, with built-in handles for hanging, but they also come in colors that naturally appeal to bugs. To make your traps, all you have to do is coat the appropriate bottles with corn syrup, petroleum jelly, or a commercial product like Tanglefoot®. Then either hang them from trees or shrubs, or stick them, upside down, on stakes that you've pounded into the ground among your troubled plants. As for the shade to choose, let this chart be your guide.

Bottle Color	Bugs That Flock to It
Blue	Thrips
Green	Walnut husk flies
Red	Fruit flies (including apple-maggot flies)
White	Flea beetles, four-lined plant bugs, plum curculios, rose chafers, tarnished plant bugs
Yellow	Most flying insects, including aphids, cabbage moths, leaf miners, psyllids, squash beetles, webworm moths, whiteflies
Yellow-orange	Carrot rust flies

ONE MORE TIME

 The sturdy (and water-proof!) plastic bottles that hold **LAUNDRY DETERGENT,** bleach, and fabric softener are some of the handiest outdoor helpers you could ask for. Here are just some of the tools you can turn those jugs into—after you've washed them thoroughly, of course:

▷ **Clothespin holder.** Cut a large hole in the side opposite the handle, so you can pop in the pins. Punch small holes in the bottom for drainage, and hang it on the clothes-line. (Either run the line through the handle, or dangle the bottle from a waterproof hook.)

▷ **Drip-irrigation system.** Poke small holes in the bottoms and sides of a whole bunch of bottles, bury them in the soil at strategic spots in your garden, and fill them with water. The moisture will flow out at a slow, steady rate, and go directly to your plants' roots.

▷ **Funnel.** Just remove the cap from a bleach bottle, and cut off the bottom half of the jug. Repeat the process with several more bottles, and keep them in your car, boat, garden shed, or anyplace else you might need a funnel for motor oil, water, antifreeze, or liquid fertilizer.

▷ **Garden-tool caddy.** Make a big hole in a giant-size bottle on the side opposite the handle. Then insert your trowel, pruning shears, dibble, and other small hand tools into the bottle through this hole.

▷ **Plant labels.** Cut the sides of white or yellow bottles into strips, write on them with an indelible marker, and shove the strips into the soil next to the appropriate plants.

▷ **Scoop.** Slice diagonally across the bottom of a bleach bottle, screw the top back on, and use it to scoop up fertilizer, compost, potting soil, sand, or just about any other non-edible substance.

▷ **Watering can.** Drill a dozen or more holes in the cap of a giant-size bottle. Fill the bottle with water, and screw the top back on. To water your plants, flip the bottle upside down, and let the H_2O flow!

▷ **Winter-weather aids.** Detergent bottles are perfect for storing and dispensing cat litter, sand, or wood ashes onto ice-covered sidewalks. Keep a few filled bottles in your car, too. Then, if you get stuck on ice or snow, pull one out and spread the contents under your wheels for instant traction.

TIP Here's a time-saving trick I learned not long ago: Always keep a plastic **LAUNDRY BASKET** in the trunk of your car. Then, when you're out shopping, put all your packages in the basket. That way, they don't get tossed all over the place, and when you get home you can tote the whole load into the house, or over to the garden shed, in one quick trip.

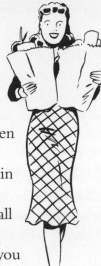

TIP What could be more welcome after a long, cold winter than a bed full of cheerful spring bulbs? And what could be more sloppy-looking than all that withering foliage after the flowers have faded? But, as tempting as it is to whack those leaves off, if you do that, you'll deprive the bulbs of the food they need to fuel next year's big show. Well, here's a simple solution to that dilemma: Plant your bulbs in plastic **LAUNDRY BASKETS.** Then, when the blooms go bust, pull up the baskets, whisk them off to a spot where the foliage can die down in private (maybe behind the toolshed or garage), and fill the vacant space with annuals.

After Jack Frost puts an end to the annuals' display, sink the bulb-filled baskets back into the garden. To use this technique, first check the proper planting depth for your bulbs (the plant label or catalog description will tell you this). Then fill the basket with enough garden soil to reach the target level. Set the bulbs in as you would in open ground, and fill the basket to the top with more soil. (Tuck the plant label in the basket so you'll know where to replant it in the fall.) Dig a hole about an inch deeper than the basket, lower the container into the hole, fill in around the basket with more soil, and water.

TIP Grandma Putt furnished her big, old-fashioned porch with white wicker. Those tables, chairs, and ottomans were the apples of her eye, and you can bet she kept them as clean as the new-fallen snow. Besides dusting on a regular basis, each spring and fall she gave each piece a deep-cleaning. Her formula still works as well as ever. Here's all you need to do: Put about 1 tablespoon of mild **LAUNDRY DETERGENT** in 4 cups of water, and mix until it's frothy. Apply the suds to the furniture with a soft cloth, working one area at a time. Then wipe with a clean, damp cloth.

TIP When messy outdoor chores leave you with greasy, grimy hands, wash them with **LAUNDRY DETERGENT** (either liquid or dry). Those mitts'll be as clean as a whistle in no time!

TIP Chinch bugs are known far and wide for sucking the life out of turfgrass. If your lawn is full of round, yellow patches that quickly turn brown and die, these lowlifes are the most likely culprits. To get rid of them quick, mix 1 cup of

MURPHY'S OIL SOAP® with 3 cups of warm water in a 20 gallon hose-end sprayer, and saturate your lawn. After it dries, apply gypsum to the area at a rate of 50 pounds per 2,500 square feet of lawn area.

TIP When it comes to sluggin' it out with slugs and snails, **PINE CLEANER** is one of the most effective weapons in your laundry-room arsenal. Either pick the slimy villains up and drop them into a bucket of water with a cup of the cleaner added to it, or pour a half-and-half batch of pine cleaner and water into a hand-held spray bottle, take aim, and let 'er rip.

TIP Anytime our concrete walkways started looking a little dingy, Grandma cleaned them with a stiff broom dipped in a solution made from 1/4 cup of **WASHING SODA** per 2 gallons of warm water. Then she rinsed with clear water from the garden hose. (This formula works just as well on patios, house foundations, and concrete-block walls.)

GRANDMA PUTT'S Secret Formulas

DOWN-HOME DECK AND PORCH CLEANER

Grandma Putt's house had big, wide, wraparound porches, and she kept them spotless with this simple formula. (It works just as well on any wooden structure, including 21st-century decks.)

1 qt. of household bleach
1/2 cup of powdered laundry detergent
2 gal. of hot water

Mix all of the ingredients in a bucket, and scrub the porch or deck using a stiff broom or brush. Then hose it down thoroughly.

Fabric-Softener Sheets

Although liquid fabric softeners have been around since the 1930s, fabric-softener *sheets*, a.k.a. dryer sheets, didn't appear until the early '70s. That's when Procter & Gamble researchers found a way to infuse nonwoven fabric with softening agents that are released gradually as clothes tumble around in the dryer. But these handy, hanky-size squares can do a lot more than keep your duds soft and static-free. They can perform a gazillion chores all through the house. Just take a gander at these possibilities:

▶ *Clean your shower door.* Wipe the glass with a dryer sheet, and soap scum will disappear.

▶ *De-electrify your hair.* When dry air leaves your locks full of static, rub a dryer sheet over your tresses, from the roots toward the ends.

▶ *De-hair your furniture (and clothes, too).* Fido and Fluffy can't help leaving hair behind, so don't scold them— but don't put up with the mess either. Just rub a dryer sheet over the fabric, and the offending strands will disappear like magic.

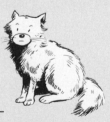

▶ *Deodorize your shoes.* When your footgear is smelling less than dainty, put a sheet into each shoe, and let it sit overnight. By morning, the unpleasant odor will be an unpleasant memory.

▶ *Dust your computer.* And all those other dust magnets around your house, like television screens and metal mini blinds. Gently rub a dryer sheet over the surface, and dirt particles will leap onto the fabric.

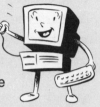

▶ *Eliminate static cling.* Run a sheet over the offending clothes, and that fabric will flow free and easy.

▶ *Freshen the air.* Tuck a dryer sheet into the bag compartment of your vacuum cleaner. As you clean the floor, the aroma will spread around the room.

▶ *Freshen the air, Take 2.* Remove the cover from each heating vent, spread a dryer sheet over the back of the cover, and replace it in the wall or floor. Besides scenting the air, the sheet will trap dust, pollen, pet hair, and other airborne debris. When the "filter" fills up with nasty particles, replace it with a new one.

(continued)

FAST FORWARD

(continued from page 235)

➤ *Keep your luggage ready to ramble.* Between trips, store a sheet or two inside each suitcase. When it's time to hit the road, you'll have a sweet-smelling home for your travelin' clothes.

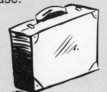

➤ *Pick up sawdust.* When you're sanding or drilling wood, use a dryer sheet as a tack cloth to pick up the dust.

➤ *Prevent odor buildup in garbage cans and wastepaper baskets.* Put a sheet or two in the bottom of each container—indoors and out.

➤ *Repel mosquitoes.* Tie a scented dryer sheet through a belt loop. The bloodthirsty skeeters will keep their distance.

➤ *Repel packing "peanuts."* Before you pack, or unpack, a box that's cushioned with those little foam nuggets, rub a sheet over your hands (and arms, too, if you're wearing short sleeves). This way the clingy devils will stay in the carton, where they belong—and not crawl all over your body.

➤ *Save your soil.* Before you "pot up" a plant, put a dryer sheet over the drainage hole. It'll keep the soil in, but let water drain out.

➤ *Scent your clothes.* And linens, too. Put dryer sheets in drawers and on shelves to keep all your fabric pieces smelling springtime fresh.

➤ *"Scrub" your pots.* To remove baked-on food, fill the pan with warm water, toss in a dryer sheet, and let it soak for an hour or so. Those stubborn spots will wipe right off.

➤ *Sew smoothly.* Before you start a hand-sewing project, run your needle and thread through a dryer sheet. This will keep the thread from clinging to the fabric, and prevent it from getting tangled.

CHAPTER SIX

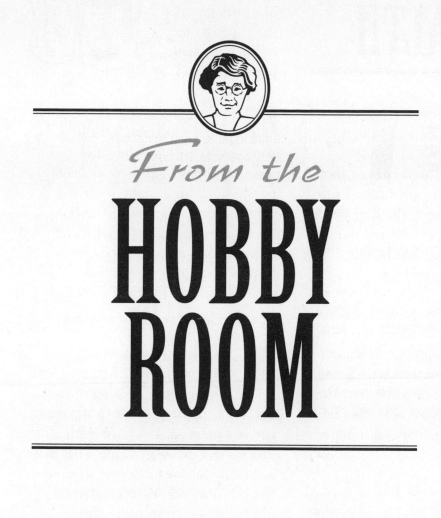

From the

HOBBY ROOM

237

To your
HEALTH

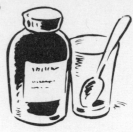

Before you take a shower or tackle a wet job like washing the car, the dishes, or the dog, protect a bandaged finger and keep the surrounding skin dry by pulling an uninflated **BALLOON** over your injured digit.

Make medicinal ointments and salves last longer by squeezing the end of the tube with a large **BINDER CLIP.** (This same trick also works for toothpaste, as well as hair gels, and even kitchen condiments that come in tubes.)

As Grandma Putt was getting on in years, she found that the directions on medicine bottles (prescription and otherwise) seemed to grow smaller and smaller. But she didn't take that shrinkage lying down! Instead, she wrote the information she needed on a piece of paper, in letters and numbers that were big enough to read—even without her spectacles on—and fastened the paper to the bottle with transparent **TAPE.**

If you take prescription drugs of any kind, the last thing you need is to have the label smeared by wet hands or defaced by the liquid medicine itself as it dribbles over the side of the bottle. So, stop trouble in its tracks. The minute you get your meds home from the drugstore, do what Grandma did, and cover the label with transparent **TAPE.**

Trying to quit smoking? Congratulations! And here's a tip to help you on the road to success: As a first step, keep your package of cancer sticks closed with **TAPE.** And use *lots* of tape. That may not stop you from taking a cigarette, but it'll slow you down and at least it'll force you to think about the consequences each time you do!

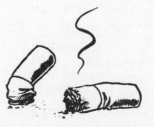

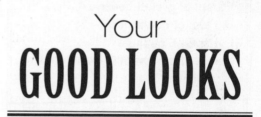
GROWN-UP PACIFIER

We all know that stress can lead to health problems—major and minor. Well, this handy little device can help ease your stress load. Of course, it won't take the place of a week or two at a lakeside cabin, or even a leisurely stroll in the woods. But it will give you a simple way to sit back and recharge your batteries any time of the day or night.

Small glass jar with a tight lid*
Baby oil
15–20 beads (either glass or plastic)
Superglue
Paint (optional)

Fill the jar with the oil to within roughly ¼ inch of the top, and add the beads. Brush or squeeze the glue onto the inside rim of the lid, and screw it onto the jar. If you like, paint the lid in your favorite color. Then, anytime daily life begins to feel like an out-of-control roller coaster, sit down in a comfortable chair, take hold of the jar, and turn it end over end. Watch the beads gliding through the oil; they will function as a visual mantra, letting your mind relax and—for a few minutes, at least—ease out of the fast lane.

* A fancy mustard or jelly jar is perfect.

TIP To coax a splinter out of your skin, try one of Grandma's first aid tricks: Cover the sliver with a thin layer of **WHITE GLUE,** and spread it over the area. Once the glue is dry, peel it off. The intruding speck will come right out.

TIP Fresh out of dental floss? Just reach into your knitting or needlepoint basket, and pull out a piece of white wool **YARN.** It's thicker than floss, but it'll do the job just as well as the commercial stuff—maybe even better!

Your
GOOD LOOKS

TIP If you have baby-fine hair, you know that it's almost impossible to find a barrette that will hold your locks in place. So, at those times when getting your hair out of your face matters more than a chic appearance—for instance, when your in-laws are coming for a visit, you have to clean the house *now*, and the thermometer is climbing—grab a **BINDER CLIP** and clamp it onto your wayward strands.

TIP Tired of paying beauty-shop prices just to have your bangs trimmed? Then close up your wallet, and cut 'em yourself, as Grandma did. Here's how: When your hair is wet, run transparent **TAPE** across your forehead, with the top edge where you want the bottom of your bangs to be. Looking in a mirror, cut just above the tape. You'll have a professional salon look for zero bucks!

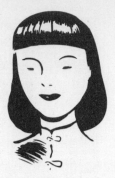

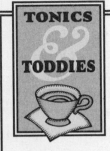

TONICS & TODDIES

LUSCIOUS LIP GLOSS

Hey, candle makers! The next time you make candles, save some beeswax and use it to whip up a batch of this smooth, tasty, and great-smelling gloss.

1 tbsp. of grated beeswax
4½ tsp. of coconut oil*
1 vitamin E capsule
⅛ tsp. of pure vanilla extract (not artificial)**

Put the beeswax and coconut oil in an ovenproof container, and add the contents of the vitamin E capsule. Put the dish in the oven, and heat it at 250°F until the wax is melted. Pour in the vanilla extract, mix well, and let cool completely. Store it in a container with a tight lid. Apply it to your lips with a lip brush or your finger.

* Available in health food stores and the cooking-oil section of many supermarkets.

** Or substitute almond extract.

TIP Grandma Putt rarely wore nail polish, but she did have this piece of advice to offer her young lady friends: When you're planning a big night on the town, and can't decide what shade of fingernail polish to wear, cover a nail or two with transparent **TAPE,** and paint the polish over that. Keep experimenting until you've reached a final decision.

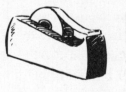

TIP Multishade eye shadow cases are a great convenience (or so my lady friends tell me), but they do have one drawback: After a while, the different-colored powders tend to mix and mingle. Fortunately, there's a simple way to clean up those little compartments. Just blot the surface of each one with a piece of **TAPE.**

Around the
HOUSE

TIP Use **ADDRESS LABELS** to make "custom-printed" notepads. Attach the labels to pages of plain-paper tablets, and use the notes for quick, informal messages.

TIP **ADDRESS LABELS** come in handy when you're invited to a potluck or picnic. Attach the labels to your dishes and to the handles of your serving utensils, and the gear is sure to find its way home to your kitchen.

TIP To keep a skin from forming on the paint in a partially used can, do what Grandpa used to do: Blow up a small **BALLOON,** and set it on top of the paint in the can before putting the lid on.

TIP Coupons can save you a lot of money on your grocery bill— if you remember to use them. The best way to do that is to keep 'em where you can see 'em. When you clip your coupons, instead of tossing them into a drawer, fasten them

In Grandma's Day

For most of Grandma Putt's life, she, and everybody else, did their letter and check writing with a fountain pen. It's not that **BALLPOINT PENS** weren't around—an American inventor named John H. Loud patented the first one in 1888. But he intended the early, fairly crude models for marking cardboard and other rough surfaces, not for genteel penmanship. The smooth-rolling ballpoint pens that we use today owe their existence to World War II technology, and to a Hungarian-born Argentine resident named Lazlo Biro. Wartime contractors had perfected the process of grinding ball bearings for machinery and weapons, and fitting them tightly in place. By adapting the techniques for use in pens, Mr. Biro produced the first instruments suitable for writing on paper.

together with a **BINDER CLIP,** and hang it on your kitchen bulletin board, or on a magnetic hook on the refrigerator door. Then, as you head for the supermarket, grab the clip and its contents, and tuck in your shopping list. When you get to the store, attach the whole shebang to your shopping cart.

It seems that every time I open my mailbox, I find at least one letter from some worthy charity or other, presenting me with a sheet of **ADDRESS LABELS** with my name and address on them. Several years ago, when these things first started streaming in, I thought, "This is ridiculous. Even if I did nothing but write letters, I'd never be able to use all these!"

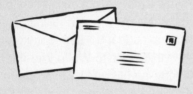

Now I realize that they're handy for a *lot* more than sticking on envelopes. In addition to the stack in my desk drawer, I keep a sheet of labels in my pocket (folded up, of course) and one in the glove compartment of my car, and I always take a supply along when I go on a trip. I use 'em in all kinds of ways. You can, too. For instance...

▷ **Announce your move.** Tuck a label into each change-of-address card that you send to friends or relatives. That way, they can simply stick the label

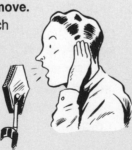

over your entry in their address books. (For this purpose, you may want to have labels printed, so you can include your new phone number.)

▷ **Claim your coat.** A lot of coats and jackets look alike when they're hanging on a rack in a restaurant or an office. To make sure you—and the owners of similar-looking garments— grab the right one, stick a label onto the outside-facing sleeve. For good measure, tuck a few labels (still on their backing) into a pocket. That way, if the grabber gets all the way home before discovering that he has the wrong coat, he'll know where to find you.

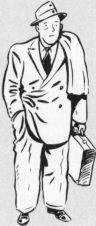

▷ **Claim your luggage.** You've collected so much stuff on your vacation that you had to buy an extra duffel bag to hold it all—and, of course, it'll need a baggage tag. Just grab a paper one at the airline ticket counter, and slap your address label on it.

▷ **Claim your rebate.** Instead of struggling to fit your name and address on the closely spaced lines they give you on the return form, stick a label in the space. Besides saving you time, it'll be easier to read than your itty-bitty writing—thus increasing the chances that you'll actually get your money back.

▷ **Enter to win.** You're on your way into the supermarket, and you see the high school drama club is raffling off a quilt to raise money for a theatergoing trip to New York. So you buy a book of tickets. Instead of writing your name and address on all those stubs, just slap a label on each one.

▷ **Get letters.** Or at least postcards. When your children or grandchildren head off to camp or college, give them stamped envelopes or postcards (or both) with your address label attached to each one. With luck, the youngsters may use them.

▷ **Hand out treats.** At Halloween, stick labels on the goodies you give out to little ghosts and goblins. When they get home with their sacks full of loot, their parents will feel more secure, knowing where the treats came from.

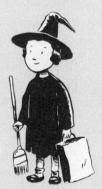

▷ **ID their stuff.** Send your kids or grandkids off to camp or school with labeled backpacks, sleeping bags and clothing (for camp), or labeled book bags, pencil cases, and whatever else they lug along to school. If they have to cover their textbooks, stick an address-label on the inside cover flap so they know which books are theirs. This is especially helpful when kids have to share lockers.

▷ **Identify yourself on the trail.** Going off alone on a hike, bicycle trip, or horseback trail ride? Put a label on the tongue, or inside the top, of each boot or shoe. That way, if

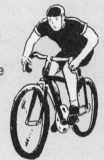

the unthinkable happens, and you meet with an accident or foul play—even if the ID you have in your pocket disappears—you'll be quickly identified.

▷ **Plan your next vacation.** If the travel magazine you're reading on the plane offers brochures for destinations you'd like to visit, just pull out the reader-service card, check off the publications you want, and stick your label in the space provided.

▷ **Tag your pet's "taxi."** Put an address label on your cat's (or small dog's) carrier. That way, when you leave Fluffy or Fido at a kennel or the vet's office, you'll be sure to get the right vehicle back when you pick up your pal.

The dilemma: You'd like to hang your favorite snapshots and postcards on a cork-board (or maybe the wall of your office cubicle), but you don't want to put holes in your treasures. 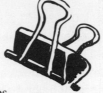 The simple solution: Stick pushpins into the board or wall, attach **BINDER CLIPS** to your pictures, and hang the clips on the pins.

 You've found a veneer-topped antique table for peanuts at a local shop, and it's priced that way for a good reason: The veneer has a dent in it. Should you buy it? My advice is yes—but fix that dent fast. Otherwise, it could split, and you'll have a bigger repair job on your hands. All you need to do is cover the dent with damp **BLOTTING PAPER,** and hold a warm (not hot!) iron on the paper until the table surface is smooth again. (How long this will take depends on the depth of the ding, so keep checking every minute or so.)

 A clear **CD CASE** makes the perfect picture frame. Cut

Chalk It Up to Cleanliness

You may think of **CHALK** as something kids use to draw on the sidewalk or write on a blackboard. Well, think again: White chalk is actually a mighty useful cleaning aid. Grandma Putt always kept a box on hand, and so should you. Here's how to put its power to use at your house.

Cleaning Challenge	How to Put Chalk to Work
Dingy metal (any kind)	Sprinkle powdered chalk on a damp, soft, cotton cloth, and rub the tarnished piece until it's shiny again. Then rinse with clear water, and dry thoroughly.
Dirty marble	Dip a damp, soft, cotton cloth in powdered chalk, and rub the marble surface until it's clean. Rinse with clear water to remove all the chalk residue, and dry thoroughly.
Grease stains on washable fabric	Rub the spots with chalk, wait until the grease has been absorbed, and launder as usual.
Ring around the collar	Rub white chalk onto the stain, and wash the shirt with your regular detergent.

two snapshots to fit, and place them back-to-back in the case. *Voilà!* A double-sided frame that's perfect for putting on a desk or table. Or insert just one photo and hang it on the wall.

 TIP Keep emergency money on hand but out of sight by tucking some bills into a music **CD** or movie **DVD CASE** (keep the liner in the case so you can't see inside and so there's a title running down the edge). Then slide it onto a shelf among others of its kind, and no one will be the wiser.

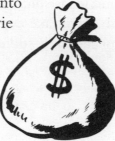

TIP Grandma Putt kept her silverware sparkly-bright by storing a couple sticks of **CHALK** in her silver chest. The chalk absorbed the moisture that caused tarnishing. Grandpa borrowed that idea to keep his tools rust-free. He tucked a few sticks of chalk in his toolbox to attract the moisture that would otherwise cling to the metal.

TIP **CHALK** can fend off moisture all through the house. Just hang muslin bags or pantyhose pouches of chalk (either powdered or

ONE MORE TIME

When it comes to giving a special glow to your dinner table, or anyplace else in the house, nothing beats good, old-fashioned **CANDLES.** But these waxy wonders can do a whole lot more than light up your life—even when they've burned down to mere stubs. Here are just a few ways you can put those nubbins to work:

▷ **Paint with pizzazz.** Draw a design with a white candle on a sheet of white paper. Then paint over the paper with watercolors. When the paint dries, the wax will show through. (*Note:* This process is fun for kids, but it's also a clever technique to use if you make your own Christmas cards.)

▷ **Unstick stuff.** To make zippers, windows, drawers, and even your car's radio antenna glide more smoothly, just rub a candle along the moving parts.

▷ **Waterproof wood.** Keep the cut edges of plywood and other lumber from absorbing moisture by rubbing them with a candle.

stick) in closets, basement and bathroom cupboards, and anyplace where dampness could be a problem.

CDs and DVDs

If there's one modern-day question you *know* Grandma Putt never had to ponder, it's this: What can you do with all those CDs and DVDs that keep arriving in the mail, pitching everything from Internet services to new supermarkets? I'll tell you one thing, 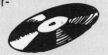 though: If Grandma *were* around today, she'd have a ball inventing clever uses for those shiny silver circles. And these just might have been some of them.

▶ *Announce your location.* To mark the entrance to your walk or driveway, nail three or four CDs to a wooden stake, and pound it into the ground in the appropriate spot.

▶ *Decorate your fridge (or let the kids do it).* Paint a picture or make a collage on one side of the disc, glue a magnet on the flip side, and stick it on the door.

▶ *Draw a perfect circle.* What better template could you ask for? (That is, as long as it's the size you need!)

▶ *Entertain a baby.* To make a mobile that will delight any infant or toddler, gather up a bunch of CDs, and drill a small hole in the edge of each one. Tie a piece of nylon fishing line through each hole, and hang the discs at varying lengths from a coat hanger (either wire or plastic will do). Attach another piece of fishing line to the top of the hanger, and suspend it from an eye hook that you've screwed into the ceiling.

▶ *Light your bike.* Provide extra reflective power by attaching a CD to your bicycle's handlebars and another one to the back of the seat.

▶ *Mark your beds.* Use a permanent marker to write the name of each crop on a CD. Then nail the discs to wooden stakes, and pound them into the ground to show what's planted where.

▶ *Protect your table-tops.* Make a coaster by cutting five 1-inch squares from felt or thin corkboard, and gluing them to the printed side of a CD. Or, if you'd prefer to display the graphic art, fasten the flat "feet" to the shiny side. Whichever side you use, space four of your squares more or less evenly around the edges, and put one over the hole in the middle. Then use your creations to catch drips from drinks, broad-based candles, or potted plants.

▶ *Save your fruit crop.* 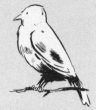 To keep hungry birds from snatching your cherries, berries, and other fruit, hang CDs from the branches of your trees and bushes. The light flashing in the sun will scare the rascals and send them elsewhere for their sweet treats.

▶ *See the light.* If you have a pull-cord light in the attic, basement, or the back of a deep closet, hang a CD from the cord. The glossy surface will reflect even dim light, making it easy for you to spot the "on switch."

▶ *Stop in time.* Hang a CD from your garage ceiling, on a cord that brings the disc level with your windshield at exactly the spot where you need to stop. That way, you'll never have to guess about whether you're in far enough to clear the door—but not so far that you might hit the wall.

▶ *Trim your Christmas tree.* Drill a hole in the rim of each disc, and decorate one or both sides with paint, sequins, fabric scraps, or other pretty stuff. When you've got a whole collection of ornaments, tie ribbons through the holes, and hang 'em up.

▶ *Trim your Christmas tree, Take 2.* Make a garland by weaving a long strand of ribbon through the center holes of as many CDs (either embellished or plain silver) as you can gather up. Then twine it around the tree, or nestle it into evergreen boughs on your mantel or stair rail.

▶ *Walk safely.* When you get the urge to take an evening stroll, and you don't have any reflective clothing on hand, thread a disc on a cord and wear it around your neck. Better yet, wear two discs: one in front and one in back.

And Don't Forget the Jewel Cases!

Those slim, trim plastic boxes (a.k.a. jewel cases) that CDs and DVDs come in are pretty darned useful in their own right. Consider these opportunities.

▶ *Check the date.* Just slide a small calendar inside a case, and stand it up on your desk.

▶ *Display your treasures.* Use them to show off your butterfly, button, coin, or stamp collection.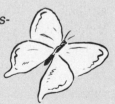

TIP It's hard to drive a screw into a board (or anything else) when the danged screwdriver keeps slipping. Fortunately, you can solve that problem in a hurry by rubbing a little **CHALK** on the tip of the screwdriver.

TIP Got a hole in a plaster wall that's too deep to fill with Spackle™ alone? Insert a stick of **CHALK** into the hole, cut it off even with the wall, and then spackle over it.

TIP When you've got a wall problem of the opposite size—namely, a hairline crack—and you're not ready to paint the whole room, try this temporary repair: Cover the line with **CHALK** in a color that matches the wall.

GRANDMA PUTT'S
Secret Formulas

BEESWAX FURNITURE POLISH

Most modern, commercial furniture polishes are made with silicone, and these products work just fine on newer wood. But they give antique pieces an unnatural (you could even say phony-looking) shine. Grandma polished her treasured tables and cabinets with this homemade formula, and I still use it on the ones she left me.

2 oz. of beeswax (available by the ounce in craft-supply stores)
⁵⁄₈ cup of turpentine*
Very hot (almost boiling) water

Coarsely grate the wax, and put it in a glass jar that has a screw-on lid. (A mayonnaise jar is perfect.) Add the turpentine, and screw the lid loosely on the jar. Stand the jar in a heat-proof bowl, and pour the water into the bowl so that it comes to or just above the level of the wax. Let the jar sit in the water until the wax has melted. Then remove the jar, and shake it gently until a paste forms. Let the mixture cool, then pour it into a wide-necked jar (like a clamp-top canning jar) for storage. If the polish hardens, soften it up again by standing the jar in warm water. To use the polish, rub it onto the wood with a clean, soft, cotton cloth, and buff with a second cloth.

* Do not use mineral spirits or turpentine substitute.

TIP If you've got a balky house or car key, try this routine: Rub some **CHALK** over the tip and along the teeth of the key. Slide it in and out of the keyhole three or four times, and you're good to go.

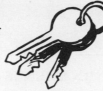

 TIP Cover spots on suede shoes or clothing by rubbing the marks with **CHALK** of the same color.

TIP Grandma Putt always said that one of the trickiest parts of sewing was getting snaps to match up on both sides of a garment. As always, though, she found a method that made it a snap (I couldn't resist). She sewed all the small, "male" parts on first, and rubbed a stick of **CHALK** over the little point on top of each one. She put the second piece of fabric over them, making sure the snaps were in the right position. Then she rubbed the back of the fabric covering each point—thereby marking the spot for the larger, "female" part of the snap.

TIP Here's a clever idea for kitchen storage that comes straight from your hobby room (or maybe your home office): Hang a **CLIPBOARD** on the inside of a cupboard or pantry door, and use the clip to hold placemats. They'll stay wrinkle-free and ready to grab at a moment's notice.

TIP Grandma Putt loved to clip recipes from newspapers and magazines. She kept them all neatly filed, so anytime she wanted to whip up a certain dish, she knew exactly where to look. And, to make it easier to follow the recipe, she had a special piece of equipment: a **CLIPBOARD** that she had attached to the wall above her kitchen counter, at her eye level. She'd clamp the cutout paper onto the board, and away she'd go.

TIP If you spend a lot of time in white shoes—whether for work or play—keep a bottle of **CORRECTION FLUID** close at hand. It's perfect for covering all those scratches and scuff marks that stand out like neon lights on pristine white leather.

TIP In a busy kitchen, it doesn't take much for white appliances to pick up scratches. It doesn't take much to cover them up, either. Just brush a little **CORRECTION FLUID** over the marks.

PAINTED EGG ORNAMENTS

At Grandma's house, we made these ornaments twice a year: in the spring to give as special Easter presents, and at Christmastime to hang on the tree. (We decorated them differently for each season, of course!)

Long carpet needle
Raw eggs, at room temperature
Acrylic paint
White glue
Decorative trimmings*
Embroidery floss
Clear acrylic fixative (available at art-supply stores)

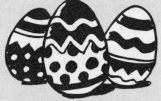

Using the carpet needle, *very* carefully poke a hole at each end of an egg, making one hole a little larger than the other. Hold the egg over a bowl, with the larger hole pointed down, and gently blow into the smaller hole, so the yolk and whites flow out. Rinse the inside of the egg thoroughly with clear water, and lay it on paper towels to dry overnight. The next day, decorate the eggs with the paint and trimmings of your choice. Then, for each ornament, thread the carpet needle with a 12-inch length of embroidery floss, and pull it through both holes in the egg. Tie a knot at the end that's outside the smaller of the two holes. At the other end, tie a loop for hanging. Spray the finished product with acrylic fixative.

* Such as sequins, stickers, or tiny pieces of fabric or paper.

TIP Whenever Grandma needed a temporary cover-up for a ding in a white wall or white-painted furniture, she used (you guessed it) **CORRECTION FLUID.**

TIP The next time you find a minor scratch in a piece of wooden furniture, color the mark gone. Find a **CRAYON** in a color that matches the tone of the wood, and rub the wax onto the blemish. Then use your fingertip to blend the color and smooth out the surface.

TIP Use an appropriately colored **CRAYON** as a substitute for shoe polish. This is an especially neat trick when you don't have any neutral-colored polish on hand, and your footwear is a nonstandard shade, like yellow, purple, or turquoise. Draw a few lines around the whole shoe, or simply color in the scuffed areas, and buff with a soft cloth or shoe brush.

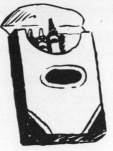

TIP Jars of dried herbs may look great in a rack hanging on a wall, or sitting on a shelf above the stove, but as Grandma Putt knew, that's actually the worst place you can store them. That's because heat and light dry up the volatile oils, making fragrance and flavor go downhill fast. If you're short on shelf space in closed cupboards, try this flavor-saving trick. Tack a strip of **ELASTIC** to each interior side of a drawer. Then tuck the little bottles and jars inside the stretchy bands. They'll stay upright, organized, and easy to reach—and they'll keep their flavor longer.

TIP Like most women I know, Grandma Putt could never bear to part with a button. (Why is that, anyway?) But, organized soul that she was, she didn't just toss

them in a box or junk drawer. Instead, she sorted them by size and color, and threaded each group onto a separate piece of **EMBROIDERY FLOSS,** matching the color of the floss to that of the buttons. That way, when she was sewing something that needed those handy closing devices, it took only seconds to find the right shade. (Yarn will also work for this trick, as long as the holes in the buttons are big enough.)

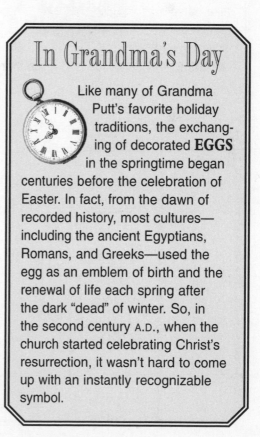

In Grandma's Day

Like many of Grandma Putt's favorite holiday traditions, the exchanging of decorated **EGGS** in the springtime began centuries before the celebration of Easter. In fact, from the dawn of recorded history, most cultures—including the ancient Egyptians, Romans, and Greeks—used the egg as an emblem of birth and the renewal of life each spring after the dark "dead" of winter. So, in the second century A.D., when the church started celebrating Christ's resurrection, it wasn't hard to come up with an instantly recognizable symbol.

ONE MORE TIME

 When you finish a sewing project, don't throw away the **FABRIC SCRAPS.** No matter how small they are, they can still lead useful "lives." Here's a sampling of possibilities:

▷ **Accessorize.** Depending on the size of your remainders, use them to make accessories like hats, scarves, ties, sashes, headbands, or hair bows.

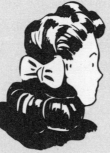

▷ **Create a collage.** Turn those snippets into a picture—either on their own or as part of a mixed-media work (as they say in artist lingo)—containing other hobby-room leftovers, such as sequins, buttons, or fancy paper. Just cut the material into shapes of your choice, and paste them onto a wood panel or a piece of archival mounting board. (If this idea sounds enticing but intimidating, check with your local community college or adult-education center; many of them offer collage-making classes for all levels of experience.)

▷ **Decorate a dollhouse.** Turn the pieces into pint-size curtains, slipcovers, tablecloths, or wall coverings.

▷ **Make a quilt.** Or give your scraps to a quilter who will turn them into a work of useful art. You can bet your bottom button they'll find a happy home, especially if the fabrics are choice silks and velvets!

▷ **Make rugs.** Cut your leftovers into strips, and turn them into either hooked or braided rugs. (Many quilting and fabric shops offer classes in this old-time pastime.)

▷ **Protect your clothes—and linens, too.** Sew little pouches, and fill them with dried lavender or other herbs that smell terrific *and* repel cloth-destroying moths.

▷ **Thrill your cat.** Cut out two pieces in the shape of (for instance) a fish, sew them front-to-front, leaving one end open. Flip the little pouch inside out, stuff it with high-quality catnip, and stitch it shut. Your resident feline will jump for joy!

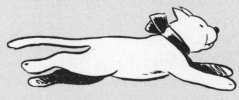

▷ **Trim your Christmas tree.** Cut out trees, stockings, or other seasonal shapes, and stitch them together, as described in "Thrill your cat" at left. But instead of stuffing your creation with catnip, use cotton batting or pantyhose. (Otherwise, you'll have Fluffy scrambling through the boughs!) Atttach a color-coordinated ribbon, and hang your creation on the tree.

▷ **Wrap presents.** Use larger pieces in place of gift-wrapping paper, and tie them with braid, rickrack, or high-quality ribbon. As a bonus, the packaging does double duty as the makings of a decorative pillow.

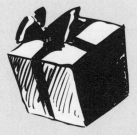

▷ **Wrap presents, Take 2.** Cut appropriately themed shapes (e.g., holiday, birthday, baby) out of smaller remnants, and glue them onto plain white or colored gift-wrapping paper.

TIP Grandma always kept an **EMBROIDERY HOOP** in her laundry room to use as a stain-removal aid. When she had to treat a spot on something really big, like a tablecloth or a sheet, she'd clamp the hoop over the soiled part of the fabric, and then go to work with the appropriate de-spotting method. (You'll find a whole lot of her favorite ways and means in Chapters 4 and 5.)

TIP In a pinch, an **ENVELOPE** makes a fine funnel for transferring dry ingredients from one container to another. Just cut a triangle from one end of the envelope, snip off the tip, and open it into a cone. Gear the size of the envelope to the size of the container you're filling. For instance, for a small jar, a standard number 10 office envelope will do fine; for a larger jar, you might need a big manila type.

TIP When the back of a chair leaves a scuff mark on the wall, take it off with a white **ERASER.** Either the soft rubber or the crumbly, gum kind will remove most scuffs without hurting the paint or wallpaper. Whichever kind you use, just make sure it's white. An eraser that's pink (or any other color) may leave a new stain on the wall.

ONE MORE TIME

 The long, sturdy cardboard tubes that **GIFT-WRAPPING PAPER** comes on are the bee's knees (as Grandma would say) for a trio of household storage tasks. The items in question are:

▷ **Christmas lights.** Just wrap the cords around the tube, wrap the whole thing in tissue paper, and tuck it away in the designated light box.

▷ **Scarves.** Instead of folding them, roll your scarves around the tube.

▷ **Tablecloths.** When you fold them, tuck a tube into each fold to keep creases from forming.

Just one word of caution: When you're using this trick for long-term storage of either scarves or tablecloths, put a layer of acid-free tissue paper between the cardboard and the fabric. You can find it at art-supply stores and in catalogs that specialize in archival storage supplies.

TIP A white **ERASER** makes a terrific tool for cleaning parchment lampshades. Dust the shade with a soft, cotton cloth, then use the eraser to take off any spots or splotches.

TIP Need a pincushion pronto? Grab an **ERASER** (any kind or color will do fine), and insert your needles and pins.

TIP Raise the nap on suede shoes, and remove surface soil, by rubbing the leather with a white **ERASER.**

TIP Use an **ERASER** to clean gold or gold-plated jewelry. It'll make dirt and smudges vanish without harming the metal.

TIP If you keep **FEATHERS** around your hobby room to use in craft projects, you've got some great housecleaning tools on hand—large, soft feathers are perfect for dusting delicate treasures, like oil paintings and fragile figurines.

TIP Although Grandma Putt never went in much for fancy kitchen gadgets, she did love her blender. There was just one problem: Soon after she got the machine, she discovered that the rubber feet made marks on her counter. She fixed that in a hurry by gluing a little piece of **FELT** to each foot.

TIP Got a table or chair leg that's just a little too short? Do what Grandma did to even things up: Cut a few pieces of **FELT** to the right size, glue them together, then glue the mini stack to the bottom of the leg.

TIP To cover scrapes and scratches on brightly colored shoes, use a waterproof, **FELT-TIP MARKER** in a matching shade.

TIP Does the foot pedal on your sewing machine tend to ramble? Then do what Grandma did: Glue a piece of **FOAM RUBBER** to the bottom of the pedal. It'll stay right where you want it.

TIP Could you do with a little extra storage space around your house? Of course you could! Who couldn't? Well, before you go out and buy expensive boxes for that purpose, consider this more creative approach: Bring home a few copy paper boxes from your office (or beg a few from the local copy shop), and cover the top and sides with colorful **GIFT-WRAPPING PAPER.** You can attach it with either white glue applied with

a brush, or a spray-on adhesive available in craft- and art-supply stores. Just one note of caution: Don't use these boxes to store good clothes or valuable textiles of any kind, because over time, the acid in the cardboard will leave brown marks, and eventually cause the fabric to deteriorate.

TIP Don't trash those **JUNK MAIL** envelopes! Instead, use them as shopping aids. Write your shopping list on the back of an envelope, and tuck your coupons inside. At the end of your shopping trip, take the unused coupons home in the envelope.

TIP If you're planning to move in the near future, hang on to sturdy **JUNK MAIL** envelopes. Then, when you disassemble a table, bookcase, or other piece of furniture, put all the nuts, bolts, and screws into an envelope, and tape it to the back or underside of the piece. When you get to your final destination, you'll have the hardware right where you need it.

ONE MORE TIME

 We all know the old pessimism-optimism test: A pessimist sees a glass as half empty; an optimist sees it as half full. Well, you could look at **JUNK MAIL** in much the same way. Some folks look at a mailbox full of the stuff and see, well, junk. Others look at that same pile of papers and see opportunity. No, make that opportunities, plural—like these, for instance:

▷ **Art material.** If you don't care to cut the stuff up and make colorful collages, give it to a day care center, senior center, art class, or creative youngster (or not-so-youngster) who'd love to have it.

▷ **Bookmarks.** For each one, cut the bottom corner off an envelope, about 2 inches from the point of the envelope, then slip the triangle over the corner of your book.

▷ **Compost.** Tear or shred the paper, and toss it onto your compost pile or into your bin. (Use only uncoated paper for this job, not catalogs or other glossy stuff.)

▷ **Entertainment, grandchild-style.** Save your unopened junk mail in a box (or better yet, a genuine mailbox) and present it to your grandchildren when they come to visit. While they busy themselves with their important correspondence, the grown-ups can chat in peace.

▷ **Packing material.** Run the unwanted sheets through your paper shredder, and use the strands to cushion breakables you send through the mail, or your household goods when you pack for a move.

▷ **Tax help.** No, you can't deduct the cost of your time for sifting through your junk mail! But you *can* use the big envelopes to organize receipts, bank statements, and other backup documents that you need to keep with your yearly tax returns. (After all, why pay good money for file folders to hold papers that are just going to stay in a closed box for umpteen years?)

TIP Sometimes, the shrink-wrap on packages can be the very dickens to remove—but not if you try this simple trick: Straighten out a **PAPER CLIP,** and use it to poke a hole in the plastic. Then shove your finger into the hole, and peel the stuff right off.

TIP When you lose the pull tab on a zipper, replace it with a small **PAPER CLIP.**

TIP Like many of Grandma Putt's favorite pastimes, knitting is all the rage again. If you've recently jumped on the knit-purl band-wagon, you may not have one of the special gadgets that pattern instructions refer to when they say, "Transfer stitches to a holder." So what do you do when you read that ominous sentence? Just grab an unsharpened **PENCIL,** and slip the stitches onto that. (*Note:* First make sure the diameter of the pencil is no larger than that of the needles you're working with.)

TIP Free up a sticking zipper by rubbing it with the point of a **PENCIL.** The graphite will lubricate the teeth so they slide smoothly.

TIP When Grandma Putt needed a stake for a floppy, young houseplant, she often used a **PEN-CIL.** She just shoved it into the soil, and tied the plant loosely to the pencil with soft yarn or string.

TIP Rub a sharpened **PENCIL** along the edges of a key to keep it from sticking in the lock.

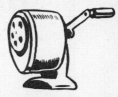

TIP Who says **PHOTO ALBUMS** are only good for storing snapshots? They're also dandy devices for organizing recipes, business cards, and other small, but important papers. Albums with clear plastic pockets work best because you can slide the contents in and out for easy rearrangement.

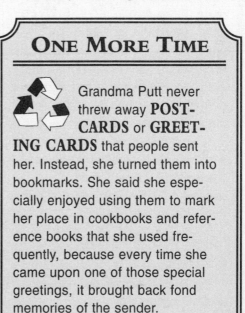

ONE MORE TIME

Grandma Putt never threw away **POST-CARDS** or **GREET-ING CARDS** that people sent her. Instead, she turned them into bookmarks. She said she especially enjoyed using them to mark her place in cookbooks and reference books that she used frequently, because every time she came upon one of those special greetings, it brought back fond memories of the sender.

SCENTED CHRISTMAS TREE ORNAMENTS

If you have an artificial tree—or a real one that's not very fragrant—trimming it with these ornaments will give it that old-time scent that says "Santa Claus is comin' to town!"

1 cup of pine-scented* potpourri
1 cup of all-purpose flour
$\frac{1}{2}$ cup of salt
Food coloring (optional)
$\frac{1}{3}$ to $\frac{1}{2}$ cup of water
Cookie cutters**
Yarn or ribbon

Combine the potpourri, flour, salt, and food coloring (if desired) in a bowl, and stir in the water until the mixture is the consistency of cookie dough. Put it in the refrigerator for 5 minutes. Roll out the dough with a lightly floured rolling pin to a thickness of about $\frac{1}{2}$ inch, and cut it with cookie cutters. Poke a hole in each ornament, and set them on a wire rack to dry overnight. Then hang them on the tree with yarn or ribbon.

* Or substitute another fragrance of your choice.

** Use open cookie cutters, not the kind with closed tops.

TIP **POTPOURRI** doesn't have to be out in the open to perform its scent-sational work. To cover up unpleasant odors in your kitchen garbage can, fill a small, resealable plastic bag to within an inch or so of the top with your favorite potpourri. Then punch a few holes in the upper part of the bag, and tape the bag to the inside lid of the can.

TIP Here's a time-saving cleaning tip, courtesy of Grandma Putt: Keep a **RUBBER BAND** around each container of furniture polish or cleanser, and use it to hold a soft, clean cloth or sponge. That way, you'll always have one when you need it!

TIP Grandma had a simple way to keep stitches from sliding off double-pointed knitting needles: She just wrapped a **RUBBER BAND** around the bottom end of each needle.

TIP When Easter rolls around, don't settle for ho-hum, solid-colored eggs. Instead, make mini works of art to tuck into your baskets. How? Just gather up some **RUBBER BANDS** of various sizes, and wrap them around each egg before you dip it into the dye. Depending on how you place the bands, the finished product will come out with stripes or diamond patterns. Best of all, it'll be a one-of-a-kind creation, because no matter how hard you try, you'll never be able to get the bands in *exactly* the same spots each time. (In Chapter 3, you'll find the lowdown on coloring Easter eggs Grandma-style. See "Old-Time Easter Egg Dye" on page 99 and "Produce to Dye For" on page 101.)

TIP Use **RUBBER BANDS** to bundle up skinny things that tend to go every which way in drawers—

chopsticks, shish kebab skewers, fondue forks, and pencils, to name just a few.

TIP To make a no-tacks-needed bulletin board in a hurry, wrap fabric around a 1-foot-square piece of ½-inch-thick wood or corkboard. Then stretch extra-long **RUBBER BANDS** (either plain brown or brightly colored) around the board in both directions to form a grid pattern. The bands will hold notes, shopping lists, or snapshots securely—and you won't have to search for thumbtacks or pushpins.

ONE MORE TIME

Grandma taught me to never throw away a perfectly good **RUBBER BAND**—she knew a ton of uses for these springy things. Here are just a few:

▷ **Get a grip.** Make screw-top jars easier to open by putting two or three rubber bands around the jar and one around the lid. This will give you better gripping action, so you can just grab hold and twist that top right off.

▷ **Light up.** If you've ever had to drill a hole or power-drive a screw in

a place where there's not much light, you know how frustrating it can be. Shed a little light on the scene by giving your drill its own version of a miner's lamp. Just attach a small flashlight to the side of the drill body using two wide rubber bands. Then flick on the light, and you're ready for action.

▷ **Stop slippage.** Prevent clothes from slipping off hangers—whether they're made of wire, plastic, or wood—by wrapping two or three rubber bands around each end of the hanger.

FAST FORWARD

Space-Age Packing Materials

Like many of the products that we use nearly every day, bubble wrap and Styrofoam™ "peanuts" came on the scene long after Grandma Putt had shipped off her last package. And—like just about all of those other new-fangled "necessities"—these sturdy, feather-weight protective materials have uses that range far beyond the ones they were intended for. Just take a look at these possibilities.

Bubble Wrap

▶ *Insulate your cold frame.* When you know a frosty night is coming, line the sides and top of your cold frame with a layer or two of bubble wrap. Remove it the next day when the air warms up.

▶ *Insulate your flush tank.* If condensation builds up on—and drips off of—your toilet's tank during hot, humid weather, there's a simple reason: The water coming into the tank with every flush keeps the tank colder than the air in your bathroom. To stop the drips, turn off the water-supply valve, flush the toilet to clear the tank, and wash and dry the interior walls. Then cut pieces of bubble wrap to fit, and glue them to the interior sides with silicone sealant, taking care that they don't interfere with any moving parts.

▶ *Sponge-paint your walls (or wooden furniture).* Instead of using a sponge or rag to create special effects on surfaces, dip a square of bubble wrap in the paint of your choice, and go to town.

▶ *Winterize outdoor container plants.* If you can't move your large pots indoors for the winter, protect the plants' roots by covering each container with two or three layers of bubble wrap, held in place with twine or duct tape. This overcoat will offer as much insulation as a couple of feet of snow would provide for in-ground plants.

▶ *Winterize your outdoor faucets.* Before the ground freezes, cut off the flow to exterior faucets, drain each spigot, and cover it completely with bubble wrap. Put a heavy-duty plastic freezer bag over that, and secure it with duct tape. Come spring, pull off the wrappings, and go with the flow.

Foam Packing Peanuts

▶ *Lighten up your potted plants—and improve drainage at the same time.* Before you add soil to a pot, spread a

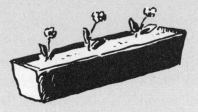

layer of foam peanuts on the bottom. How deep should the layer be? It all depends. For a small pot or hanging basket that's anywhere from 8 to 14 inches across, an inch or so will do the trick. When you're planting in a large container—especially if it will be resting on a deck or balcony, where weight is a critical factor—fill the pot one-fourth to one-third of the way with peanuts, then pour in a lightweight potting mix. (Use this trick only for annuals and shallow-rooted perennials, not for pot trees, shrubs, or deep-rooted perennials, which need every bit of soil a big pot can hold.) *Note:* Whether you're working with small or large containers, use plastic-foam peanuts, *not* the kind made from cornstarch, which will melt into a gooey mess after one or two waterings.

➡ *Make a bath pillow.* Pour 3 to 4 cups of peanuts (plastic, not cornstarch) into a large zip-top plastic freezer bag. Then, to make the cushion easy on your neck, sew a cover from a soft towel. Put snaps or Velcro® tape on one end, so you can remove the cover for washing.

➡ *Make a beanbag chair.* Just sew a pouch that's as large as you want your chair to be, with a zipper or Velcro® closure on one side. Pop in the peanuts and close up the opening. Then sit back and relax (or give the creation to a child who's been begging for just such a lounging aid).

➡ *Make Christmas ornaments.* Using white glue, fasten peanuts together to form snowmen, snowflakes, animals, Santa Clauses, or anything else you or your young helpers would like to see on the tree. Then, glue a loop of ribbon to the top of each ornament, and hang 'em up.

➡ *Make collages.* Glue peanuts to paper or a piece of board in designs of your choice—either alone or in conjunction with other material. You can paint the little chunks, or leave them in their natural, white state. If you do decide to go the colorful route, steer clear of the cornstarch peanut versions, which won't stand up under a coat of paint.

➡ *Safeguard hook earrings.* Keep a peanut or two in your gym bag. Then, when you get to the pool or the health club, take off your earrings, poke the hooks through the foam, and pop the nugget back into your bag.

TIP Has a young artist been using your wallpaper as a coloring book? Don't worry (as long as the paper is washable). Just brush a light coat of **RUBBER CEMENT** onto the crayon marks, let it dry, then use your fingers to roll it—and the colorful wax—right off.

TIP When your vacuum cleaner gets string, thread, or strands of long hair wound around its rollers, that twining stuff can be the very dickens to get unstuck. But not for Grandma Putt. She used a **SEAM RIPPER** to cut through the tangled mess. (Before you try this trick at home, be sure to unplug your vacuum cleaner!)

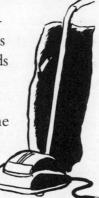

TIP To make candles shine almost as brightly as the flame they produce, polish them with a scrap of **SILK** left over from a sewing project.

TIP Grandma loved flowers of all kinds, but her favorites for indoor arrangements were big, floppy blooms like tulips, mums, and dahlias. Sometimes, though, too many of the posies in a vase flopped a little too much for her liking. To straighten them up, she stuck a **STRAIGHT PIN** vertically into the stem, just below the bottom of the flower.

TIP Is a dripping faucet keeping you awake all night? Halt the noise by tying a piece of **STRING** around the spout, so that the end dangles into the drain. The water will flow silently down the string, while you lie in bed cuttin' Z's.

TIP When you want to hand-paint small objects, attach double-faced **TAPE** to a piece of cardboard, and stick the little things in place. They'll stay put—and your fingers will stay clean.

TIP Grandma believed that everybody—man, woman, or child—should know how to sew on a button, and she taught me that useful skill very early in my life. She also taught me how to keep the thing from sliding every which way as I worked on it. You just attach the button to the fabric with a piece of transparent **TAPE,** and make your first couple of stitches right through it. Then you pull off the tape, and continue stitching.

TIP Use a variation on that theme when you want to

sew narrow ribbon, rickrack, or other trim onto a piece of fabric. Line the trim up so it's nice and straight, and fasten it in place with transparent **TAPE.** Stitch right through the tape, and when you're finished, pull it off.

TIP Instead of writing your friends' contact information in your address book or on Rolodex® cards, clip their return addresses off envelopes, and attach them to the appropriate pages or cards with transparent **TAPE.**

ONE MORE TIME

 If you do even half as much sewing as Grandma Putt did, you pile up a lot of empty **THREAD SPOOLS.** Grandma's supply was made of wood, of course, but even the 21st-century plastic versions can go on to lead useful and creative lives. To put your stash to work, just use your imagination—with this second-career list as a jumping-off point:

▷ **Costume jewelry.** String spools together to make necklaces. Unadorned, they make great play jewels for kids. But creatively painted and trimmed with sequins, mini buttons, or what-have-you, they become wearable art—something you'd be proud to wear around town or even sell at the local craft fair.

▷ **Decorative storage.** Glue them (painted or as-is) to a board or the frame of a mirror, and use them to hang (and display) your collection of necklaces and bracelets, scarves, or small fabric purses and evening bags.

▷ **Dollhouse furniture.** Paint them, or cover them with fabric or contact paper, and presto—you've got stools, ottomans, nightstands, and end tables.

▷ **Mop and broom hangers.** Screw two spools into the wall, just far enough apart to support the business end of each cleaning tool.

▷ **Small-pet toys.** Give a spool to a gerbil, hamster, guinea pig, or kitten, and you'll be a genuine superhero! You'll also have hours of fun watching your pal frolic with this small piece of would-have-been trash.

▷ **"Thumbprint" cookie molds.** Instead of pressing your thumb into a cookie to create a mini basin for frosting or jam, use a clean spool to make your impression. (It'll hold more of the sweet stuff.)

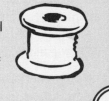

TIP To retrieve a lightweight object from a hard-to-reach place—for instance, under the sofa or behind a heavy dresser—use this old trick of Grandma's: Wrap double-faced **TAPE** around a broomstick

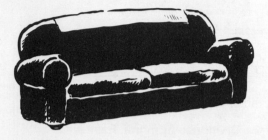

or yardstick, and go fishin'. (If you don't have double-faced tape on hand, use the one-sided kind, sticky side out.)

TIP When a plastic tile falls off a wall and you need a quick, but temporary fix, use double-faced **TAPE.** Put a strip along each side of the tile and one in the middle, remove the paper backing, and push the tile into place. (*Note:* Use a premium brand of tape for this repair.)

GRANDMA PUTT'S
Secret Formulas

OLD-FASHIONED SADDLE SOAP

This was Grandma's favorite formula for cleaning gardening shoes, work boots, and any other leather that didn't need a high polish. (It works great for dog collars and leashes, too.)

3$^{1}/_{2}$ cups of water
$^{3}/_{4}$ cup of soap flakes (such as Ivory Snow®—don't use detergent)
$^{1}/_{2}$ cup of beeswax
$^{1}/_{4}$ cup of neat's-foot oil*

Heat the water to boiling, then reduce the heat to simmer. Slowly add the soap flakes, stirring gently. Remove from the heat. Mix the beeswax and neat's-foot oil in the top of a double boiler until melted. Slowly add the wax and oil combo to the soapy water, stirring until the mixture thickens. Pour the formula into heat-proof containers, and let it cool. To use the saddle soap, rub it onto the leather surface with a damp sponge, and buff dry with a clean, soft cloth.

* Neat's-foot oil darkens some types of leather, so test it first in an inconspicuous spot.

TIP Before you start dismantling a small appliance, or anything else that has a lot of teeny-tiny parts, do what Grandpa always did: Spread a length of wide, double-faced **TAPE** on your workbench. Then, as you remove each little piece from its home, stick it on the tape. The pieces will stay right there until you're ready to put the gizmo back together again.

TIP Grandpa covered the labels on his hardware containers with transparent **TAPE.** It protected the labels from grease, water, and grimy hands—keeping the writing clear and readable. And that meant Grandpa never reached for the wood-screw bin when he wanted finishing nails.

TIP Whenever you finish a painting project, put a piece of **TAPE** (any kind will do) on the outside of 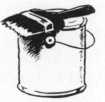 the can to show how much paint is left inside. Then, when you need to make touch-ups, or you're ready to work on another room, you can tell how much paint you have left without opening the can.

TIP The registers that banks send out with checkbooks are

ONE MORE TIME

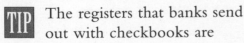 If you have an extra **YARDSTICK** or two in your hobby room, don't let those measuring sticks just lie there taking up space. Instead, cut them into 1-foot sections, and use them as lawn-mowing guide sticks. Sink the sticks into the soil at several spots in your yard (because grass grows at various rates, depending on shade, moisture, and other factors). Then mark each one at the line that's one-third over the optimum mowing height for your grass. (That's because you never want to remove more than one-third of a grass blade at any one time.) So, for instance, if your lawn is Kentucky bluegrass, which should be kept at 2 inches in cool weather, mark your sticks at the 3-inch line. When those green blades start brushing the line, haul out the old mower, and cut off the top inch.

---

awfully small. If the space feels too cramped, record your transactions on regular notebook paper, and put them in a **THREE-RING BINDER.** The full-size sheets will give you plenty of room to write, and you can keep your statements (hole-punched, of course) in the same binder.

TIP Use a **THREE-RING BINDER** to corral the owner's manuals and warranties for appliances, furniture, and electronic gear. That way, you'll always know exactly where they are when a problem crops up.

TIP If you like to sew with sheer fabrics (to make curtains, for instance), you know that the seams tend to pucker. But you can stop that nonsense by putting a strip of **TISSUE PAPER** under each seam, and stitching through it. The fabric will stay in place, and when you're finished you can pull the paper right off.

TIP A felt hat is one of the best head-warmers you can find (Grandma Putt had several of them). They're not waterproof, though, so when you get caught in the rain or snow, you need to give that topper a little special treatment. First, blot up the water spots

with paper towels or facial tissue. Then wad up a handful of **TISSUE PAPER,** and rub it over the marks in a circular motion.

TIP When you need to fill a hole in a hurry, and there's no Spackle™ on hand, make your own by mixing baking soda and **WHITE GLUE.** (Start with roughly equal parts, and add more glue or soda until you get the consistency you want.)

TIP Grandma Putt had a neat trick for keeping my Boy Scout badges in place while she sewed them onto my uniform. She fastened the badge on with **WHITE GLUE** before she started stitching. Then, the next time she washed my uniform, the glue came right out, without leaving a trace.

TIP As you're getting dressed for an outing, you discover that the little plastic cover has come off one of your shoelace tips. Of course, you have no spare laces on hand—and no time to rush out and buy more. So what do you do? Just dip the naked end in **WHITE GLUE.** That'll stop the fabric from fraying until you can get a new pair of laces.

TIP To clean underneath the icebox and other tight spaces, Grandma Putt wrapped a dust cloth around a **YARDSTICK,** shoved it into the opening, and swished it around a few times. Easy as pie!

Family and
FRIENDS

TIP As a boy, one of my favorite rainy-day projects was making things out of papier-mâché. One day, I was searching high and low for something to use as a mold for a mask. As usual, Grandma Putt came through with *just* the thing: She blew up a **BALLOON,** and told me to lay my paper strips over the surface (leaving an opening in the back, of course). When the paper had dried, I simply burst the balloon and peeled it away from the paper.

TIP Here's an idea for party invitations with pizzazz: Write them on **BALLOONS.** Just blow them up, and hold—don't tie—them, while you write the relevant details on the side with a felt-tip pen in a contrasting color. Then carefully deflate the balloons, slide them into envelopes, and mail them to your guests. When they blow up the balloons, they'll read your message.

TIP For a young, budding musician, learning to play an instrument is challenging enough, without having to worry about the sheet music sliding off the stand. Here's an easy way to solve that problem: Just attach the sheet to a **CLIPBOARD,** and prop that up on the stand.

TIP Has your family played the same board game so many times that the board is starting to fall apart? Don't call the game on account of a broken playing "field"! Cover the board with a sheet of clear **CONTACT® PAPER,** and resume the action.

TIP Grandma Putt was a great believer in simple—and useful—gifts. If they were homemade, so much the better. For instance, here's one that she always took to bridal showers and housewarming parties: stacks of 6- and 9-inch-diameter circles that she cut from **FELT** using pinking shears. "What on earth would anyone do with those?" 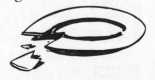 you may ask. Well, you'd put them between plates to keep the bottom of one from scratching the top of the one below.

WALKING JACK-O'-LANTERN COSTUME

When I was a boy, the thought of going out and *buying* a Halloween costume never occurred to anybody—at least nobody I knew. My pals and I (and even party-going grown-ups) made our own outfits using things we had around the house, or could get ahold of easily. This was one of my favorite getups.

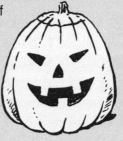

2 pieces of ½-inch-thick foam*
Orange spray paint**
Black brush-on paint**
1- or 2-inch-wide orange ribbon or cotton webbing
Rubber cement (optional)

Cut the foam into two circles that are big enough to cover the child—or yourself — from the shoulders to the knees, front and back. Spray the circles with the orange paint. When it's dry, use the black paint to make Jack's eyes, nose, and mouth. Hold the circles (one at a time) up to the child, and mark a spot above each shoulder, about 1½ inches from the edge of the foam. Poke a hole at each spot, lay the foam back-to-back, and thread the ribbon through the holes to form shoulder straps. Either tie the ribbon, or glue it in place with rubber cement. To complete the costume, have the child wear a green shirt and pants (to represent leaves) and a brown knit cap (for a stem).

This "sandwich board" technique isn't limited to pumpkins. Using the same basic method and materials, you can create just about any object you and your trick-or-treaters can think of. Try stars, candles, Christmas trees—the sky's the limit!

* How much foam you need will depend on the size of the costume wearer.

** Some paints dissolve foam, so ask the folks at your local hardware store to recommend a suitable brand.

TIP Here's a surefire—and attractive—way to keep liquor, cleaning potions, and other no-no products safely away from little hands and paws: Find a low **FILING CABINET** with at least one locking drawer, paint the cabinet in a color to suit your decor, and stash your off-limits substances inside. Use any unlockable drawers to hold nonhazardous consumables, like soft drinks and snacks, or cleanup supplies, such as cloths and sponges.

TIP You say you'd like to have a nautical backdrop for your aquarium, but your pet shop doesn't have one that appeals to you (or you don't want to pay the price)? Then find a roll of **GIFT-WRAPPING PAPER** with a design you like, and tape it outside the back of the tank, with the decorated side facing in.

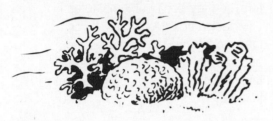

TIP Even for children who like to travel, a long drive on inter-state highways can be mighty bor-ing. To make the trip more fun, give the youngsters a **MAP** of the United States and a marking pen (washable, of course!). Then, as they play the classic game of spot-the-license-plate, they can mark their finds on the appropriate states—getting a good geography lesson in the process.

TIP If you're about to give a bon voyage present to someone who's moving to another part of the

country, or maybe headed for col-lege in a faraway place, make the package suit the occasion: Wrap your gift in a **MAP** of the traveler's destination.

TIP As a boy, there was nothing I loved better than hopping in the car and taking off on a long road trip with Grandma and Grandpa Putt. In fact, I had such an intense case of wanderlust that (with Grandma's okay), I wallpapered my room with **MAPS.**

I know that digital photography is all the rage these days, but I still take my pictures with the 35-millimeter camera Grandma Putt gave me as a graduation present. Over the years, I've collected a lot of those little plastic **FILM CANISTERS,**

and take it from me, they come in mighty handy. Here's a sampling of the jobs they can do:

▷ **Candleholders.** Paint them, or wrap them in foil—either plain old aluminum or fancier stuff from the craft store—and stick tall candles inside.

▷ **Candle molds.** Film canisters are just the size of votive candles. So, if you're the crafty type, tuck in a wick, pour in some melted wax, and there you are!

▷ **Cat toys.** Put a few dried beans or peas inside, snap the lid on tight, and watch Fluffy go to town!

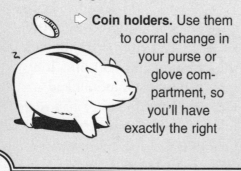

▷ **Coin holders.** Use them to corral change in your purse or glove compartment, so you'll have exactly the right amount you'll need for bus fare, rapid-transit token machines, or highway toll booths—or to give the youngsters for lunch money.

▷ **Containers for craft and sewing supplies.** They're just the ticket for corralling pins and needles or tiny buttons, bangles, and beads.

▷ **Fishing-tackle organizers.** Stash your lead weights and hooks in canisters, so they don't get jumbled up in your tackle box. (As a plus, if you take along any very young fishing buddies, it's unlikely that their small fingers will be able to open the containers.)

▷ **Gym-bag jewelry box.** Keep a film canister in your bag, and use it to hold your rings, earrings, or other small baubles while you swim or work out.

▷ **Lip gloss holders.** When you make homemade gloss (like the recipe on page 240), pack it in film canisters.

▷ **Mini paperweights.** Let the kids decorate the outside with paint, contact paper, or fabric, and fill the container with sand. Presto—a stocking stuffer for Grandma or Grandpa!

▷ **On-the-go sewing kits.** Put a needle or two inside, along with a bobbin of colorless nylon thread, a couple of buttons, and a few safety pins. Then toss the canister into your purse or suitcase, and you're all set to make emergency repairs.

▷ **Pill packages.** Rather than carry multiple bottles of medicines or vitamins when you travel, put daily doses in one or more film canisters.

▷ **Portable pantry.** When you're heading off on a picnic or an overnight camping trip, use film canisters to hold small quantities of salt, pepper, herbs, or condiments.

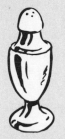

▷ **Travel-size cosmetic jars.** Pour in your favorite shampoo, conditioner, hand lotion, or whatever, and you're good to go—at a fraction of the price you'd pay for trial-size bottles.

▷ **Workshop organizers.** Tuck screws, tacks, and other small hardware inside, and write the contents on the lid using an indelible felt-tip pen.

TIP Sometimes, it's all but impossible for little fingers to manage the zipper pulls on coats and jackets. Grandma made that job easier for me by attaching a small **NOTEBOOK RING** to my zipper pulls. (*Note:* This maneuver works just as well for not-so-little fingers with injuries or stiff joints.)

TIP The next time you fly off on a vacation (or take a cruise or a train trip) make your luggage stand out from all the rest. How? Get some brightly colored **PAINT** and brushes, and turn those bags into works of art. The kind of paint you need will depend on what your suitcases are made of, so ask the folks at an art-supply store what they'd recommend. And, if you don't feel comfortable doing your own freehand designs, pick up a book of stencils while you're at the shop.

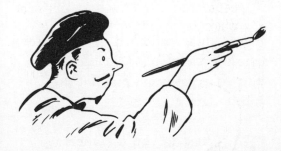

TIP At my birthday parties, my little pals and I always played a game called Gone Fishin'. Grandma Putt made all the preparations, of course—and they couldn't be simpler. First, cut fish shapes from cardboard, and write a different number on each one. Slide a metal **PAPER CLIP** onto the snout of each fish, and toss them all into a big, empty tub. To make a fishing pole, tack a string to the end of a dowel or an old broomstick, and tie a large magnet on the loose end of the string. Then let the party guests take turns casting the line into the bucket and "reeling in" a numbered fish. When the bucket's empty, tally up the numbers. The fisherman with the highest score wins.

TIP Anytime you go off on a trip, take along a container of **SAFETY PINS** in assorted sizes. Then, if (for instance) the zipper on your tote bag breaks, your skirt hem comes unstitched, or the motel curtains just won't stay closed, reach into your stash, and pull out the appropriate pin.

TIP What do you do when a child wants to help around the kitchen, but isn't old enough to handle sharp tools? Do what Grandma Putt did: Hand the budding chef a pair of clean, blunt **SCISSORS,** and have him cut up salad greens for dinner.

TIP Keep small children from pushing things (including their fingers) into electrical outlets by covering the openings with transparent packing **TAPE.**

TIP Marking the height of a growing child (or even a dog) on a wall every so often is a

ONE MORE TIME

When you get your new **TELEPHONE DIRECTORY,** you could send your old one off to your town's recycling center. Or you could turn it into a booster seat for a very young diner. Just cover the book (or two or three, or even four, depending on the size of your town) with fabric or textured wallpaper, and you've got a way to elevate a small visitor at your dinner table—or at a restaurant that doesn't happen to have a booster seat on hand.

classic way to record life's milestones. There's just one problem with this system: When you move on to your next home, those treasured historical records will have to stay behind. But here's a simple way to take them with you: Each time you measure your young 'un, write the numbers on a piece of **TAPE** that you've attached to the wall. Be sure to include the date as well as the inches. Then, either right away, or sometime before moving day, strip off the tape, and put it in a scrapbook.

TIP Uh-oh! The kids are all set to play a board game, but one of the playing tokens is missing. No problem—just replace it with a **THIMBLE.**

TIP Before you put a christening dress (or anything else made of delicate, white fabric) into long-term storage, give it the extra-special treatment Grandma used. Carefully fold white, acid-free **TISSUE PAPER** around the little garment to protect it from dust and dirt, and tuck in a lavender sachet to repel moths. Then, wrap dark blue tissue paper—again, acid-free—around the package to block out light, which can turn the fabric yellow. Keep your treasure in

a cedar-lined chest, or in a box that's specially designed for heirloom storage. (You can find acid-free paper and archival boxes at art-supply stores and in catalogs that specialize in storage products.)

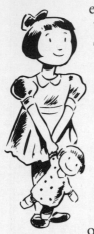

TIP When you take to the open road (or even the local amusement park) with preschoolers, make each one a personal ID bracelet using a strip of **TWILL TAPE,** cut to the size of the child's wrist. Write the youngster's full name and your contact information on the fabric with a permanent, waterproof marker. Then fasten the band on with snaps or Velcro®, and—of course—tell the young traveler in no uncertain terms that the bracelet has to stay on.

TIP Christmas was the happiest time of the year around our house, and as far as I was concerned, one of the best parts was making gift-wrapping paper. Grandma would spread white butcher paper out on the kitchen table, and we'd use **WHITE GLUE** to "draw" pictures of snowmen, stars, Santas, and so forth. Then, we'd sprinkle glitter over the glue. My grandchildren still get a kick out of making their own "designer" wrappings, not only for Christmas, but also birthdays, Mother's Day, and other gift-giving occasions.

The Great OUTDOORS

TIP Hanging tools and other gear on the wall is a great way to keep your garden shed neat. But what do you do with things like gloves and floppy sun hats that don't have holes in them? Just attach them to extra-large **BINDER CLIPS,** and slide the clip handles over wall or Peg-Board™ hooks—that's what!

TIP When I was first learning to play golf, the pro at my course taught me a simple way to build up the strength in my left wrist—which is the body part that powers your swing if you're right-handed, as I am. All you do is grasp the handles of a giant-size **BINDER CLIP** with your left hand, and keep squeezing them to open and close the clip. (Of course, if you're a left-handed golfer, you'll want to do this with your right hand.)

TIP Grandma Putt's apples were the tastiest treats in town— except, that is, for the cider, cobblers, and pies she made from them. And you can bet your bottom Braeburn she wasn't going to let apple worms (a.k.a. codling moth larvae) spoil her harvest. Anytime trouble reared its ugly head, she'd fight back with this surefire strategy: In early summer, wrap an 18-inch-wide band of corrugated **CARDBOARD** around the tree trunk, about 3 feet above the ground. As the larvae crawl down the trunk to pupate into egg-laying moths, they'll be trapped in the cardboard's nooks and crannies. Then, all you have to do is peel off the cardboard and drop it into a bucket of soapy water.

TIP Say "Keep out!" to slugs and snails with one of Grandma Putt's favorite tactics: Sprinkle powdered **CHALK** around the perimeter of your planting beds. The slimy thugs won't cross the line!

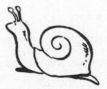

TIP **CHALK** deters ants, too. If the little rascals are "farming" aphids in your trees, shrubs, or other plants, sprinkle powdered chalk on the ground around the trunk or the whole planting bed.

TIP Keep ants out of your garden shed by sprinkling a powdered **CHALK** line around exterior door and window frames.

TIP Time for a road trip? Take along one of my favorite pieces of travel gear: a **CLIPBOARD.** Fold your map to show the area you're traveling through, and attach it to the board. Then you won't have to fumble with a whole state's worth of paper to find your next turn.

GRANDMA PUTT'S
Secret Formulas

LEATHER WATERPROOFING COMPOUND

When you treat your hiking boots or shoes with this old-time conditioner, they'll stand up to anything the great outdoors can deliver.

2 parts beeswax
1 part mutton fat*

Melt the wax and fat together, stirring well. Rub the mixture onto your shoes or boots in the evening, and let them sit overnight. In the morning, buff them with a soft, cotton cloth.

* The meat department manager should be able to order mutton fat; if not, substitute high-quality beef fat.

TIP Before you leave for a round of golf, tuck an **ERASER** into your bag. It's perfect for removing dirt and scuffs from golf balls.

TIP It's frustrating, all right: You're heading off on a camping trip and can't find hide nor hair of your tent pegs. Well, if there's a knitter in the house, don't fret. Heavy-gauge **KNITTING NEEDLES** (number 8 or higher) make fine stand-ins.

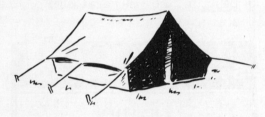

TIP Whether you use monofilament fishing line for its intended purpose, or (as Grandma did) for giving annual vines a way to climb the fence, here's a helpful hint: To keep the slippery stuff from unraveling, wrap an extra-wide **RUBBER BAND** around the spool.

TIP If you grow hot chili peppers, keep a supply on hand right through the winter by making a *ristra*. Just string the stems together, using a regular **SEWING NEEDLE**

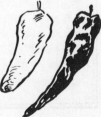

and thread, and hang the peppers in a sunny window. They'll be dry in no time. Then, just clip off a chili anytime you want to cook up something hot and spicy.

TIP If you grow a lot of flower seedlings, and you have your color scheme all planned, don't risk getting those still-green babies in the wrong beds on planting day. Instead, color-code your flats, using **STICK-ON DOTS.** (If you don't have any in your hobby room, you can buy them at any office-supply store, in every color of the rainbow.) Just assign a dot color to each flat, and make up a master list showing what each shade represents. (The dots don't have to be the same color as the future flowers; all that matters is that you know what's in the starter pots.)

TIP As Grandma knew, **TAPE** of any kind makes a fine pest-control tool. Make a trap by wrapping it, sticky side out, around a tree trunk or branch. To handpick bad-guy bugs (especially tiny ones like aphids and whiteflies), wrap the tape around your hand—again, adhesive side out—and go get 'em!

TIP When the ants in your yard are driving you crazy, put a piece of **TAPE** over the hole in the bottom of a flowerpot, and set the pot upside down on top of the anthill. When the little fellas emerge from the nest, they'll scramble up the sides of the pot. Then all you have to do is pick it up and dunk it into a bucket of boiling water.

TIP Grandma Putt used double-faced **TAPE** to keep ants from robbing the nectar in her hummingbird feeders. She wrapped the sticky stuff around the hanger's support, and it stopped the little thieves in their tracks. (If you don't have double-faced tape on hand, use the regular kind, adhesive side out.)

GRANDMA PUTT'S
Secret Formulas

GO-GO GLUE TRAP

A massive invasion of all-but-invisible pests like mites and scale insects can be mighty hard to control—that is, unless you stick it to 'em with this fabulous formula.

1 8-oz. bottle of white glue (such as Elmer's®)
2 gal. of warm water

Mix the glue and water together, pour the mixture into a hand-held spray bottle, and spray all the twigs and leaves of your stricken plant. The bugs will be caught in the glue, and when it dries, it'll flake off, taking the tiny terrors with it.

TIP Here's the dilemma: You're going to do some exterior painting, or maybe messy yard work. You want to keep track of the time, but you don't want to ruin your watch. Here's the ultrasimple solution: Cover the face with transparent **TAPE.** You'll still be able to see the numbers, and the crystal will stay crystal clear.

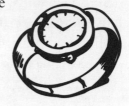

TIP When you start to open your car's trunk, and your key breaks off in the lock, don't call a locksmith. Instead, grab a curved **TAPESTRY NEEDLE** from your sewing basket, and use it to fish the broken part out of the lock.

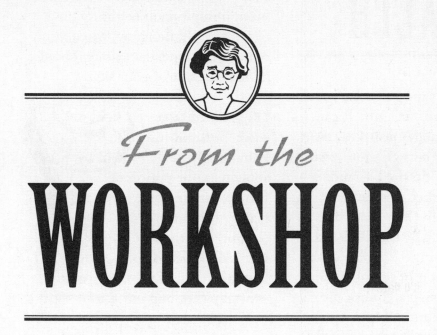

CHAPTER SEVEN

From the WORKSHOP

Buckets

Car wax

Charcoal briquettes

Chicken wire

Drop cloths

Garbage cans

Hardware cloth

Ice scrapers

Kerosene

Linseed oil

Lubricating oil

Masking tape

Nails

Paintbrushes

Sandpaper

Shellac

Steel wool

Tires

Turpentine

Varnish

 and more...

To your
HEALTH

TIP Getting a ring stuck on your finger is no fun—and it can be downright dangerous if that tight piece of jewelry cuts off your circulation. So take a tip from Grandma Putt (and a number of prestigious medical journals): Grab a can of

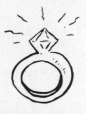

LUBRICATING OIL, aim the nozzle at the top of the offending ring, and push the button. Hold your finger upright for a few seconds, so the oil can trickle down and penetrate faster. Then the stubborn piece of precious metal will slide right off.

TIP In a pinch, make a bandage with **MASKING TAPE.** Just cover the cut with whatever clean, absorbent material you have on hand, such as facial tissue, a folded paper towel, or a scrap of fabric, then use the tape to hold it in place.

TIP To get a splinter out the easy way, cover it with a piece of

MASKING TAPE (the stronger the sticking power, the better). Wait an hour or so, and pull it off. If the sliver stays behind, apply a fresh piece of tape, and keep it on overnight. By morning, when you remove the tape, the splinter should glide right out of your skin.

TIP Need to treat a rash, burn, or insect bite? Baby your sore, itchy skin by applying your potion of choice (either homemade or drugstore-bought) with a new, soft **PAINTBRUSH.**

Around the
HOUSE

TIP Grandma Putt had a simple method for removing white rings left on her wooden furniture by wet glasses or cups. She just dipped a soft cloth in **CAR WAX,** and gently rubbed the marks away.

TIP **CAR WAX** was also Grandma's favorite polish for her Formica® countertops and kitchen table. She rubbed it on with a soft cloth, and buffed with a second cloth.

TIP If you're lucky enough to have leaded or stained glass windows in your house, keep the lead around the glass looking its best by shining it with **CAR WAX.** Just remove any residue from the glass.

TIP After you clean the ceramic tiles on your bathroom walls, rub them down with **CAR WAX.** That will make it all but impossible for soap scum to take hold—and your next cleaning job will be a whole lot easier.

TIP Before you sweep dirt into a dustpan, coat the surface of the pan with **CAR WAX.** That way, it will be a breeze to clean when you're finished.

TIP Drawer runners and window glides will move smoothly, without sticking, if you rub them with **CAR WAX.**

TIP To give leather shoes or boots a shine you can see your face in, use **CAR WAX.** Just rub it on with a soft, clean cloth as you would regular shoe polish, and buff with a second, similar cloth.

ONE MORE TIME

You've got a single, lonely **CONCRETE BLOCK** left over from a building project. What on earth can you do with it? Well, one clever thing you can do is make a portable, but sturdy step. Just wrap the block in thick foam rubber or felt, and cover it with sturdy fabric or textured wallpaper (to provide traction). Then set it wherever you need a little height boost—for instance, in front of the sink in a child's bathroom, or in a closet that has a shelf that's just a tad too high to reach.

TIP If you think of a **CHAMOIS** as just another part of your car-wash kit, think again. These soft, leather marvels are also perfect, scratchless dust cloths for delicate surfaces, like telescope and camera lenses, or even photographs.

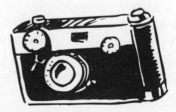

ONE MORE TIME

 After you've installed new **CARPET** in your home, stash the remnants in your workshop. Even the smallest pieces can come in mighty handy. Here are just some of the ways you can use them:

▷ **Cover your cold frame.** When frigid weather heads your way, toss a piece of carpet over your mini green-house to keep your tender plants warm and cozy.

▷ **Cushion your gear.** Cut scraps to the right size, and use them to line shelves, drawers, toolbox-es, or anyplace else you keep heavy or delicate tools and equipment. The thick mat will protect both your belongings and the container.

▷ **Cushion your knees.** Anytime you have down-and-dirty work to do, like painting a hard-surface floor or weeding your garden, slide a carpet scrap, soft side up, under your knees.

▷ **Dampen noise.** To quiet the noisy vibrations of a portable sewing machine, cut a piece of carpet to the right size, and slide it under the machine. (For all you low-tech types, this same trick works with typewriters.)

▷ **Grow weed-free tomatoes.** Before you plant your tomatoes, lay a piece of carpet over the prepared bed, and cut about a 6-inch-diameter hole for each seedling. Then set your plants into the holes. To disguise the rug (after all, this *is* a garden, not your living room!), cover it with your choice of mulch, such as grass clippings, chopped leaves, or shredded bark. Besides stopping weeds in their tracks, the carpet will conserve moisture and attract soil-building earthworms by the zillions.

▷ **Grow wormless apples.** In early summer, wrap a band of carpet around the trunk of your apple tree, about 3 feet off the ground, and fasten it tightly with twine or tape. As codling moth lar-vae crawl down the trunk to pupate in the soil, they'll be trapped in the car-pet. Then all you need to do is peel off the trap and dump it in a tub of soapy water. Or, if you'd prefer, slide it into a big trash bag, lay the bag on the ground, and stomp on it until the worms are history.

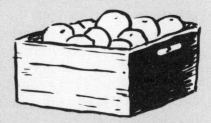

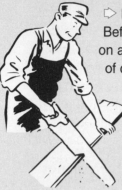

▷ **Hold your wood.** Before placing a board on a sawhorse, lay a strip of carpet under each end. This will keep the board from sliding around as you're cutting.

▷ **Keep moving.** At the start of winter, stash some good-size carpet scraps in the trunk of your car to provide traction if you get stuck on icy pavement.

▷ **Make an exercise mat.** Cut a strip of carpet that's roughly 3 feet wide and about 1 foot longer than your height (because your body tends to slide when you're doing lying-down maneuvers). In between your aerobics, Pilates, or yoga sessions, roll up the rug and stash it in a closet or under your bed.

▷ **Protect your bedroom wall.** To prevent a metal bed frame from gouging the plaster, glue small pieces of carpet to the frame's sharp corners.

▷ **Protect your car's paint job.** If you have to be *very* careful not to bang the garage wall when you open your car door, eliminate that item from your worry list. Give the door a soft crash pad by attaching carpet scraps to the garage wall.

▷ **Protect wood and tile floors.** Glue tiny pieces of carpet, soft side down, to the bottoms of chair and table legs, so they'll glide easily, without leaving scratches or black marks.

▷ **Save your tools.** If you hang your rakes, shovels, and hoes (or any other tools) on a wall made of cinder block or concrete, guard against rust by putting a barrier of carpet between the metal parts and the wall. Depending on the tools you need to protect and the amount of carpet you have on hand (or care to gather up), you have a choice of two methods: Either cut a piece that's just big enough to cover the metal portion of each tool, or cut a 2-foot-wide strip that, attached to the wall, will cover the business ends of all the tools you want to hang in that area. In either case, fasten the carpet to the masonry with construction adhesive, which you can find at your local hardware store.

TIP Not long ago, I found a great old trunk marked down to practically nothing at a secondhand store. It seems no one else wanted it because when you opened the lid, you got hit with a musty odor that just about knocked your socks off. I shouted "Sold!" Then I took it home and "de-mustified" it with an old trick of Grandma's. I put half a dozen **CHARCOAL BRIQUETTES** inside the trunk and closed it up. Then every few days, I took out the charcoal and replaced it with a new supply. After several weeks of this treatment, that vintage holdall smelled as fresh as a daisy! (Just two notes here: One, you need to use plain, old-fashioned charcoal, not the kind that's been doused with lighter fluid. And two, depending on how aromatic your piece is, the deodorizing process could take more or less time.)

TIP To get rid of odors in a closet, fill a coffee can to the top with **CHARCOAL BRIQUETTES,** and set it inside.

TIP **CHARCOAL BRIQUETTES** can also absorb aromas that make your refrigerator smell, shall we say, less than appetizing. Just put a few bri-quettes in a clean cottage cheese or margarine con-tainer (leave the lid off), and set the container at the back of a shelf.

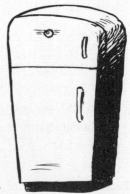

GRANDMA PUTT'S
Secret Formulas

GRANDMA PUTT'S WICKER PRESERVATIVE

Grandma rocked all her babies, grandbabies, and great-grandbabies to sleep in a big, old wicker rocking chair. She used this formula once a year to keep it—and all her other wicker furniture—in tip-top condition. It worked, too. I know that for a fact, because my wife and I have rocked all our babies and grandbabies to sleep in that very same chair!

1 part boiled linseed oil
1 part turpentine

First, remove all dust with a soft brush. Then mix the linseed oil and turpentine in a wide-mouthed glass jar. Rub the solution into the wicker with a soft cloth, paying special attention to all the nooks and cran-nies. Remove any excess formula with a clean, dry cloth, and let the furniture air-dry before you use it.

TIP When you close up a summer house for the season, take a tip from Grandma: Set a shallow box of **CHARCOAL BRIQUETTES** (a dozen or so should do the trick) in each room. That way, when you open up the place next spring, you won't be hit with a wave of damp, stale-smelling air.

TIP Keep a **CHARCOAL BRI-QUETTE** in your toolbox to sop up any moisture and keep the metal parts from rusting.

TIP Anytime Grandma Putt needed a steady base for arranging cut flowers, she bent a piece of **CHICKEN WIRE** into a ball and put it in the bottom of a vase (a nontransparent one, of course, so the wire didn't show). Then she poked the stems through the openings.

TIP Looking for a simple—and attractive—way to add storage space in your kitchen? Well, look no farther than your work-shop (or maybe the local plumb-ing-supply store). Just get some ³/₄-inch-diameter **COPPER TUB-ING,** cut it to the length you need, and fasten it horizontally to the wall with screw-in hooks. Then get some S-hooks that are big enough to go over the pipe and hold your pots, pans, and kitchen gadgets. Presto! You're in business.

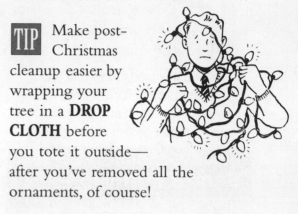

TIP Make post-Christmas cleanup easier by wrapping your tree in a **DROP CLOTH** before you tote it outside—after you've removed all the ornaments, of course!

TIP When you need to cover a *lot* of glass in a hurry (for instance, if you've just moved into a house that has enormous windows or glass doors, and they're as bare as a new baby's bottom), use canvas **DROP CLOTHS.** They come in sizes up to 12 by 15 feet, they cost a whole lot less than even bargain-basement sheets, and the neutral color will blend in with any surroundings.

ONE MORE TIME

When your magnetic **FLASHLIGHT** "dies," toss out the lightbulb end, but hang on to the magnetic body. Then stick it onto your refrigerator or a metal shelf in your office or workshop to hold pens and pencils.

Duct Tape

It's probably safe to say that few workshops in our country are without at least one roll of duct tape. But like many of our modern-day staples, this super-tough, super-sticky, super-waterproof—and super-versatile—tape was not originally intended for home use. Johnson & Johnson developed it during World War II so GIs could make emergency repairs to their battle gear. The soldiers called the stuff "duck tape" because water rolled right off. Later, during the post-war housing boom of the 1950s, heating contractors used the tape to seal (you guessed it) heating ducts, and except for one famous brand, the name evolved from *duck* to *duct*. Now, most heating and cooling systems are coated on the inside with a high-tech spray, but American consumers buy more and more duct tape every year—and find so many clever ways to use it that sometimes I think Grandma must be whispering ideas in their ears! Like these, maybe.

Indoors

▶ *Get rid of warts.* Put a piece of duct tape over the blemish, and leave it on for six days. (If it falls off during that period, replace it with a fresh piece.) At the end of the sixth day, remove the tape, soak the wart in water, and gently rub the spot with an emery board or pumice stone. Leave the area bare overnight, and apply more tape in the morning. Repeat this routine for two months—unless the wart disappears sooner, which it very well may.

▶ *Make coasters.* Put strips of tape together to form a square that's about 1/2 inch bigger all around than you want your coaster to be. Make a second square of the same size, and put the two together, sticky sides in. Then draw an outline on the tape, and cut it out. Finish by "binding" the cut edges with thin strips of tape. (Of course, you *could* use a regular coaster as a template, but why not be creative? For instance, use large cookie cutters in animal shapes, or draw a free-form shape. As long as the surface is big enough to cushion a glass, anything goes!)

▶ *Splint an injured finger.* Just wrap duct tape firmly around your hurt digit and one next to it. Then, depending on the extent of the injury, either continue what you were doing, or hightail it to the emergency room.

Outdoors

► *Claim your luggage.* Decorate your suitcase with brightly colored duct tape, so you can pick it out instantly in a jumble of plain black, navy blue, and teal green bags.

► *Clean your deck.* Leaves, branches, and other yard debris that lodge in between the boards on a deck are more than a nuisance—they're also an invitation to moisture and decay. To get that junk out easily, use duct tape to attach a putty knife or screwdriver to an old broom or mop handle, and poke the stuff through the cracks and onto the ground.

► *Cushion your knees.* Before you start a chore that you have to do on your knees—for instance, weeding the garden or painting the porch—put on your work pants, and fasten a rectangular sponge to each knee with duct tape. (Go easy with the tape so you'll be able to remove it, and the sponges, before you wash your trousers.)

► *Have a picnic—even on a windy day.* Fold the tablecloth under the table, and hold it there with strips of duct tape.

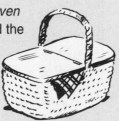

► *Keep shovels on the job.* When a shovel handle splits (maybe because you've used it to pry out rocks or move a heavy shrub), wrap duct tape around the break. Then save that tool for lighter chores, like loosening soil in the vegetable garden, or tossing compost on a flower bed.

► *Keep the welcome mat out for purple martins.* If you've ever put up an apartment house for purple martins, you know house sparrows often move into the cozy quarters before the martins return from their winter homes in the South. Solve that problem by putting a piece of duct tape over each entrance hole until you spot the first martin of the season shopping for real estate. Then pull off the tape so the prodigious purple pest controllers can move in!

► *Play ball!* Crumble a sponge or a wad of paper into a ball, and wind duct tape around it until it's the size you want. Then let the game begin!

► *Repair your tent.* Or your backpack, rubber boots, bicycle seat, kayak, rubber raft, rain slicker, or any other gear that tears or springs a leak when you're far from home—in other words, exactly the job "duck" tape was invented for!

TIP Ladies, if you keep your fingernails long and sharp, this tip's for you: Before you pull on a pair of rubber gloves, put a strip of **ELECTRICAL TAPE** over each nail. This way, no matter how much *oomph* you put into your cleaning job, you won't puncture the fingers of your gloves.

TIP Ice is ice, whether it's on the windshield of your car or the walls of your freezer. So, the next time you defrost that cold-food keeper, use an **ICE SCRAPER** from your workshop to remove the ice without damaging the freezer's surface.

TIP But wait! Ice isn't the only thing an **ICE SCRAPER** can scrape. Its nonscratching plastic blade is perfect for getting dried paint splatters off ceramic tile, wood, or other easily scarred surfaces.

TIP An **ICE SCRAPER** is also a dandy addition to your kitchen utensil basket. How so? Well, that broad blade makes smooth work of moving sticky blobs of dough from a countertop or pastry board.

TIP Grandma Putt always washed her windows from the top down, to avoid leaving them with water spots. Every once in a while, though, she did wind up with water spots here and there. When that happened, she wiped **KEROSENE**

GRANDMA PUTT'S
Secret Formulas

SUPER-DUPER DUST CLOTH

Grandma Putt used these powerful picker-uppers to dust all her wooden furniture, and even her stair railings. I still use 'em to this day. Besides making the wood gleam, they help condition it with every wipe.

2 tbsp. of boiled linseed oil
1 tbsp. of ammonia
1 tbsp. of mild soap powder (like Ivory Snow®)
1 qt. of warm water
1 soft, cotton cloth*

Mix the linseed oil, ammonia, soap, and water in a small bucket, and soak the cloth in the mixture for four or five minutes. Wring out the cloth, hang it up to dry, and store it in a glass jar or plastic container with a tight lid. After you've used it for dusting, wash it as you would any rag, and re-treat it with the formula.

* A cloth diaper or a piece of an all-cotton flannel sheet is perfect.

onto the marks with a soft, cotton cloth, then rubbed them with crumpled newspaper. Bingo! No more spots!

TIP Have you just bought a new house with a brick fireplace? Or maybe built a new fireplace in your old house? Then, chances are, the masonry looks pretty raw. But I know a trick that will make it look as though Santa's been coming down your chimney for years. Just brush the bricks with boiled **LINSEED OIL.** Let it sit for a few hours, and wipe off any excess oil with old rags. Then set those flammable, oil-soaked cloths outdoors to dry thoroughly before you toss 'em in the trash. If you don't have boiled linseed oil in your workshop, you can buy it at your neighborhood hardware store. Whatever you do, don't try to make your own supply by boiling plain linseed oil—it's strictly an industrial process.

TIP To get a cigarette burn off a wooden tabletop, rub the mark with a paste made of boiled **LINSEED OIL** and baking soda, working with the grain until the spot disappears.

TIP You may not cry over spilled milk, but spilled paint could be another story—especially if the paint is oil-based, the "victim" is your favorite wooden table, and you didn't reach the scene until the spots had dried. Well, stiffen up that upper lip, and reach for a bottle of boiled **LINSEED OIL.** Brush a generous coat onto the marks, and let it stand until the paint has softened (how long this takes will depend on how long the paint has been there). Then remove it with a soft cloth soaked in more boiled linseed oil. Finally, scrape off any residue with a plastic scraper or a credit card. Whatever you do, don't use paint remover or thinner, or you'll ruin the wood's finish.

TIP By the time spray **LUBRICATING OIL** arrived on the scene, Grandma Putt had a passel of great-grandchildren. And when those budding Picassos and Georgia O'Keefes filled the walls with crayon drawings, Grandma knew exactly what to do: She reached for her can of oil, sprayed the marks lightly, and wiped the wall clean. (Of course, she took a snapshot of the artwork first!)

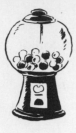 **TIP** Got a wad of chewing gum stuck to the bottom of your shoe? Just spray the lump with **LUBRICATING OIL,** and give it a couple of minutes to penetrate. The sticky stuff will pull right off.

 TIP When it comes to removing stubborn, no-skid stickers from a bathtub, nothing beats **LUBRICATING OIL.** Just saturate the stickers, making sure to spray the edges, and go about your business for two or three hours. When you come back, pull the rubber doodads right off.

TIP Silence a pair of squeaky shoes by spritzing **LUBRICATING OIL** on the source of the sound (most often, it's the point where the shoe upper meets the sole). Buff away any excess oil, and walk on. (If you get any oil on the sole, remember to wipe it off before you track it onto the carpet!)

TIP If you still have the kind of old-fashioned box springs that held up Grandma Putt's mattress, here's a tip to keep in the back of your mind: Anytime those springs start squeaking, remove the fabric from the bottom of the box (it's only held on with staples), and spray the springs with **LUBRICATING OIL.** Then staple the fabric back on, and drift off to dreamland.

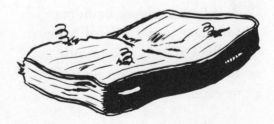

GRANDMA PUTT'S
Secret Formulas

WOOD CABINET POLISH

Don't let the name fool you—this potent potion will shine any wooden surface in your house, whether it's painted, varnished, or lacquered. (In fact, the glow will be so bright, you may need to put on your sunglasses when you walk into the room!)

½ cup of linseed oil (not boiled)
½ cup of malt vinegar
1½ tsp. of lemon juice

Combine the linseed oil and vinegar in a small jar or bowl. Add the lemon juice for a fresh scent. Apply the polish with a soft, cotton cloth, adding a little elbow grease, and your cabinets will be the talk of the town (or, at least, of your house)!

TIP I have a confession to make: Even though I use a computer for most of my writing work, I still keep Grandma Putt's old typewriter in my office for typing labels and envelopes. When the letters and numbers on the paper start looking dim, I spray the ribbon lightly with **LUBRICATING OIL.** That renews the supply of oil contained in the ink, and I'm back in business.

TIP Steel wool is great for all kinds of household chores, from refinishing furniture to sharpening scissors. But after you're through, what do you do with all those tiny specks of steel dust? The answer is simple: Wrap a piece of cloth around a **MAGNET,** and slide it over your work area to pick up all the particles. Then, to get rid of them, shake the cloth over the trash can.

TIP Here's a handy household hint I learned from Grandma Putt: Always keep a **MAGNET** in your junk drawer. It'll automatically corral little metallic clutter-causers like paper clips, safety pins, and screws.

In Grandma's Day

To us, it seems as though **MASKING TAPE** has been around forever, but it was a bright, new star in the workshop when Grandma Putt was a young woman. We owe this Mama Bear of the tape world (not too strong, not too weak) to a 3M employee named Dick Drew, who came up with the idea in the early '20s. Back then, the Minnesota Mining and Manufacturing Company made abrasives—not the gazillion kinds of tape that we know and love. One day, Mr. Drew visited an auto body shop in St. Paul, Minnesota, to test a new batch of sandpaper. There, he found a group of workers painting a two-tone car.

Unfortunately, the only way they had to mask parts of the body was to apply a combination of strong adhesive tape and butcher paper. When they took it off, part of the new paint came with it.

Mr. Drew went back to his lab, did a little tinkering with some ingredients he had on hand—namely the backing and adhesive used to make sandpaper, minus the abrasive material—and produced just what the car painters needed: a tape with a little less sticking power. Painting hasn't been the same since. Nor has 3M.

TIP Even for an experienced do-it-yourselfer, it can be hard to hit a tiny nail on the head—as I know from painful experience! But I haven't banged my fingers with a hammer even once since I learned this simple trick: Use a small **MAGNET** to hold the nail in place, and use your free hand to hold the magnet. Then pound away—at a safe distance from your fingers!

ONE MORE TIME

Is there a jumbled mess of rubber bands lurking in your junk drawer? Well, dismantle that elastic "nest," and snap the bands around an empty reel from a roll of wide **MASKING TAPE.** Bingo—the beginning of the end of your war on clutter!

TIP Are you packing up for a move? Then use **MASKING TAPE** to help protect mirrors, glass cabinet doors, and picture glass during the trip. For small-to-medium-size panes, a single *X* across the surface should do the trick. For larger pieces, add two or three more strips of tape across the glass. *Helpful hint:* Unless your moving budget's really tight, don't try to pinch pennies by using a cheap brand of tape—it'll safeguard the glass just fine, but when you remove it, you'll have a lot of sticky gunk to get rid of. Instead, look for the kind of easy-off tape professional painters use. The friendly folks at your neighborhood paint or hardware store will be happy to recommend a winner.

TIP *Crash!* Your Little League superstars were playing catch in the yard, and one of them threw a wild pitch that sailed right through your window. Now the trick is to get the broken glass out of the pane without cutting yourself. Here's how Grandpa went about that chore when a fastball of mine went astray: First, crisscross lengths of **MASKING TAPE** over the breaks (don't worry about making the strips reach all the way across the pane; just try to make sure each crack has a piece of tape crossing it). Next, cover the inside of the window with a heavy cloth, like a drop cloth or old blanket. Lay another heavy cloth on the ground outside the window. Then, from the inside,

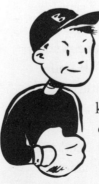

gently tap the glass with a hammer or rubber mallet. The pieces will fall onto the ground without splintering. Then you can gather them up and—very carefully—dump them into the trash can.

TIP If you share Grandma Putt's passion for needlepoint, this advice may be old hat, but novice stitchers, take notice: Before you start a project, always bind the edges of your canvas with high-quality **MASKING TAPE.** It'll prevent the yarn from catching and fraying on the unfinished edges, and will also keep the strands of canvas from unraveling. For best results, make sure you choose a tape that won't leave gummy residue behind to mar your masterpiece.

TIP You've hung a painting exactly where you want it on the wall, but no matter what you do, the danged picture keeps slipping to one side. Here's how to solve that problem in a hurry: Take the artwork down, and cover the center 2 inches or so of the wire with **MASKING TAPE.** This will enable the wire to get a better grip on the hook.

TIP The next time you need to clean a fabric lampshade, do what Grandma always did: Wrap a piece of **MASKING TAPE,** sticky side out, around your hand, and gently dab the surface of the shade. Dust and dirt will cling to the tape. This masking tape "mitten" is also the perfect tool for getting lint or pet hair off clothes and upholstered furniture.

GRANDMA PUTT'S Secret Formulas

SOLID-TRACTION FLOOR POLISH

Grandma kept her wood floors shiny bright with this nonslip formula. (This recipe makes enough to polish roughly 144 square feet of floor area—in other words, a room that measures about 12 by 12 feet.)

½ **cup of orange shellac**
2 **tbsp. of gum arabic (available at hardware stores)**
2 **tbsp. of turpentine**
1 **pint of denatured (not rubbing) alcohol**

Mix the shellac, gum arabic, and turpentine until the gum arabic is dissolved. Add the denatured alcohol, and store the polish in a glass jar with a tight lid. Apply the polish to the floor with a soft, cotton cloth. Wait half an hour, then buff with a second soft, cotton cloth.

ONE MORE TIME

 If you change your car's oil yourself, you have guaranteed rust protection for your garden tools—even through the toughest, wettest winter. Just pour that used **MOTOR OIL** into a plastic garbage can filled with sand, and plunge the metal business ends of your shovels, rakes, hoes, and weeders into the mix. They'll stay as clean and sharp as they were when you put them to bed.

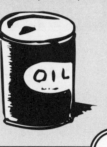

TIP Are your candles a little too narrow for the candlesticks you want to use? Just wrap **MASKING TAPE** around the bottoms of the candles. They'll stay firm and steady in the holders.

TIP When you're running around the house taking a lot of measurements—say, for new curtains or built-in bookshelves—it's all but impossible to keep track of the numbers. Of course, you *could* carry a pad and pencil with you. Or you could do what Grandma

Putt always did: Stick a piece of **MASKING TAPE** to your yardstick 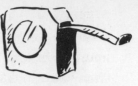 or the case of your tape measure, and jot down the numbers on that.

TIP Here's the problem: You need to paint the stairway that leads to your second floor, but if you have to declare the wet surface off limits, your family will have to bunk in the living room until the treads are dry enough to bear the foot traffic. Here's the simple solution: Run a strip of **MASKING TAPE** down the center of the stairs, and paint the right half. When it's thoroughly dry, remove the tape, then paint the left side.

TIP Grease stains can be tough to get out of a wooden table, but this technique always worked for Grandma. Saturate the area with **MINERAL SPIRITS**—*not* paint thinner, which could damage the finish (and smell up the house, to boot). Then put an old, clean, cotton cloth over it to soak up the grease. (Be sure it's 100 percent cotton, because synthetics don't absorb worth beans.) You may have to repeat the procedure a couple of times, but I guarantee it'll send that grease packin' for good!

TIP Correction fluid comes in mighty handy around the house—even if you don't own a typewriter. But what do you do when you spill some of that thick, white liquid on your clothes or upholstered furniture? Just dampen a cloth with **MINERAL SPIRITS,** and wipe the spots away! (In Chapter 6, you'll find a whole lot of clever uses for this old-time office product.)

TIP The house you just bought has an aluminum storm door that's in fine shape, except for one thing: Corrosion has built up on the surface. Well, don't rush out and replace the door! Instead, remove the ugly deposits by rubbing them with steel wool dipped in **MINERAL SPIRITS.**

TIP Got some shoes that are looking as dull as used dishwater? Then try this trick I learned from Grandma Putt: Saturate a new, clean powder puff with unused **MOTOR OIL,** and let it dry overnight. In the morning, give your footgear a good rubdown with the oiled puff, and buff with a soft, clean cloth. Then stand back, and admire your reflection in the leather! *Note:* This same technique will make leather handbags and briefcases sparkle like the dew.

GRANDMA PUTT'S Secret Formulas

SHELLAC SHAPE-UP

You don't see shellac finishes on newer furniture, but it was commonplace when Grandma Putt was keeping house—and today it's hot stuff in vintage-furniture stores. If you've got some shellacked treasures at your place, give them a coat of this fabulous formula once a year or so. (In between coats, dust the pieces with a dry cloth or the dusting brush attachment of your vacuum cleaner. Don't ever clean the pieces with water, because moisture—even high humidity—tends to make shellac sticky.)

1 part boiled linseed oil
1 part mineral spirits

Mix the ingredients in a small bucket, then dip a sponge or soft, cotton cloth into the solution, and rub it evenly over the wood surface. (Make sure you wear gloves.) Wipe away the excess with a soft, dry cloth. If it's been more than a year since you've cleaned the furniture—or if you've just acquired a piece that hasn't seen loving care in a while—you may need to repeat the process to remove all of the dirt. When you're through, wash your gloves and cleaning cloths in hot, soapy water.

TIP If you love fresh salmon as much as I do, you know how annoying—and even dangerous—those little pin bones can be. (They're the tiny, needle-sharp slivers they don't remove at the seafood market.) Fortunately, it's a snap to take them out yourself. Just grab a pair of **NEEDLE-NOSE PLIERS** and wash them well. Then rub your fingers over the flesh side of the raw fish. As you encounter each bone, grip it firmly with the pliers, and pull it out in the direction it's pointing. Don't rip it straight up, or you'll rough up the flesh.

TIP Whenever Grandma dusted any furniture that had intricate carvings in the wood, she set her dust rag aside and reached for a soft **PAINTBRUSH.** It got into all the little nooks and crannies that a cloth-covered finger could never reach.

TIP Got a grease spot on one of your favorite leather shoes? No problem—if you're a bicyclist,

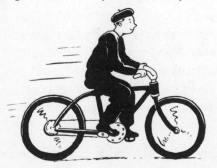

that is. Just mosey into your workshop, cut a piece of **PUNCTURE REPAIR ADHESIVE,** and stick it on the stain. Let it sit overnight, peel off the patch, and shine your shoes with your usual polish.

TIP Before you wear a new pair of leather-soled shoes for the first time, do what Grandma always

GRANDMA PUTT'S
Secret Formulas

PAINT has been around for more than 20,000 years, but for most of that time, painters had to mix the stuff by hand, adding the pigments to carrying agents like white lead, linseed oil, and turpentine. It wasn't until 1880, during Grandma Putt's lifetime, that the Sherwin-Williams Company of Cleveland, Ohio, introduced ready-mixed paint to the home consumer. A decorating craze swept the country, with people rushing to cover up and color up every surface in their homes, indoors and out, including intricately carved woodwork, and furniture made of rich woods like ebony, teak, and mahogany. Today, of course, many descendants of those amateur decorators find themselves up to their ears in paint stripper, asking, "Why on earth would *anyone* paint *this*?!"

did: Roughen up that smooth-surfaced sole with **SANDPAPER.** That way, you won't find yourself slipping and sliding across the carpet the first time you wear them.

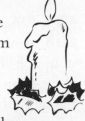

TIP Remove a cigarette or candle burn from a carpet by rubbing the mark with fine **SANDPAPER.** Work with a light, circular motion, and keep at it until the spot disappears.

TIP When you need to open a jar lid that just won't budge, try this trick: Put a piece of **SANDPAPER,** rough side down, over the lid, and twist. It should come right off. (The larger the grit, the firmer your grip will be.)

TIP Don't toss out a perfectly good glass if it gets a little chip in the rim! Just rub the ding, and the surrounding area, with extra-fine **SANDPAPER** until that edge is smooth again.

TIP Anytime Grandma Putt got a spot or two on her good suede shoes, she rubbed the marks away with fine-grade **SANDPAPER.**

TIP Here's a question for you: How can a **SCREWDRIVER**

help keep your house clean? The answer: Keep one (a sturdy, flat-tip model) by the door, and suggest—firmly—that everyone in the family use it to scrape out caked mud from the treads of their shoes or boots before venturing indoors.

TIP There's no doubt about it: Wooden hangers are a lot easier on your clothes than the metal and plastic types. Granted, sometimes, the wood can snag fabric, but you can solve that problem by sanding the prickly hanger and giving it a coat of clear **SHELLAC.**

TIP Grandma Putt sharpened dull scissors by cutting a pad of **STEEL WOOL** into small pieces. (I should say, this was her method of choice for sharpening *everyday* scissors. She kept her treasured sewing shears razor sharp by taking them to a professional knife sharpener at the first hint of dullness.)

TIP Make a stained wooden spoon look like new again by rubbing along the grain with fine **STEEL WOOL** until the marks disappear. (Make sure you wear rubber gloves for this job.) Then pour a teaspoon or so of vegetable oil onto a soft cloth, and rub it into the wood.

Extend Yourself

Or at least your reach. How? Simply find a long **TOOL HANDLE** (either a new one, or one that you've saved from a broken tool), and screw or tape the appropriate gizmo to the end. Here's a trio of possibilities.

Attach This	And Do This
Large cup hook	Reach down behind the dryer or radiator to retrieve a dropped sock, or up to a high shelf to grab a basket or pillow (but nothing heavy, please!).
Paintbrush	Get at all those narrow places your arm won't fit (for instance, behind appliances or radiators), or high spots where you want to use a brush, not a roller.
Squeegee	Wash high windows without a ladder.

TIP Uh-oh! You were giving yourself a manicure at the kitchen table, and you spilled nail polish on the wooden tabletop. No problem—you'll just wipe it off with nail polish remover, right? *Wrong!* That stuff'll ruin the finish in a New York minute! Instead, blot up as much of the polish as you can with a soft, cotton cloth. Then rub the spot with extra-fine **STEEL WOOL** dipped in furniture wax, and wipe dry.

TIP "Mouse-proof" your house by stuffing **STEEL WOOL** into the gaps around gas and water pipes, and any other nooks and crannies the rodents could squeeze through.

TIP When you need to fill a hole that's too big for Spackle™ alone to work, stuff **STEEL WOOL** into the opening so that it comes to about $1/16$ to $1/8$ inch shy of the wall. Then, spackle over the steel wool. Its grabbing power will hold the covering firmly in place.

TIP Even with a light on, basement stairs can be tricky—and dangerous—to navigate. Make the up-and-down trek simpler by adding a strip of brightly colored adhesive **TAPE** to each step, about 1 inch in from the edge. Use either fluorescent tape, or a shade that contrasts strongly with the color of the stairway.

TIP If the inside of your sewing box looks like an earthquake hit it, transfer your gear to a **TOOLBOX,** and assign all the little odds and ends to separate compartments. That way, it'll be a snap to find exactly what you're looking for.

TIP Marks on bronze will vanish if you wipe them with a soft cloth dampened with **TURPENTINE.** (To avoid irritating your skin, wear rubber gloves when you work with turpentine or other solvents.)

TIP Rats! You didn't see the "Wet Paint" sign, and now you've got spots on your clothes. What's worse, it's oil-based paint! Well, don't worry—there's hope for those spattered duds (as long as they're washable, that is). Just pour a half-and-half mixture of **TURPENTINE** and sudsy ammonia onto the marks, let the garment sit overnight, then wash it as usual.

TIP In the summertime, Grandma Putt always put her leather handbag away, and brought out her straw purse. It held its good looks for donkey's years because when it was new, Grandma painted it with a coat of clear **VARNISH.** That kept the fiber from splitting and made cleaning a breeze.

GRANDMA PUTT'S
Secret Formulas

OILED FURNITURE FORMULA

Grandma Putt knew that the worst thing you can do to a piece of furniture with an oil finish* is to treat it with furniture polish or wax. For routine cleaning, she just wiped away the dust with a soft, cotton cloth. Then, every few months, she used this formula.

2 cups of gum turpentine
2 cups of boiled linseed oil
³⁄₄ cup of white vinegar

Combine all the ingredients in a small bucket. Then dip a sponge into the solution, and gently wipe the surface of the furniture. (Wear gloves—this stuff will irritate even the toughest skin!) Let the formula stand for five minutes or so to loosen any tough dirt. Then wipe away the excess with a clean, soft cloth, and buff to a shine with another soft cloth. (Make sure you get all of the formula off the wood, or you could wind up with a gummy residue.) Wash out the sponge, and your gloves, with hot, soapy water.

* If you're not sure what kind of finish your furniture has, drop a little boiled linseed oil onto the surface. If the oil soaks in, the wood has an oil finish. If it beads up, the wood has a hard finish.

TIP I don't know about you, but there's nothing I love better than coming across an old, neglected table or cabinet, and bringing it back to "life." It's a pastime I learned from Grandpa Putt, whose favorite hobby was refinishing furniture. He also taught me to make one of the essential tools of the trade: a tack cloth. You can do it, too—in less time than it will take you to run down to the hardware store and buy one. First, find a lint-free cloth, like cheesecloth or a piece of an old, all-cotton sheet. Soak it in water, and wring it out until it's barely damp. Then lay the fabric out flat, and spatter it with **VARNISH** (I use a paintbrush for this job). Gather it up, and roll it around in your hands to distribute the varnish. Store your tack cloth in a glass jar with a tight lid, so it won't dry out. Anytime you need to renew the stickiness, sprinkle the cloth lightly with water, and shake out any excess.

ONE MORE TIME

Nothing went to waste at Grandma's house—not even scraps of **WALLPAPER.** Once, after Grandpa finished papering the kitchen, he had just a little bit of the covering left. Grandma used it to make a press for her best linen napkins. First, she cut two pieces of illustration board and two pieces of wallpaper, so they were about half an inch bigger all around than the unfolded napkins. Then she glued one sheet of the paper to each board, and laid the napkins inside the squares, with the covered sides facing out. She tied the whole thing together with a big, pretty ribbon, and stashed them in the dining room sideboard. Then, when she wanted to use the linen napkins for Christmas dinner or some other special occasion, she just pulled them out—all neatly pressed and ready to go.

TIP To make an aluminum door shine like new, rub it with **WHITEWALL TIRE CLEANER** on a soft, cotton cloth. Rinse with a second cloth dipped in clear water, and dry with a third cloth.

TIP Clean dirty grout in a brick or stone fireplace by spraying **WHITEWALL TIRE CLEANER** directly onto the grout, and rubbing with newspaper. Finish by wiping with a cloth dipped in a solution of 1 tablespoon of vinegar per 2 cups of water (no need to rinse).

TIP Getting ready to paint? Before you start, tape a piece of

WIRE (any kind will do) across the top of the opened paint can at the center. Then wipe your paint-loaded brush against the wire, rather than the side of the can. This way, paint won't collect in the rim and make the lid stick when you close the can.

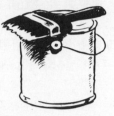

TIP It's happened again: You've lost the cap to a tube of glue, and it's still half full. Well, don't toss that tube away. Just replace the cap with a **WIRE NUT.** (Those are the little plastic doodads that hold electric wires together inside a light fixture.)

Family and
FRIENDS

TIP Keep cupboards and drawers off-limits to small children and pets by stretching a short **BUNGEE CORD** between two door-knobs or drawer pulls.

TIP Attention, church organists! Do you ever wish you had eyes in the back of your head, so you could keep tabs on the congregation, or the choir director while you're playing? Well, here's the next best thing to an extra set of peepers. Screw a **CAR MIRROR,** complete with its adjusting bracket, to a wooden block, and set the contraption on your console, where you can see the mirror and your music at the same time.

TIP If your youngsters or grand-children like to build model boats, cars, or airplanes, here's a tip they'll be glad to hear: When you accidentally get model cement on the clear plastic pieces of your little vehicle, you can polish it away by rubbing with a little **CAR WAX** on a soft cloth.

TIP In the winter, before I headed for the neighborhood sledding hill, Grandma always rubbed **CAR WAX** on my sled's runners. I flew down the trail faster than a speeding bullet!

TIP Make a sliding board more slippery by coating the surface with **CAR WAX.** Give it two coats, buffing in between.

TIP To prevent playing cards from sticking together, rub the backs lightly with a few drops of **CAR WAX** on a soft cloth.

TIP When your dog gets caught in the rain, dry him off with a **CHAMOIS.** The soft leather will absorb water faster than a towel, and feel nice and soft on Fido's coat.

TIP To give the youngsters some real fun on a rainy day—or even a whole rainy week—spread a sturdy plastic **DROP CLOTH** over the floor. Then hand out markers

GRANDMA PUTT'S
Secret Formulas

AT-THE-READY POTTY TRAINING KIT

Grandma Putt knew that a puppy doesn't have full bladder control until he's at least five or six months old. That's why, no matter how well he understands that his bathroom is outside, and no matter how hard he tries to contain himself, accidents happen—often on your carpet. Whenever a new baby dog arrived at our house, Grandma assembled several of these kits and stashed them around the house, so there was always one close at hand. (Use a 5-gallon plastic bucket to hold and tote the items.)*

Roll of paper towels
Spray bottle filled with water
Spray bottle filled with hydrogen peroxide**
Pot-scrubbing sponge

Blot up as much of the urine as you can with the paper towels. Don't rub! Next, spray the spot with water, and blot again. Finally, spray with peroxide, and gently rub it into the carpet fibers with the pot-scrubbing sponge.

* The minute you see the pup start to tinkle, say "Outside!" and rush him there. (Don't scold him; he's only doing what comes naturally.) Wait for him to finish his business, and praise him for his superstar behavior. *Then* rush inside to erase the evidence.

** Test your carpet first; if it's not colorfast, use white vinegar. Whatever you do, don't use ammonia: You'll only be asking for more trouble, because to a dog, ammonia smells just like urine.

(the washable kind, of course!) in a rainbow of colors, and let the kids go to town.

TIP If you have small children or grandchildren who ride their bikes, trikes, or pedal cars in your driveway, here's a super safety tip: Lay an **EXTENSION LADDER** across the end of the drive to keep the youngsters from riding into the street.

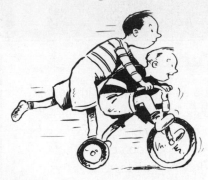

TIP Would you like to find a sturdy, good-looking—and pet-proof—container for dog or cat food? Use a clean, new galvanized **GARBAGE CAN.** The metal blends right in with chrome and stainless steel kitchen gear, and the cans come in sizes that hold everything from a 6-pound bag of cat chow to a giant, 50-pound sack of dog food.

TIP Is there a young artist in the house? When you run out of hanging space on the walls, here's a clever way to store your growing collection of masterpieces (as long as

In Grandma's Day

Grandma Putt always said that the only superstition she knew of that made good, practical sense was the one that claimed it was bad luck to walk under a **LADDER.** After all, if you happen to bump the thing, even lightly, there's a good chance that some heavy tool could come tumbling down on your head! Well, it turns out that, unlike many ancient superstitions, the possibility of physical harm had nothing to do with the ladder taboo. Rather, the belief stemmed from the fact that a ladder leaning against a wall forms a triangle. Since the beginning of recorded history in many cultures, that shape has represented a sacred trinity of gods, and folks who strolled through any triangular arch were showing defiance of sanctified territory—and surely that could only bring trouble!

they're works on paper). Buy some mailing tubes at an office-supply store, and label them in whatever way makes sense—for instance, by school year or subject matter. Roll up a stack of pictures, and stuff it into the appropriate tube. Then stand all the tubes in a small, new galvanized **GARBAGE CAN.**

In the summertime, keep wading-pool or sandbox toys near the scene of the action by storing them in a clean, new plastic **GARBAGE CAN.**

Mother Nature has just dropped a deep blanket of perfect sledding snow, and you've got an anxious youngster in the house. Unfortunately, you don't have a sled on hand. But there's a good chance you have a terrific stand-in: a clean, plastic **GARBAGE CAN LID** with the handles on the sides.

GRANDMA PUTT'S
Secret Formulas

BICYCLE WHEEL TRELLIS

Got an old bicycle wheel in your workshop? Then do what Grandma did for me one summer: Make a trellis that'll delight the daylights out of your kids or grand-kids. Here's all there is to it.

8-foot wooden stake*
Bicycle wheel
Four 2-inch wood screws
10–12 short stakes (either metal or wood)
String or twine
Seeds for the annual vine of your choice**

Sink the 8-foot wooden stake about 1 to 1½ feet into the ground in a prepared planting bed, and slide the wheel over the top. Install the screws just under the wheel to make sure it stays put. Next, pound the short stakes into the soil around the perimeter of the wheel. Run lengths of string or twine from the wheel spokes to the ground, and tie each one to a stake. Plant two or three seeds beside each stake. In no time flat, the vines will scramble up the strings and over the wheel.

* Use a stake that's just wide enough to fit tightly inside the hole in the middle of the wheel.

** Choose a lightweight flowering vine such as morning glories or sweet peas, or a vin-ing vegetable crop, like peas or beans. Avoid perennial vines like wisteria, or heavy vegetables such as squash or indeterminate tomatoes, which will break your trellis.

TIP Time to strike up the band, kid-style? Give the percussion section a couple of clean, galvanized **GARBAGE CAN LIDS** to use as cymbals.

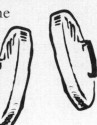

TIP It's time to change the cat litter in Fluffy's box, and you're fresh out of the stuff. Don't rush off to the store. Just mosey into your workshop and scoop out some clay-based **INDUSTRIAL ABSORBENT** (it's made from exactly the same kind of clay used in commercial cat litter).

TIP When the self-stick tab on a disposable diaper doesn't stick, use **MASKING TAPE** instead.

TIP Whenever you head off to the beach with a carload of youngsters, take along a clean, soft **PAINTBRUSH.** It's the perfect tool for de-sanding little (or even not-so-little) feet before they track sand into the car.

TIP Here's another great use for a **PAINT-BRUSH:** Use it to get beach sand off buckets, balls, or even shell collections.

TIP Like any little kid, I always wanted to help with whatever work Grandma and Grandpa were doing around the house. They encouraged my enthusiasm—even when it came time to paint the front porch. Grandma just gave me a clean **PAINTBRUSH** and a small pail filled with water, and let me "paint" the steps. Because the water made the wood look darker, I thought I was really accomplishing something. By the time the stairs had dried to their normal color, Grandma had put me to work "painting" the fence.

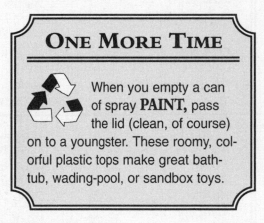

ONE MORE TIME

When you empty a can of spray **PAINT,** pass the lid (clean, of course) on to a youngster. These roomy, colorful plastic tops make great bathtub, wading-pool, or sandbox toys.

TIP Help guard the toddlers in your life from hard knocks by covering sharp-edged chair and table legs with foam **PIPE INSULATION.** Just cut it to the right length, and slip it around the leg. If the stuff doesn't want to stay put, secure it with electrical tape.

Ah, Those Scraps!

Sometimes, when you finish a home-improvement project, you find yourself with **SCRAPS** that seem too small or too few to bother with, so you think you might as well toss 'em. Well, think again! You never know when those little odds and ends might come in handy. Here's a sampling of for-instances.

Workshop Leftovers	What to Do with Them	How to Go About It
Ceramic tiles	Give them to children to use as art material.	Have the kids draw pictures on paper, and glue them to the tiles. Then spray the surface with clear acrylic paint to protect the art. The result: paperweights or coasters.
Concrete paver or stepping stone (at least 12 inches across)	Get rid of gophers.	Put the paver in the middle of your lawn. Then, using the handle of a rake or shovel, pound on the paver for two or three minutes twice a day. After three or four days of this onslaught, the underground vibrations will drive the gophers to calmer territory.
Drywall	Make a message board.	Find an old (or new) picture frame, and cut the drywall to fit inside. Then cut a piece of fabric that's 4 inches larger, on all sides, than the drywall. (Heavy cotton, linen, or burlap is a good choice.) Wrap the fabric around the drywall, and attach it to the back with a staple gun. Put the cloth-covered board inside the frame, and hang it up. Use thumbtacks or pushpins to post messages.
Hardware cloth	Keep your gardening shoes dry.	Set a 12- to 14-inch square piece of mesh on the ground under your outdoor water spigot. The screen will let the water pass into the soil without puddling up and making a mucky mess for you to step in.
Hardware cloth, Take 2	Sift your compost.	Nail 1- by 2-inch strips of wood together to make a frame that reaches across your wheelbarrow. Then cut your piece of hardware cloth to fit, and fasten it to the frame with rustproof brads.

Workshop Leftovers	What to Do with Them	How to Go About It
Rubber stair tread	Cover a swing seat.	To help swing riders get better traction on a metal swing, and avoid splinters from a wooden one, just glue the tread to the seat.
Vinyl floor tiles	Make heavy-duty coverings for shelves or drawers.	Cut the tiles to fit, peel off the backing, and set them in place.
Wood chips	Deodorize your sneakers.	Put a handful of chips into each shoe, then seal them up in a plastic bag, and leave them for a week.

TIP Every dog or cat gets an upset tummy now and then. The cleanup process is never pleasant, but it will be faster and easier if you use a broad plastic **SCRAPER** (instead of paper towels or an old rag) to pick up the tossed "cookies."

TIP Does Fluffy insist on using your potted plants as a litter box? Or maybe she just gets a kick out of digging up the soil. Either way, protect your green friends by laying pieces of fine-mesh **SCREEN** over the soil. Water and air will get through, but kitty's claws won't.

TIP We played a *lot* of board games around our house. And the boards stood right up to all the wear and tear, because when each one was new, Grandma coated it with clear **SHELLAC.**

The great
OUTDOORS

TIP You chose blackwalled tires over whitewalls because you thought they'd stay clean longer. And they do—but they *don't* stay that way forever. Here's a simple trick to keep those babies looking as good the day you drove them out of the tire store: Just rub on a thin coat of **BRAKE FLUID,** using a clean, soft cloth. Then wipe it dry with a second soft cloth.

SLUG BARRIER CLEANER

A mini fence of copper strips, or even copper tubing laid on its side, is one of the best slug and snail defenses you could ask for. That's because, when the pests try to slink over the barricade, something in their body slime reacts with the metal to deliver a fatal jolt. There's just one minor catch: Once verdigris builds up on the copper, it prevents the lethal charge from getting through. That's why, at the first hint of a green tinge, Grandma Putt cleaned her anti-slug barriers with this simple formula.

1 tbsp. of kerosene*
1 tbsp. of baking soda

Mix the ingredients, dip a sponge or soft cloth in the mixture, and scour away the green. Then rinse with clear water, and dry with a clean cloth.

* This formula works wonders on virtually any copper surface. But if you use it indoors (for instance, on copper cookware), use deodorized kerosene and rinse really well.

TIP If you need a place to hang your garden hose, you could go out and buy a special hanger—or you could try this simple trick I learned from Grandpa Putt. Just drill three holes, in a triangular pattern, in the bottom of a galvanized steel **BUCKET.** Then either screw or bolt it to the wall of your garage or shed, with the open end of the bucket pointing out. Coil your hose around the pail, and use the inside to store extra nozzles and hose-end sprayers.

TIP You say you've got no room for a compost pile, or even a bin? Sure you have! Just make an on-site composting bin from a 5-gallon (or larger) plastic **BUCKET** with a lid. Here's how it works. If the bucket has been used before, clean it thoroughly. Then cut off the bottom, and push the container about a foot into the soil in one of your garden beds. Add a few cups of compost (homemade or store-bought) to jump-start the "cooking" process. Then, every day toss in whatever organic matter you have on hand, such as spent flowers, grass clippings, fruit and vegetable scraps, coffee grounds, or tea bags—but no meats, fats, or sauces. In between toss-in sessions, keep the lid on tight to avoid attracting flies and other hungry scavengers. When the bucket is nearly full, pull it up. You'll have a little pile of partially

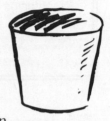

finished compost. Just cover it with soil, and it will continue to break down, providing your plants with essential nutrients. (This trick is especially effective for big eaters like tomatoes and winter squash.)

TIP Here's another space-saving garden tip: If you don't have room to grow tomatoes in the ground, grow them upside down in 5-gallon plastic **BUCKETS.** For each plant, cut a 3-inch-diameter hole in the bottom of a bucket, and insert a seedling so the leaves are coming out the hole. Fill the bucket with a half-and-half mix of commercial potting mix and compost, and hang the container by the handle. Before you know it, you'll have a hanging garden of tomatoes! (*Note:* For best results, use a small, determinate variety that's bred for containers. 'Pixie', 'Tiny Tim', or 'Tumbler' are good choices.)

TIP Control invasive plants like mint, catnip, and bamboo with 5-gallon plastic **BUCKETS.** First, dig a hole that's big enough to hold a bucket. Then cut off the bottom, and remove the handle. Set the pail into the hole, fill it to the proper planting depth with soil, and plant your would-be rambler. The roots will grow straight down instead of galli-vanting through your garden.

TIP Trap plant-munching mice with 5-gallon plastic **BUCK-ETS.** Set each bucket upright near a shrub or other handy climbing device, and put your bait in the bottom. (It seems that almost everybody has a different idea about top-notch mouse bait, but Grandma Putt favored chunky peanut butter for this job.) The mice will scramble up and over the edge, jump in to get the goodies, and stay put. Unless you release them, they'll quickly die of starva-tion or be eaten by predators.

TIP Before you head out to mow the lawn, coat your mower's underside with a little **CAR WAX.** It'll keep grass clippings from stick-ing to the blades and the bottom of the deck—and save you a whole lot of scraping.

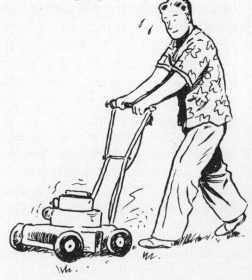

A BUCKET OF STEPPING STONES

Grandma Putt put stepping stones in all her large flower and vegetable beds, so she could work among her plants without tramping on their fluffed-up soil. Of course, stepping stones also make terrific walkways for informal settings. You can buy these useful pieces of pavement at any big garden center—or you can make your own with this simple formula. (This recipe makes enough for five stones.)

Tape measure
5-gallon plastic bucket with straight sides
Band saw or sharp utility knife
Plastic drop cloth
Lubricating oil
60-lb. bag of concrete mix
Wooden stirring paddle
Straight edge
Old pencil or sharp stick, or decorative material, such as marbles or ceramic shards (optional)

Measure the height of your bucket, and divide that number by five. (It should come out to roughly 3 inches.) Make a mark on the side of the bucket at each of those intervals, and repeat the process at three more places around the bucket's circumference. At each of those intervals, cut or saw through the bucket crosswise, to produce five rings. Spread the drop cloth across a flat surface (like a patio or sidewalk), and lay the rings, a.k.a. molds, on top of the cloth. Spray lubricating oil on the inside of each one to make the finished stones easier to slide out. Then mix the concrete according to the instructions on the bag, and pour it into the molds to a depth of roughly 1 inch (or a third of the way up the side).

Now comes the fun part—use a straight edge to level the surface of each stone, and add whatever embellishments you like. For instance, write messages, draw designs, or push ceramic shards or marbles into the soft concrete. When the concrete has hardened, push the stones out of the molds. Then, either fill 'em up again to make another batch, or stash them away for a later pouring.

TIP Cast-iron outdoor furniture wears like, well, iron. Of course, you do have to guard against its number one enemy—rust. Fortunately, you can accomplish that maneuver the way Grandma did. At the start of each season, clean your furniture thoroughly. Then dip a soft cloth in **CAR WAX,** and rub each piece from top to bottom.

TIP An annual coat of **CAR WAX** will also keep gate hinges, latches, and other outdoor hardware free of rust.

TIP Before you put your garden tools to bed for the winter, wipe them lightly with **CAR WAX** to prevent rust and corrosion from setting in.

TIP Remove tar from whitewall tires by applying paste-type **CAR WAX** to the spots with a cloth or sponge, and polishing with a soft cloth.

TIP When I was a boy, one of my regular winter chores was keeping our driveway and walkways cleared of snow—and

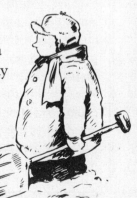

where we lived, there was *plenty* of it! Lucky for me, Grandma knew how to make my load a little lighter: She told me to rub **CAR WAX** onto the shovel blade, so the snow would slide right off the metal surface. (It works just as well on plastic shovels, but of course, they didn't exist back then.)

ONE MORE TIME

Turn an old **DOWN-SPOUT**—or even a piece of one—into a vertical planter. Cut roughly 2-inch-diameter holes in one side of the spout, about 6 inches apart, and attach the other side of the spout to a wall or fence. (Make sure the open end touches the ground so the soil doesn't spill out). Then begin filling the holes with planting mix. When the soil reaches the level of the first hole, set a seedling in on its side, so the top pokes out the hole. Continue filling and planting until you reach the top of the spout. Then water well. The best plants for this high-rise container are ones that naturally trail and tumble. Your local garden center will have dozens to choose from, but some choice winners are strawberries, creeping thyme, lobelia, ivy, and million bells.

TIP Grandpa Putt always kept a small sack of **CEMENT** in his workshop for emergency patch-up jobs. If you do that, too—or if you have some left over from a larger project— you've got a great grease cleaner-upper. Whenever something greasy leaves unsightly marks on your driveway, patio, or any other concrete surface, cover the spot with dry cement, wait 20 minutes or so, and sweep it up. If any trace of the stain remains, repeat the process.

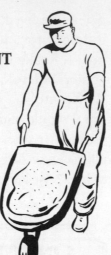

TIP It's finally happened: Your favorite leather garden gloves are beginning to show the results of years of hard labor. Well, don't toss 'em out. Just cut patches from a **CHAMOIS,** and glue or stitch them to the worn spots. Then get back to work!

TIP If raccoons are gunnin' for your corn crop, foil the rascals by laying strips of **CHICKEN WIRE** between the stalks. Raccoons have sensitive, hairless feet, and they don't like to walk on anything that feels sharp, or even the least bit strange.

TIP You say your problem isn't 'coons snitching your corn, but felines frolicking in your flower garden—and leaving fragrant souvenirs behind? In that case, try this old trick of Grandma Putt's. First, plant seeds of an attractive, low-growing groundcover, like creeping thyme or sweet alyssum, in a 2- to 3-foot-wide strip around the perimeter of the garden. Then, cover that fresh seedbed with **CHICKEN WIRE.** When the plants

In Grandma's Day

As a lad, I figured that **CONCRETE**—the stuff of which sidewalks, house foundations, and superhighways are made—had come on the scene during Grandma Putt's lifetime, or at most only half a century or so before her birth. How wrong I was! It turns out that the Romans invented the stuff in the early years A.D. They started with cement, which they made from a volcanic ash called *pozzuolana*, but they quickly found that by mixing the stuff with water, lime, and chunks of stone, they could build strong walls and lay down roads that crisscrossed their whole empire. And, of course, they proceeded to do just that.

grow up, they'll conceal the flat fencing, so you won't notice it. But when the cats' sensitive paws touch that wire, they'll scurry in a hurry!

TIP It's no secret that tomatoes are some of the heaviest eaters in the vegetable garden. But here's a secret you may not know: You don't have to feed your crop at all—not, that is, if you build this 24-hour diner. Here's all there is to it: First, dig a hole that's 3 feet in diameter and 10 inches deep. Next, put a 2-foot-high cylinder of **CHICKEN WIRE** around the hole, and fill it up with compost or well-rotted manure. Then set six tomato plants in a circle around the cylinder, about 1 foot away from it. When you water the plants, water the food supply, too. You'll have the biggest, tastiest tomatoes in town!

TIP One of the most potent weapons in the never-ending war on weeds is hanging right in your workshop. What is it? A **CLAW HAMMER.** Just slide that claw around the stem of a dandelion, or other deep-rooted weed, at ground level. Then rock the hammer's head back just as though you were prying up a nail. That bad-guy plant will pop right out, root and all (at least *most* of the time).

TIP When raccoons want something—whether it's your corn crop, the seed in your bird feeder, or the contents of your garbage can—they'll stop at almost nothing to get their greedy little hands on it. If you've tried every trick in the book, and nothing's worked, here's one that should do the job: Gather up all the electric **FANS** you can beg, borrow, or buy, and set them in place around the 'coons' target. (Be sure to use outdoor-grade extension cords.) Then, just before you go to bed, turn on the fans. Repeat this

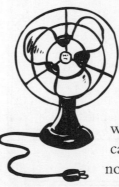

procedure every night for a week or so, and your troubles should be over. (I say "should" because with these wily rascals, there simply are no guarantees!)

TIP Before Grandma put her garden tools to bed for the winter, she cleaned them well, and sharpened the blades. Then she filled a **GARBAGE CAN** about halfway with sand, poured in a quart of mineral oil, and shoved each tool, business end first, into the sand. That kept them all sharp and free of rust and corrosion until spring rolled around.

When you need some extra-sturdy plant stakes for your blockbuster tomatoes, don't run out and buy them—at least not before you've taken a good look around your workshop. Chances are, you've got some **PROJECT LEFTOVERS** or used material that will work just fine. Here's a half dozen possibilities:

▷ Concrete reinforcing rod, a.k.a. rebar

▷ Copper tubing

▷ Galvanized steel pipe

▷ Handles from broken tools

▷ Metal fence posts

▷ Wood strips (sizes of either 1 by 1, 2 by 2, or 1 by 2 inches will work fine)

TIP Tool storage isn't the only wintertime chore in a **GARBAGE CAN's** repertoire. These metal or plastic barrels also make perfect containers for salt, sand, cat litter, or whatever substance you use to keep your stairs and walkways free of ice. Just empty your melter of choice into the can, toss in a big scoop, and you're good to go—with no leaky, messy bags to fumble with.

TIP I learned at Grandma Putt's knee that a big root cellar is the best place to store many kinds of vegetables—not just root crops like potatoes, onions, and beets, but also cabbages, Brussels sprouts, and winter squash. But these days, who has room for a built-in root cellar? I sure don't! But I do have room for a fine stand-in: a plastic **GARBAGE CAN.** And the "construction" process couldn't be simpler. Before the ground freezes, dig a hole that's about 2 inches shallower than the can you want to use. That way, you'll have room to put the lid on. Set the can (a clean, new one, of course!) into the hole, lay your produce inside, and put the lid on. Then cover it with a thick layer of insulation that's easy to remove when you want to get at your treasure—evergreen boughs, a burlap bag filled with straw, or even a piece of carpet will work fine. Finally, mark the location of your mini cellar, so you'll be able to find it easily in the snow.

TIP Looking for an inexpensive birdbath or tray feeder? Use a clean **GARBAGE CAN LID** (either plastic or galvanized metal will work). For a ground-level bath or feeder, set the lid, upside down, on bricks placed far enough apart to hold the curved portion. Or, for a hanging version, drill three holes in the sides of the lid, run rustproof wire or nylon fishing line through the holes, and hang your feathered friends' comfort station from a tree branch.

TIP Groundhogs may be cute as all get-out, but the damage they can do in a garden is anything *but* cute. Fortunately, when Punxsutawney Phil and his pals showed up for dinner at Grandma's house, she knew a simple way to say "This restaurant's closed!" She just set a soup-size can of **GASOLINE** at each of the critters' tunnel openings. It didn't take the woodchucks long to pack up and move to less aromatic quarters. (The rascals may not move far on the first try. There's a good chance you'll have to use this tactic several times before they take off for the far horizons.)

TIP Crops that grow on sprawling vines, like cucumbers and winter squash, are prime targets for crawling pests and soilborne fungi. So lift your harvest out of harm's way with these simple supports that Grandma used to make. For each one, cut **HARDWARE CLOTH** into a roughly 3- by 5-foot rectangle, bend it into an arch, and set it, open side down, in your prepared garden bed. If you like, put a few stakes or concrete blocks in the center of the arch for added support. Then plant your seeds along the sides, and as the seedlings grow, train them up the wire mesh. Besides holding the plants off the ground, the metal supports will draw static electricity from the air—providing an extra supply of nitrogen. (Using this process is called electroculture. See "In Grandma's Day" on page 230.)

ONE MORE TIME

If you've got some old lengths of **GUTTER** lying around, you've got the makings of a first-class slug barrier. Just dig a trench around your planting bed, set in the gutters so their rims just reach the soil surface, and pour about a $1/2$-inch layer of salt or vinegar in the bottom. When slugs (or snails) try to slither over to your plants, they'll fall into the trench and die.

TIP What do you use an **ICE SCRAPER** for? To scrape ice off your car windows, of course! But that's not the limit of its talents. It's also the perfect tool for taking old wax off the bottom of your skis.

TIP When an overnight ice storm leaves you stranded in your driveway—and you happen to have some clay-based **INDUSTRIAL ABSORBENT** in your workshop—you're in luck. Just spread a layer of

Do Fence 'Em Out

When you need to guard your garden against munching critters, **HARDWARE CLOTH** can come in mighty handy. Exactly how you use this metallic defense measure depends on who the varmints are, and what they're gunnin' for. Here's a rundown. (*Note:* In each case, use hardware cloth with openings that are no more than 1/4 inch across.)

Mischief Makers	Targets	Your Defense Strategy
Chipmunks and squirrels	Bulbs	Lay a piece over the bed at planting time. Once the ground has settled, the varmints will lose interest, and you can remove the screen and put it away until next year.
	Seeds	Lay a piece over the bed at planting time. Remove it at the first sign of little green shoots.
Gophers	Bulbs	Line the bottom and sides of the holes (or the entire planting bed). To keep the screen from restricting root growth, set it about 3 inches below the deepest-planted bulbs.
	Flowers or vegetables	Lay the screen on the bottoms of individual planting holes, or entire beds, at a depth of at least 2 feet under the soil surface. Line the sides all the way up to 3 or 4 inches above the surface.
Rabbits	Flowers or vegetables	Dig a trench around the area you want to protect, and install the screen so that it extends at least 3 feet above the ground and 6 inches below, with another 6 inches bent out underground at a 90-degree angle from the garden. Then, if looks matter, disguise the wire with a more decorative fence.

the crunchy stuff under your tires to give them traction, and go on your merry way.

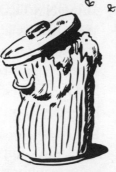

TIP **INDUSTRIAL ABSORBENT** (the clay-based kind) can make your outdoor garbage can less of a "nosesore." Sprinkle a half inch or so of the material on the bottom of the can to absorb odor-causing grease and moisture.

TIP Add a touch of rustic style to your garden with this trick of Grandma's: Lay a wooden **LADDER** (or even two or three) on your prepared planting bed, and plant herbs, flowers, or salad greens between the rungs. (Don't worry if the wood looks a little raw; Mother Nature will weather it in no time!)

TIP Need to load some heavy things into a pickup truck or van? Don't risk injuring your back by lifting them! Instead, make a

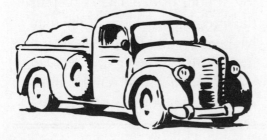

GRANDMA PUTT'S
Secret Formulas

ROAD-SALT REMOVER

If you live in snowy-winter territory, you know that the road salt that builds up on your car can shorten its life span considerably. So keep this simple recipe handy, and use it every time you come home from a drive on wet, salt-treated roads.

1 cup of kerosene
1 cup of dishwashing liquid
Water

Mix the kerosene and dishwashing liquid in a bucket of water, and use a sponge to rub the salt deposits away. (But remember: This stuff is flammable, so use it with caution!)

loading ramp by leaning a **LADDER** against the back of the vehicle, and covering the ladder with a strong board or two. Then set your cargo on the ramp, and slide it right along.

TIP Before you take off on a long bicycle ride, spray your bike from stem to stern with **LUBRICATING OIL.** Just a light coat of the slippery stuff will keep dirt and mud from building up on the metal.

TIP If tree pruning leaves your clippers covered with sap, clean off the goo by spraying the blades with **LUBRICATING OIL,** and wiping them with a soft cloth.

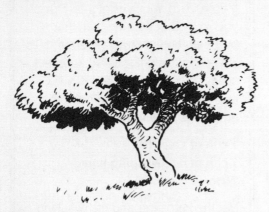

TIP **LUBRICATING OIL** on a soft cloth is just the ticket for getting tar off tools, your car, or anything else that's made of metal.

TIP Dang! It's a warm winter day, you're about to head out cross-country skiing, and you realize you're fresh out of ski wax—that sticky, melting snow could stop you in your tracks! Don't worry. Just grab your spray can of **LUBRICATING OIL,** and lightly spritz the bottoms of your skis. You'll glide right along.

TIP Keep squirrels out of a stationary birdhouse or feeder by spraying the pole with **LUBRICATING OIL.** It'll prevent the critters from scampering up.

TIP One of Grandma Putt's favorite garden tools was a weeder that Grandpa made from a **MASON'S TROWEL.** He just put the triangular head in a vise and bent the handle to a 90-degree angle. Presto: a pull-toward-you weeder like the ones they sell in garden centers—for about a fifth of the cost. (If you don't have a mason's trowel in your workshop, you can buy one at your neighborhood hardware store for just a few dollars.)

TIP When you need to get oil or grease off a concrete surface, don't rush out and buy a fancy masonry cleaner. Instead, grab a can of **MINERAL SPIRITS** from your workshop, and pour the fluid onto the concrete, saturating the spots and an area 8 to 12 inches beyond them. Then cover the whole shebang with a layer of cat litter—thick enough so that you can't see the concrete underneath. (Although old-fashioned clay litter will work for this job, the newer, clumping kinds will absorb the grease better and faster.) Let it sit for an hour or two. Then sweep up the litter with a broom. If the stain has been around for a while, you may need to repeat the procedure. *One note of caution:* Good ventilation is essential, so if you're working inside the garage, keep the door open.

You've just finished a building project, and you've got a whole lot of **SAWDUST** on your hands—or rather, on your workshop floor. After you sweep the stuff up, what can you do with it? Plenty! Here are some ideas to get your creative juices flowing:

▷ **Lower your soil's pH.** Besides making the soil more acidic, aged sawdust will add valuable organic matter to it.

▷ **Make compost.** Sawdust is a first-class brown, a.k.a. high-carbon, ingredient.

▷ **Make fire-starters.** Mix $1\frac{1}{2}$ cups of sawdust with 1 cup of melted paraffin. Pour the mixture into an egg carton or small paper cups (the size used for bathroom dispensers is perfect), and let it harden. Then, when it's time to light your fireplace or barbecue grill, set one of the pellets onto the kindling or coals, and hold a match to it.

▷ **Mend a broken handle.** To replace a handle that has broken off a mug, fill a shoebox about halfway with sawdust. Push the mug, handle side up, far enough into the sawdust so that it won't roll around. Then glue the handle in place, and let it dry overnight. (This trick works just as well with teacups and pitchers.)

▷ **Store apples for the winter.** After you harvest your fruit, dry it thoroughly (without washing), and pack it in boxes filled with dry sawdust. Keep them in a cool, dry place.

▷ **Sweep a concrete floor.** Mix 6 cups of sifted sawdust with 2 cups of rock salt and $1\frac{1}{2}$ cups of mineral oil, and store the mixture in a plastic garbage can with a tight lid. To use this as a cleaning aid, just dip it out with a scoop, sprinkle it on the floor, and sweep it up—along with a whole lot of dust and dirt.

What Not to Do with Sawdust

Some folks like to use sawdust as a mulch for newly sown grass seed, but my advice is to avoid it like the plague. How come? Because when sawdust gets wet, it tends to form a crust that can be very difficult—and sometimes darn near impossible—for little grass seedlings to penetrate.

TIP Before you pour concrete into a new wooden frame, brush **MOTOR OIL** onto the wood. You'll end up with cleaner frames and neater concrete.

TIP Iron deficiency can cause problems in plants, just as it can in people—although the symptoms are different, of course. Plants that aren't getting enough of the stuff tend to attract mildew or an overabundance of insect pests (or sometimes both). Grandma's method of delivering a health-giving dose of iron was to throw a handful of rusty **NAILS** around the roots of the malnourished victim. If you don't have any rusty nails on hand, just douse some new ones with water, and bury them half an inch or so under the soil. They'll rust up and start "bleeding" their Fe into the soil in no time!

GRANDMA PUTT'S
Secret Formulas

WOOD-SCRATCH REMOVER

Grandma Putt had an old-fashioned porch swing made of varnished wood, and anytime it picked up a scratch or two, she got those marks off with this wonderful recipe.

1 part boiled linseed oil
1 part turpentine
1 part white vinegar

Mix the ingredients together in a wide-mouthed glass jar. Then dip some extra-fine steel wool into the mixture, and gently rub the scratches away. (This formula also removes scratches from any shellacked or waxed wooden surface, including floors and furniture.)

TIP You've been itchin' to set up a horseshoe court in your yard, and you've just found a set of great shoes at a yard sale. There's just one problem: The stakes are missing. So make some! All you need is two pieces of ½-inch-diameter galvanized **PIPE,** each piece about 2½ feet long. Pound the pipes about 10 inches into the ground, and you're good to go.

TIP Grandma Putt used to grow a lot of plants in clay drainage pipes. (They make great containers for plants that are typically grown in hanging baskets, like fuchsias, ivy-leaved geraniums, and tuberous begonias.) To keep bugs from coming up through the open bottom, Grandma put a piece of fine-mesh **SCREEN** under each pipe.

ONE MORE TIME

Outfitting your car with new **TIRES** can make a pinch in the pocketbook—but it won't hurt so much if you think about all the things you can do with the old ones. Consider these possibilities:

▷ **Cushion your arrival.** Attach one to the end wall of your garage to soften the blow when you don't remember to stop in time.

▷ **Grow pest-free squash and cucumbers.** Set tires on top of your prepared planting bed, and tuck two or three seeds in each. (Later, thin the seedlings to one per tire—choosing the strongest one, of course.) No one is quite sure why, but something in the rubber repels both squash bugs and cucumber beetles.

▷ **Grow terrific tomatoes.** In a spot that gets at least eight hours a day of sun at the height of summer, stack up three tires per plant. Fill the inside of this mini tower with a half-and-half mixture of good garden loam and compost. In the middle, insert a sturdy wooden stake or, better yet, a metal pole that rises at least 6 feet above soil level. Then plant your seedling (only one per planter). The tires will collect and hold the

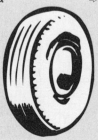

sun's heat, thereby providing the warmth tomatoes crave. Furthermore, the rubber planter will store water for days, releasing it to the plant as needed.

▷ **Make a sandbox for a small child.** Just set the tire on its side, fill it up with clean, beach-type sand, and turn the tyke loose. (If you can lay your hands on an old tire from a farm tractor or—wow!—an airplane, you'll be a superhero of the under-seven set.)

▷ **Make a stand.** For what? For all sorts of things. Fill the center of the tire with cement and, while it's still wet, insert a pipe that's 3 to 4 inches in diameter. Then insert whatever you need to hold up—for instance, a flagpole, post for a mailbox, kid-size basketball hoop, tether ball, or bird feeder. *Note:* If you want to make your stand easier to move, cut a piece of heavy-duty plastic to the size of the tire, and glue it to the bottom before you pour in the cement.

▷ **Make a swing.** Grandma grew up swinging on a tire, and it's just as much fun today as it was back then. Just tie one end of a rope to the tire, and the other end to a sturdy tree limb, and climb aboard!

TIP Grandma's strawberries were the toast of the town (and the main attraction at her church's annual strawberry ice cream social). So you can bet your boots she babied those babies! At planting time, she wrapped each root ball in fine-mesh **SCREEN** before she set the plant in its hole. The roots could grow right through the wires, but greedy grubs (the larvae of strawberry crown moths and strawberry root weevils) couldn't get through.

TIP Head off cutworms by surrounding each seedling with a barrier made from fine mesh **SCREEN.** For each mini corral, cut a strip that's roughly 5 inches wide by 6 inches long—that's long enough to produce an opening about 2 inches in diameter. Sink the mesh 2 inches into the soil with about 3 inches showing above. (Although either metal or nylon screen will work for this trick, nylon has one distinct advantage: Because it doesn't rust, you can save your collars and use them year after year.)

TIP One of the fastest ways to remove rust from metal is to pop a wire wheel on the end of an electric drill, and whirl the stuff

away. But what if you've just found a treasure, like an old iron garden gate, and you don't have a wire wheel? Of course, you could run down to your local hardware store and buy one. Or you could make a bunch of the things from one piece of metal **SCREEN**—for a whole lot less money than the commercial versions. For each wheel, cut about 12 5-inch-diameter circles from the screen, and drill a ¼-inch hole in

ONE MORE TIME

If you've replaced some **WINDOWS** in your house recently, now's your chance to make that cold frame you've been wanting. Just save one of the old windows (or more if you want to build a few of these handy season extenders), and take the glass out. You'll also need enough heavy, clear plastic to cover the frame, four wooden boards, and rustproof nails.

To build your frame, cut the boards to the right size, and nail them together to make a box that's just half an inch or so smaller all around than the window frame. Tack the plastic over the frame, set it on top of the wood box, and you're ready to grow!

the center of each one. Slip the stack of discs onto a bolt, with a washer at each side, and hold them in place with a nut. Put the end of the bolt into the opening where your drill bit would go, and tighten it. Then go to town on your fabulous find!

TIP Here's a simple, foolproof way to tell whether it's time to water your lawn: Just push a long **SCREWDRIVER** into the ground. If you have to struggle to get the tool 6 inches or so into the soil, turn on the sprinklers and give that turf some liquid refreshment.

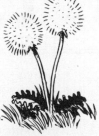

TIP When it comes to prying stubborn weeds out of hard-to-get-at spaces, like the gaps between stepping stones, or cracks in a sidewalk, nothing beats a sturdy, flat-tip **SCREWDRIVER.**

TIP There's nothing a roaming cat loves to do better—or can do faster—than climb up a thick, wooden post that has a birdhouse or feeder on top of it. If you've got one of these feline hot spots in your yard, here's something you should know: You can put an end to Fluffy's fun by covering part of the post with **STOVEPIPE.** For a 4-inch-square post, use a length of standard 6-inch-diameter pipe that's about 24 inches long and has an open seam (most of them do). Just slip the pipe around the post about 8 inches to 1 foot below the house or feeder, and fasten it to the wood with rustproof nails. If you like, paint the metal to match the post. When Fluffy starts to shinny up for dinner, she'll get as far as that smooth surface, and slide right back down.

TIP Grandma always kept a few fresh, clean **WINDOW SCREENS** in the workshop. Then, whenever she wanted to dry herbs or flowers, she hauled out the screens, propped them up on bricks or concrete blocks, and set her plant materials on them.

TIP Older, not-so-clean **WINDOW SCREENS**—set on blocks—are perfect for sifting clumps of topsoil in the garden.

TIP Are the neighborhood raccoons or opossums stealing your corn and tomatoes? If so, try this: Prop old **WINDOW SCREENS** against the cornstalks or staked tomato vines. The hungry varmints will dine elsewhere.

CHAPTER EIGHT

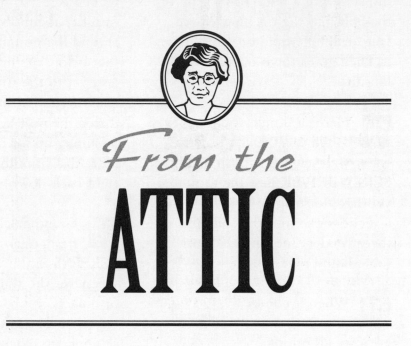

From the
ATTIC

To your
HEALTH

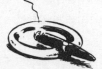

TIP Grandma Putt would be delighted to see that there are far fewer smokers around today than there were in her time. But she'd be sad to know how many beautiful **ASHTRAYS** are lying, hidden and forgotten, in attics and storerooms. So why not gather up some small, pretty ashtrays, and put them on the shelves of your medicine cabinet? Then fill 'em up with pill bottles, tubes of antiseptic ointment, small quantities of bandages, and other tiny, health-giving odds and ends.

TIP You've a bad case of athlete's foot, or maybe just dog-tired dogs, and you've whipped up one of Grandma's potions to give yourself some relief. There's just one thing you overlooked: You don't have a pan that's big enough to hold a pair of feet. Well, before you quadruple the recipe and pour it into your bathtub, limp up to the attic. If you're in luck, you'll find an old **BABY BATHTUB** that'll work just fine. (You'll find some terrific tootsie-soothing treatments in Chapters 3 and 4.)

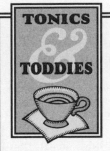

TONICS & TODDIES

FOAMING BATH CRYSTALS

When you're feeling stressed to the limit, down in the dumps, or just tired and achy all over, it's good to have a big, beautiful jar of these colorful crystals on hand. (They make great gifts, too.)

6 cups of rock salt
½ cup of liquid hand soap or mild dishwashing liquid
1 tbsp. of vegetable oil
4–5 drops of food coloring

Put the rock salt in a bowl. In another bowl, mix the liquid soap, vegetable oil, and food coloring together, and pour the solution over the salt. Stir to coat the crystals, and spread them out on wax paper. When they're completely dry (usually in about 24 hours), put them in a jar. At bath time, pour ¼ cup of the crystals into the tub under running water.

TIP Are you prone to tired, sore, or achy feet? Then always keep a couple of old **BASEBALLS** or tennis balls close at hand. When discomfort strikes, roll a bare foot over each ball for three to five minutes, or until your "back paws" feel better.

TIP As Grandma knew, nothing soothes frayed nerves, relaxes aching muscles, or lifts lagging spirits like a long soak in a hot bath. If you have some big, lovely old **GLASS JARS** stored away, bring them out of hiding, and fill them up with "Grandma's Foaming Bath Crystals" (see page 325). With the combination of the colorful crystals in the old glass, you'll have something beautiful to look at, even when you're not relaxing in the tub. And, as Grandma always said, a thing of beauty is a joy forever.

TIP If you can't get a good, restful night's sleep because your spouse is a snorer (as Grandpa Putt was), solve that problem the way Grandma did. At just about the midpoint on the back of each of Grandpa's

pajama tops, she sewed a patch pocket about 8 inches square. Then before he put on his jammies at bedtime, Grandpa popped an old **TENNIS BALL** into the pocket. That made it all but impossible for him to sleep on his back, so he was forced to snooze on his side—a position in which even the most vocal snorers rarely sound off.

TIP Ease your, or someone else's, achin' back with **TENNIS BALLS.** Stuff three or four balls into a kneesock, and knot or stitch the end closed. Then lie face down or, if that's not possible, sit backwards on a chair, leaning your arms against the back, and have a pal roll the sock over *your* back. You'll feel your muscles heave a sigh of relief (so to speak).

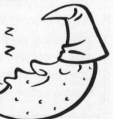

TIP If you use a walker, or have a friend or relative who does, then you know how difficult it is to carry anything from one room to another. But here's a nifty solution to that problem: Find an old **WICKER BICYCLE BASKET** (the kind that attaches to the handle-bars), and hang it from the front bar of the walker. Then toss in your book, newspaper, reading glasses, dog biscuits, or anything else you need to tote around the house.

Your
GOOD LOOKS

TIP It's probably safe to say that every attic (or the equivalent storage space) has at least a few small, pretty **BOWLS** that never even get looked at, much less used. Well, why not put them to work as part of your regular beauty routine? Make them your designated vessels for preparing and applying home-made cleansing and skin-softening potions (like the Berry Good Facial Masque at right).

TIP If you use kitchen-counter cosmetics like baking powder, baking soda, and cornstarch, keep these old-time beauty aids in vin-tage **CASTORS**—glass jars with hole-filled lids, designed for sprin-kling sugar on cookies and cakes. (In Chapter 4, you'll find a whole lot of

Grandma's tips for making lotions, potions, and powders with fresh-from-the-kitchen ingredients.)

TIP No law says **CRYSTAL DECANTERS** have to hold liquor. They also make beautiful containers for mouthwash, bath oil, or cosmetic lotions in the bathroom or on your bedroom dressing table. (Just don't use them in a bathroom that you share with small children!)

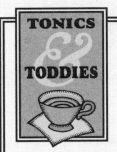

TONICS & TODDIES

BERRY GOOD FACIAL MASQUE

When your skin is craving nourish-ment and moisture, this masque's the berries!

3–4 ripe, medium-sized strawberries
1 tbsp. of evaporated milk
1 tbsp. of honey
1 tsp. of cornstarch (optional)

Puree the berries in a blender or food processor. In a pretty bowl, mix the puree with the milk and honey. If it's too runny, add the cornstarch. With your hands, spread the mixture onto your face and neck, leave it on for 10 minutes, and rinse with luke-warm water.

JEWELRY BOX IN A FRAME

Don't keep a beautiful, old (and empty) picture frame locked away in the attic. Turn it into artful storage for your costume jewelry collection. Here's how.

Picture frame
Tape measure
Tin snips or wire cutters
Hardware cloth or chicken wire
Staple gun and staples
Spray paint (optional)
2 eye hooks
Picture wire and hook
S-hooks (optional)

Remove any glass from the frame, along with any hardware that has held it in place. Measure the inside opening at the back, cut the wire mesh to fit, and staple it in place (painting it first, if you'd like). Screw the eye hooks into the back of the frame, about one-third of the way down from the top on either side, stretch picture wire between them, and hang the frame as you would any painting. Attach the catches of necklaces, bracelets, and earrings to the wire mesh, or dangle them from S-hooks.

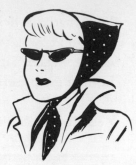

TIP When my cousin Betsy found a lot of old **NAPKIN RINGS** in Grandma Putt's attic, she put them right to work—organizing her collection of silk scarves in a dresser drawer. She just looped each scarf loosely through a ring, thereby keeping her stash free of creases, and easy to grab at a moment's notice.

TIP Does it seem as though there's never enough space in the bathroom to store all your cosmetic supplies? Here's a novel idea: Scavenge around for an old **WICKER BICYCLE BASKET.** Hang the loops from a towel bar, or from two hooks that you've screwed into the wall. Then pop your hair dryer, combs and brushes, or what-have–you, inside.

Around the
HOUSE

TIP When you're searching for containers to organize supplies in your home office or hobby room, don't overlook retired **ASHTRAYS.** They're perfect for holding small necessities like paper clips, pushpins, tubes of glue, and rolls of tape.

TIP If there's a long-outgrown **BABY GATE** languishing in your attic (the expandable kind, with a crisscross pattern), turn it into a wall rack in the kitchen, entryway, or anyplace else you could use extra storage space. Paint the gate if you'd like, and attach a 1-inch-thick piece of wood to the back of each corner, so the rack

will stand out from the wall—thereby giving you enough depth to accommodate S-hooks. Fasten the whole thing to the wall by driving screws through the corners. Then add hooks, and hang up your gear.

TIP When Grandma no longer needed her **BABY GATE** to corral visiting great-grandchildren, she turned it into a sweater dryer. If you want to copy this idea, just lay the gate across a bathtub or laundry sink, and spread your fine washables on top.

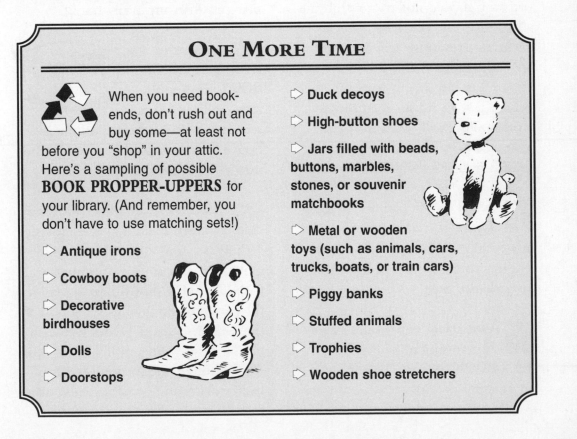

ONE MORE TIME

When you need book-ends, don't rush out and buy some—at least not before you "shop" in your attic. Here's a sampling of possible **BOOK PROPPER-UPPERS** for your library. (And remember, you don't have to use matching sets!)

▷ **Antique irons**

▷ **Cowboy boots**

▷ **Decorative birdhouses**

▷ **Dolls**

▷ **Doorstops**

▷ **Duck decoys**

▷ **High-button shoes**

▷ **Jars filled with beads, buttons, marbles, stones, or souvenir matchbooks**

▷ **Metal or wooden toys (such as animals, cars, trucks, boats, or train cars)**

▷ **Piggy banks**

▷ **Stuffed animals**

▷ **Trophies**

▷ **Wooden shoe stretchers**

TIP Even if your Little Leaguers have gone on to the Majors (or to nonsporting careers), you have a good reason to keep at least one **BASEBALL BAT** out of the attic: It makes a great defensive weapon against burglars and other invading bad guys. You need to wield it the right way, though. My friends on the police force tell me that, when someone is attacking you, you should not try to club the villain over the head, because his instinctive response will be to reach up with his hand and stop the bat in midair. Instead, swing your big stick as hard as you can in an upward motion. This will take him by surprise, and you'll stand a better chance of landing a stunning blow.

TIP Need a new laundry basket? Don't go out and buy one. Instead, do what Grandma did, and reassign your babies' old **BASSINET** to wash-day duty.

TIP One thing you would never find in Grandma Putt's attic was a **BOOK.** No, sir. All her volumes were lined up, neat as can be, on shelves in every room in the house. But if you're like a lot of folks, chances are you have at least a couple of boxes of books moldering away in the attic. If that's so, you just might want to haul them downstairs and unpack them—even if you don't intend to read them. Why do I say that? Well, for starters, besides adding a warm, lived-in look to a home, book-filled shelves provide some of the best insulation you can find anywhere. On exterior walls, they help keep heat in and cold out. On inside walls, they muffle sound between one room and the next. And that's a first-class bargain in my book!

TIP Rescue a big, shallow **BOWL** from your attic, and set it on a table in your entryway to corral house keys, outgoing mail, and other not-to-be-forgotten stuff.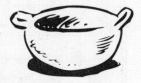

TIP Some people collect souvenir T-shirts from places they visit. Others go in for shot glasses, snow globes, or, as a cousin of mine does, **CANVAS TOTE BAGS** bearing colorful graphics and sayings such as "I ♥ the Grand Canyon." Does she stash her fabric treasures in her attic? No, *sir*—although she did find some of her favorites in Grandma Putt's attic. Instead, she makes throw pillows

BOOKED-SOLID SAFE

Turn an extra-thick book into a hiding place for small valuables. Here's the simple how-to routine.

Hardcover book, 3 to 4 inches thick
Pencil or pen
Straight edge
Craft knife
Glue

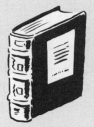

Open the book and on page 5, draw a rectangle in the center of the page, with a 1- to 2-inch border all around. Working a few pages at a time, use the craft knife to cut around the rectangle, removing the cut-outs as you go, and using a previous page as a template. Continue cutting until you reach the back cover. Glue the back cover closed. Then, if you like, for added stability, glue the pages together in ¼-inch layers. Put your emergency money or other small valuables in the center compartment, and set your literary safe on a shelf with other books. To make it as inconspicuous as possible, include it among volumes of roughly the same subject matter, or the same place in the alphabet (depending on how you organize your library).

from them. The process couldn't be simpler. She just cuts off the handles, stitches Velcro® tape onto the open end of the sack, and stuffs a ready-made pillow form inside. She keeps her ever-growing collection in her kitchen, on a gigantic bench that she rescued from an abandoned railroad station. (For more ideas for creative cushion makings, see the One More Time box on page 342.)

TIP Looking for a place to store your fireplace kindling? Rescue a big, old **CERAMIC PLANTER,** and assign it to that vital task.

TIP What's that? You don't have a need to corral kindling, but you *do* have a **CERAMIC PLANTER** that's looking for a new career? Turn it into a wastebasket for your living room, bedroom, bathroom, or office. (Better yet, make it a paper-only recycling "bin," so its good looks won't be marred by messy garbage or an ugly plastic bag.)

TIP The **CHENILLE BEDSPREAD** you grew up with might have a few holes in it, but it can still give you years of enjoyment. Just do what Grandma did: Cut out the holey pieces, and use the good parts to upholster a chair, bench, or other small piece of furniture.

TIP Your **CHILD-SIZE TABLE AND CHAIRS** saw a *lot* of tea parties in their day. But now that munchkin furniture is just sitting in the attic collecting dust. Well, it doesn't have to. For instance, it makes a perfect setting for displaying a grown-up's collection of teddy bears, dolls, or miniature china (or even all of the above).

TIP Not a collector? Then you could borrow this idea from a friend of mine who has a small apartment. She "rechristened" her old **CHILD-SIZE TABLE** as a coffee table, and she uses the **CHAIRS** to hold plants, books, and a piece of folk-art sculpture.

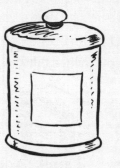

TIP When my niece found a box full of old **COOKIE JARS** in Grandma's attic, she knew exactly what to do with them. She took

---

ONE MORE TIME

 You've found a box of old **COOKIE CUTTERS** in the attic, but you've got plenty of them in the kitchen—so turn your booty into one of these handy helpers:

▷ **Christmas tree ornaments.** Tie a ribbon around each one, and hang 'em on the tree. Or wind a longer strand of ribbon through the cutters to form a garland.

▷ **Gift tags plus.** Write your to-and-from greeting on the metal (in washable marker!), and tie the cutter to the package with ribbon.

▷ **Ornament cutters.** Use them to make decorations from dough or clay. (See "Scented Christmas Tree Ornaments" on page 258.)

▷ **Stencils.** Trace around them to make designs on paper, fabric, metal, or even wet concrete. Or set a cutter in place, and lightly spray-paint over it. Let the paint dry, then lift off the stencil. If you've used a closed-top cutter, you'll have a silhouette. The open type will give you a thin outline against a wash of color (as they say in art lingo).

Go to the Head of the Bed

If you want a one-of-a-kind headboard for your bed, chances are you can find a **FAMILY HEIRLOOM** that's just the ticket. Here are some examples of possible treasures, and how to transform them into part of the furniture.

Future Headboard	Transformation Method

Old softies, such as:
  Hooked rug
  Oriental rug
  Painted floorcloth
  Patchwork quilt
  Tapestry
  Vintage tablecloth
	Stitch a 2-inch-wide strip of muslin to the back of the fabric, along the top edge. If the piece is a valuable textile, make sure the stitches catch only the back of the material and don't show in the front. (Unless you're skilled at hand-sewing, have a pro do this job.) Then push a curtain rod through the sleeve, and fasten it to the wall at the head of your bed with curtain brackets.

More substantial stuff, like:
  Decorative folding screen
  Doors from an antique cabinet
  Fancy shutters
  Lattice panels
  Ornate ironwork from old
    balcony railings
  Piece of picket fencing
	Bolt or screw the piece to the wall at the head of your bed.

them home and lined them up on a wide windowsill, with their tops by their sides. Then she set a small, potted houseplant into each jar. (First, though, she sprinkled gravel on the bottom to provide drainage, and to bring the inner pot up to just below the rim of the jar.) For more creative container ideas, see the One More Time box on page 341.

TIP You opened an old box of papers and found, among other things, a few canceled **CREDIT CARDS?** Well, don't cut them up and throw them away. Save them to use as mini scrapers. They're just the ticket for clearing paint or dried wax drippings from glass or wooden tabletops, or other delicate surfaces, like the inside walls of your freezer.

In Grandma's Day

In a way, you could say that one of Grandpa Putt's favorite pastimes—**POOL**—launched the entire American plastics industry. It happened back in 1868, when a New York company called Phelan and Collender was having a hard time getting enough ivory to make its major product, billiard balls. The firm offered a prize of $10,000 to anyone who could come up with a suitable substitute. Up stepped John Wesley Hyatt, a young inventor who presented a substance he called Celluloid. It wasn't precisely his brainchild. A British professor named Alexander Parkes had come up with its forerunner in 1850. When the product failed to take off in the marketplace, Parkes sold the patent to Hyatt, who grabbed the ball and ran with it. He opened his own billiard-ball manufacturing company in Newark, New Jersey, but quickly broadened his horizons. By 1890 the world's first plastic had taken the country by storm, with people swarming to buy everything Celluloid, from shirt collars to dentures. I guess you could say that young Mr. Hyatt was really on the ball!

TIP There was nothing Grandpa Putt loved more than an after-dinner game of darts. When Uncle Art gave him a new **DARTBOARD** for Christmas one year, Grandpa put the old one in the attic. Soon after that, it came back down to the kitchen—because Grandma realized it made a perfect trivet for the casseroles she served at our big, casual family get-togethers.

TIP If your **DEMITASSE CUPS** haven't seen the light of day since you opened the box at your bridal shower, take those pretty things out of storage, and give them a new name: candleholders. Set each petite cup on its little saucer, stick a fat candle into each one, and group them on a tabletop, or line them up on a windowsill or along a fireplace mantel.

TIP Your latest foray into the attic turned up a bunch of ancient, threadbare **DOWN JACKETS.** Why on earth did you hang on to *those* things? Maybe because you're a kindred spirit of Grandma Putt, who would say, "Do you have any idea how much down-filled furniture costs? Cut away that slick fabric, and use the stuffing to reupholster your sofa—or at least a bench cushion!"

TIP Do you ever wish you could sleep in a garden? Well, you can (more or less) if you turn a beautiful, well-used **GARDEN GATE** into a headboard for your bed. Just clean up the gate if necessary, paint it if you'd like, and bolt it to the wall behind your bed. Then go to sleep and dream of hollyhocks and roses. For more creative headboard options, see "Go to the Head of the Bed" on page 333.

TIP Do you have an old net **HAMMOCK** stashed away? Hang it from the ceiling in your basement, garage, or attic, and use it to store lightweight, nonbreakable stuff like sleeping bags, pillows, and out-of-season clothes.

TIP When Grandma Putt made her special jams, jellies, and preserves, she stored them in a tall, narrow, wooden **JELLY CUPBOARD** in her kitchen. Now that beautiful piece of furniture stands in my living room, where it holds CDs and videos. (They fit on the shelves so well, you'd think the cabinet had been custom-made for them!)

TIP If you have an old wooden **LADDER**—the kind with rounded rungs—and you could use an overhead pot rack in your kitchen, you're in luck. Just insert sturdy eye hooks in the ladder and the ceiling. Then hang the ladder (after you've cleaned it up, of course) using lengths of chain with an S-hook on each end. Suspend your pots and pans from the rungs, using large hooks available in cookware stores and catalogs. (*Note:* The number of eye hooks and chains you need will depend on the size of your ladder and the weight of the gear you intend to hang. If you're not sure about how to install the ladder, have an experienced carpenter do the job.)

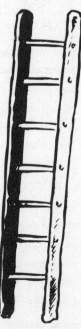

TIP Not so many years ago, a lot of old wooden **MEDICINE CABINETS** got stuffed into attics all over the country. If you're fortunate enough to have one of these treasures, and you don't want to use it for medicinal purposes, hang it up in another room in the house. The narrow shelves are just the right size for holding dried herbs and spices in the kitchen; small supplies in your office; or coasters, candles, and matches in the living room or den.

TIP Put an out-of-work **MESH PLAYPEN** into service by using it as a hamper at the bottom of your laundry chute.

TIP You say your grandma's beautiful **PINE HUTCH** has been sitting in the attic for years because there's no room for it in your kitchen or dining room? Shame on you! Just use your imagination. That heirloom doesn't have to hold glassware and china. Move it to a spot where you

GRANDMA PUTT'S
Secret Formulas

PINS FROM THE PAST

Here's a fun, easy way to turn potential trash into treasured mementos.

Wire mesh file (available in hardware and building-supply stores)
Flat, lightweight ceramic shards, about the size of a half-dollar
Pin backs (available in craft-supply stores)
Pencil
Super-strength, quick-drying glue
Acrylic paint
Small artist's paintbrush

Using the file, rub the edges of each shard until they're smooth. Position a pin back so the metal piece is centered from side to side, and just below the top edge of the shard. Mark the spot with a pencil. Apply a drop of glue to the metal, press it onto the ceramic, and hold it in place for the time specified on the label. When the glue has dried, paint the ceramic edges.

   If you'd like to expand your repertoire beyond pins, check with your local art center or community college. Many of them offer classes in making bits-and-pieces mosaics, a.k.a. memoryware.

can admire it every day, and fill it up with whatever you need to store in that room, such as clothes, books, CDs and videos, office supplies, or even towels and toiletries.

TIP As you might imagine, Grandma Putt had quite a few **PLANT STANDS**—both wicker and iron. Some of them still perform their original jobs for Grandma's descendants. But at my house, we use one to store extra towels in the guest bathroom, and another to hold keys, gloves, and dog leashes by the front door. (Before you put an iron plant stand in a bathroom, give it a coat of rustproof paint or clear sealer.)

TIP Grandma turned a cast-off **POOL CUE** of Grandpa's into a quicker picker-upper. Glue a small magnet onto the narrow end. Then, anytime you drop paper clips, nails, straight pins, or other small, metal objects, just point your stick in the right direction and gather up the goods.

TIP It's always heartbreaking to open a long-stored box and find a pile of **PORCELAIN SHARDS,** when you'd expected to see (for instance) your parents' wedding china, your childhood collection of ceramic horses, or maybe souvenir plates from your big cross-country road trip. Well, chin up. All is not lost—in fact, you just might find that you'll get more pleasure out of those little odds and ends if you transform them into mosaic masterpieces, either to keep for yourself or to give as gifts. For an easy starter project, see "Pins from the Past" at left.

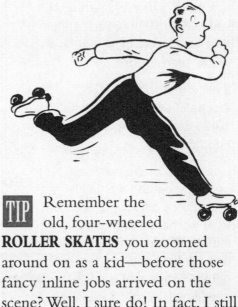

TIP Remember the old, four-wheeled **ROLLER SKATES** you zoomed around on as a kid—before those fancy inline jobs arrived on the scene? Well, I sure do! In fact, I still have my old skates, and I haul them out every time I need to move a big, heavy box or piece of furniture. I cover each skate with a folded towel, so the surface is even. I lift up one end of (let's say) the bookcase, slide one of the improvised "dollies" underneath, and lower the case onto it. Then, after repeating the process on the other end, I roll the load to its destination.

GEL AIR FRESHENER

Just about everybody has at least one box of drinking glasses stashed in the attic. Whether yours are unused wedding presents, jelly glasses with Howdy Doody prancing across the sides, or souvenirs of your 1966 road trip, you can turn them into clever gifts with the help of this simple recipe.

2 cups of distilled water
4 cups of unflavored gelatin
10–20 drops of fragrance oil
Food coloring

Heat 1 cup of the water almost to boiling, then add the gelatin and stir until it's dissolved. Remove from the heat and add the remaining cup of water, the fragrance oil, and the food coloring (enough to get the shade you want). Pour the mixture into clean glasses, and let them sit at room temperature until they've fully gelled. (While it's true that they'll set faster in the refrigerator, in the process, they'll share their scent with your food, so it's best to have patience and cool them at room temperature.)

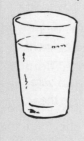

TIP The old **RUBBER BALL** that you found in the attic may have lost its bounce, but it can come in mighty handy if you're planning to brush-paint a ceiling or overhead woodwork (that is, assuming the ball is hollow). Just slice the sphere in half, cut a slit in one of the halves, and slide it over your paintbrush handle, hollow side up. It'll catch the drips that fall from above, leaving you with paint-free hair and arms.

TIP After searching for ages, some friends of mine finally found a lakeside cabin they loved at a price they could afford. There was just one problem: They knew they'd have a lot of visitors, and the guest room had no closet. The solution came straight from their attic at home. They found several louvered **SHUTTERS,** attached them to the wall, and hung wooden coat hangers in the openings between the slats. Bingo—plenty of room for weekend guests to hang shirts, jackets, and dresses.

ONE MORE TIME

 If you're like most folks I know, you've got at least a couple of those **GIANT-SIZE GIFT TINS** that once held popcorn or other snack treats. Well, don't keep 'em stashed in the attic taking up space! Even if they are covered with snowmen, Halloween goblins, or other seasonal images, they can still perform plenty of good work all year long. Just cover the tin and its lid with paint, fabric, or contact paper, and assign them one of these supporting roles:

▷ **Cat litter canister.** If you're short on closed storage space, and you don't care to keep a bag or box of cat litter on display, pour the contents into a tin. Add an old measuring cup or plastic mug for scooping.

▷ **Holiday storage organizers.** Use tins to hold seasonal trimmings, such as Christmas tree ornaments, painted Easter eggs, or the makings for Halloween costumes. Don't tamper with the tin's surface—leave it as a can't-mistake-it label for the contents.

▷ **Hose caddy.** Drill three or four holes in the bottom of the tin, and screw it to the wall in your garage or shed. Roll your hose around the outside of the container, and stash spray nozzles and other gear inside.

▷ **Kindling container.** Set a tin beside your fireplace or woodstove, and stand your sticks and twigs inside.

▷ **Pet-food canister.** 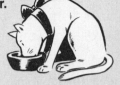 Just open the sack and pour the dry chow into the container. Besides looking neater than a floppy old bag, the tin will keep Fido's or Fluffy's crunchies fresh longer.

▷ **Planter.** Spray the inside with a waterproof sealer. Then proceed in one of two ways. Either drill five or six $1/2$-inch holes in the bottom of the tin, add potting mix, and tuck in your plants, or pour an inch or two of gravel in the bottom, and set a potted plant on top of the gravel.

▷ **Umbrella stand.** Start with a tin that's at least 18 inches high. Spray the inside with a waterproof sealer. Line the bottom with a plastic bag, or set in a plastic plant saucer that fits snugly. Pour in 2 to 3 inches of sand or gravel, and set your stand by the door.

▷ **Wastebasket.** If you plan to use the container for messy refuse, line it with a medium-size garbage bag. Otherwise, just spray the inside with a waterproof sealer, and forget the throwaway liner.

TIP Some of those old, wall-hung **SOAP DISHES** are just too attractive to sit moldering away in a box—especially when they can perform important work as message-board accessories. All you need to do is screw the dish to the board's frame, or the wall beside it. Presto—you've got a handy place to keep your pushpins. (If you have a metal-wire soap dish, rather than the ceramic kind, cover the center grid with a small, shallow bowl or basket.)

TIP In Grandma's later years, her favorite pincushion was a little **STUFFED RABBIT** that once upon a time had been *my* favorite toy. She said she'd found it in a box in her attic one day, and it seemed so lonesome, she just had to take it downstairs and put it to good use.

TIP One day, as Grandma Putt was poking around in her attic, she came across an old **TEAPOT** that had belonged to *her* grandma. She was tickled pink! There was just one minor problem: The old china pot had a hairline crack. Well, that didn't stop my grandma from keeping the heirloom on the job. She turned it into a twine holder. She popped the ball inside the pot, and threaded the end through the spout. Then any-time she needed to tie up a package or truss a turkey, she pulled out as much twine as she needed, and snipped it off.

TIP Can't find your jar wrench? Cut an old **TENNIS BALL** in half, and use it to grip that hard-to-twist lid.

TIP Hang on to that **TENNIS BALL** half because you may need it again soon. It'll make a dandy hand protector if you need to change a burned-out lightbulb that's still hot.

TIP When you put a down-filled jacket in the clothes dryer, toss in a couple of old **TENNIS BALLS.** They'll fluff up the feathers as the garment tumbles around. (This trick also works with down or feather pillows.)

TIP At spring-cleaning time (and in the fall, too), Grandma Putt used to hang her area rugs on the clothesline, and whack the dust off them with a carpet beater. Those things are hard to come by today, but you probably have a tool that will do the job just as well: an old **TENNIS RACKET**.

ONE MORE TIME

Some of the most use-ful—and decorative—storage containers were never designed for household storage at all. Here's a sampling of well-used **HOLD-ALLS** that can corral anything from out-of-season clothes to your TV remote:

▷ **Cast-iron or enamel kettles**

▷ **Cigar boxes**

▷ **Doctor's bags**

▷ **Doll-size (not dollhouse) dressers and cupboards**

▷ **Hatboxes**

▷ **Jewelry boxes**

▷ **Military footlockers or ammunition boxes**

▷ **Produce boxes with original labels**

▷ **Steamer trunks**

▷ **Suitcases (If they have vintage travel decals or baggage tags attached, so much the better!)**

TIP What do you get when you combine an out-of-service **UMBRELLA** with a crystal chandelier? A match made in heaven—at least that's what Grandma called the combo on cleaning day! She simply opened the umbrella, and hooked the handle over the center of the light fixture. Then she mixed 2 teaspoons of rubbing alcohol in 2 cups of warm water in a hand-held spray bottle, sprayed the solution onto the chandelier, and let the drips fall where they might.

TIP Remember that little red (or maybe wood-framed) **WAGON** you loved as a kid? Well, if it's still lurking in your attic, why not give it a new career in the decorative storage "business"? For instance, you could use it to hold towels in a bathroom, magazines or CDs in the living room, or extra pillows in a bedroom.

TIP If a **WAGON** doesn't suit your taste in home decor, give that wheeled wonder a less visible job: Load it up with rags, sponges, sprays, and powders, and stash it in your broom closet. Then, on cleaning day, instead of carrying all your gear from room to room, just roll it along behind you.

One-of-a-kind throw pillows add a personal touch to any room. You can buy some mighty fancy ones in craft galleries, but that can be expensive. You can make your own by piecing together odds and ends of fabric, braid, and ribbon, but that's time-consuming. Or you can comb your attic for **VINTAGE FABRIC ITEMS** that are already pillow size and suit your style, whether it's elegant, rustic, or tongue-in-cheek. Lay two pieces of same-size fabric front-to-front, stitch around three sides, and add a zipper, snaps, or Velcro® tape to the fourth side. Flip the pouch inside out, insert a pillow form, and fasten the closure. That's all there is to it! Here are some all-but-instant covers to search for:

▷ **Bandannas**

▷ **Crocheted or lace doilies (stitch these to a solid fabric backing)**

▷ **Dish towels**

▷ **Handkerchiefs**

▷ **Napkins**

▷ **Silk, linen, or wool challis scarves**

▷ **Unpieced quilt blocks**

Cut 'Em Up

If, in your quest for old fabric, you find a beautiful piece (vintage or otherwise) that's riddled with moth holes, or splotched with the brown stains that paper wrappings can cause, don't assume it can't be used. Even if you can't use *all* of the material, most likely you can cut out enough sections to make pillow covers. Here are some damaged goods worth salvaging:

▷ **Bedspreads (especially chenille with ornate designs)**

▷ **Blankets made of cashmere or lightweight wool**

▷ **Crocheted or handwoven throws and afghans**

▷ **Curtains and draperies**

▷ **Dresses made of silk brocade or other substantial fabric**

▷ **Lace veils or curtain panels**

▷ **Oriental or Navajo rugs**

▷ **Quilts and unfinished quilt tops**

▷ **Silk kimonos, dressing gowns, or smoking jackets**

▷ **Tablecloths**

TIP If you have an old **WINDOW FRAME** (preferably one that has multiple openings, or "lites," as they're known in the trade), do what Grandma Putt did with a frame from her old childhood home: Make a one-of-a-kind bulletin board. Just cut a piece of corkboard to the size of the overall frame, and glue or tack it to the back. Then hang your creation on the wall, and tuck your postcards, snapshots, and messages under the edges—no tacks necessary.

TIP Your remodeled kitchen sports a new, built-in **WINE RACK.** So what do you do with your old one? Use it to store rolled-up towels in a bathroom.

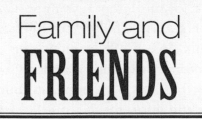

Family and
FRIENDS

TIP Attention, former smokers (and close relatives of former smokers)! Do you still have some **ASHTRAYS** tucked away? Those glass or ceramic containers make

dandy pet-food dishes. Just round up some in the appropriate size, wash them well, and pass them on to your resident canine, feline, or even rabbit or guinea pig.

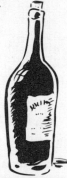

TIP What can you do with no-longer-used rattles, teething rings, and similar **BABY TOYS?** I'll tell you what Grandma Putt did with the ones she came by: She gave them to her parrot, Jake—a big baby if there ever was one! He shook, rattled, and gnawed on those playthings for hours on end.

TIP When a young friend of mine refinished a bureau for her toddler's room, she used some old wooden toy **BLOCKS** as drawer handles. If you want to borrow this neat idea, just drill a hole in the center of each block, and screw it on in place of the original knob.

TIP When your baby leaves home to set up her first apartment, surprise her by converting her **CRIB** into a loveseat. Just remove the sliding side rail, replace the mattress with a softer seat cushion if you'd like, and add throw pillows for the back.

DAZZLING BASIL POTPOURRI

When I found a box of clamp-lid canning jars in Grandma's attic, it brought back memories of this potpourri that she used to make with dried herbs and flowers from her garden.

4 cups of sweet basil leaves and flower spikes
2 cups of dark opal basil leaves and flower spikes
2 cups of rosebuds
2 cups of rose petals
2 cups of rose geranium leaves
1 cup of lavender blossoms
1 oz. of orrisroot*
1 oz. of sweet flag powder*

Put the dried leaves and flowers in a big bowl, and toss them gently. Add the orrisroot and sweet flag powder, and toss the mixture again. Scoop the potpourri into clamp-lid canning jars or other airtight containers, and store them in a cool, dark place. To use your colorful, sweet-smelling creation, pour it into a basket or bowl, and set it out to be admired.

*Available in craft-supply stores, herb shops, and nurseries that specialize in herbs.

TIP A while back, I came across one of Grandpa Putt's old **FISHING POLES.** Now it's my cat's favorite toy. And all I had to do was tie a feathery, catnip-filled fish onto the end of the line (first making sure the hook was gone, of course!). When I'm home, I cast the line, and Fluffy has a ball romping after the "bait." When I go out, she fishes on her own. I just lay the pole on a table, weight it down with a couple stacks of magazines, and let the fish dangle over the side.

TIP We all know that small children love to imitate whatever they see their parents doing—even sitting down at a desk to pay bills or catch up on paperwork. Grandma Putt found a nifty way to help me along on that score. She brought an old **PIANO BENCH** down from the attic and turned it into a lift-top desk for me. I kept my "important papers" inside, and one of my little chairs close by. Then, whenever Grandma or Grandpa sat down at their big desk, I sat down at mine, too, and got right to work.

TIP The table, net, and paddles are long gone, but you still have a box of **PING-PONG™ BALLS.** Correction: If you look at it the way Grandma would have, you've got a box of cat toys in the making. For each one, cut a 6- to 8-inch square of cellophane, and sprinkle ¼ teaspoon or so of catnip in the center. Wrap the cellophane around the ball, and twist the end closed. Tie it tightly with a ribbon or piece of yarn, and present it to your resident feline. Then stand back and watch the fun begin. (Cats go bonkers over the combination of their favorite scent and the crackly sound of the cellophane.)

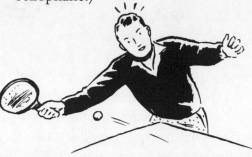

Made of These

Hey, pack rats! Does your attic have a sizable supply of **GAMES, PUZZLES, AND TOYS** with crucial parts that have gone AWOL? Well, don't throw them out—and don't even *think* of keeping them tucked away in boxes. Instead, get creative. Use gun power (*glue* gun power, that is) to turn those little bits of trash into treasured memories for someone on your birthday or Christmas gift list. How? Just pull out appropriately themed nuggets, and attach them to a picture frame that has a broad, flat surface. Then insert a mirror. (The folks at your neighborhood glass company will be happy to cut one to size.) Here's a handful of for-instances.

If the Recipient Is a (n)...	These Bits and Pieces Fill the Bill
Architect or builder	LEGO® pieces, Lincoln Logs®, or Monopoly® hotels and houses
Banker or gung-ho investor	Monopoly money
Canasta, bridge, or poker player	Playing cards, poker chips
Fashion fiend or clothing-store owner	Clothes and accessories from a long-gone Barbie® doll
Interior designer or new, house-proud homeowner	Dollhouse furniture and accessories
Jigsaw-puzzle enthusiast	Pieces from a jigsaw puzzle (of course!)
Writer, editor, or voracious reader	Scrabble® letters

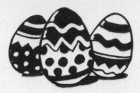

TIP You used to buy pantyhose that came packaged in big **PLASTIC EGGS,** and you kept every single one of them because you knew they'd come in handy one day. Well, that day is here! Haul those things out of the attic, and decorate them with paint, paper, fabric, or spangles. Then fill them with jelly beans, marshmallow bunnies, and tiny treasures, and tuck them into Easter baskets. Or use them as clever small-gift boxes at any time of the year. (After all, no law says that eggs are *only* for Easter!)

TIP Grandma turned a lot of our old clothes into **RAG RUGS.** Of course, as new rugs came along, the old ones generally wound up in the attic. But anytime young children came to visit, Grandma

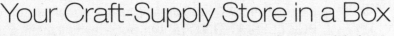

Your Craft-Supply Store in a Box

How many times have you had to scramble to find materials for your child's school project—or, worse yet, had to drive off to the craft-supply store when you had a thousand and one other things to do? Well don't let that happen again! Find an old **TRUNK,** and make it your designated craft "closet." Put it in a spot where the kids can get at it easily, and fill it up with supplies, both store-bought staples and all those odds and ends you don't quite know what to do with. Here's a suggested starter inventory, but remember, the sky's the limit!

Staples	Odds and Ends
Acrylic paints and brushes	Broken costume jewelry
Construction paper	Bubble wrap and packing peanuts
Crayons and felt-tip markers	Buttons and broken zippers
Glue (both white and super-strength)	Colorful junk mail
Glue stick	Duplicate or not-so-great snapshots
Pens and pencils	Fabric scraps
Rulers	Greeting cards
Scissors	Maps and old road atlases
Sheets of cardboard and poster board	Old postage stamps
Stencils	Small springs, metal fasteners, and
Tape	other nifty-looking hardware

brought down an old rug or two, in the brightest colors she could find, so the youngsters could go on a magic carpet ride.

TIP As you know if you have a tall dog, like a Great Dane or an Irish wolfhound, these big guys should eat from bowls that are roughly at the height of their chests. That's because bending down to the ground to scarf up food is not only hard on their leg and neck muscles, but can also cause severe digestive problems. Even smaller breeds benefit from an elevated dining arrangement. You can buy canine tables, a.k.a. feeders, in pet-supply stores and catalogs, but it's a snap to make one from an old wooden **TRUNK.** Just measure Fido's dishes, and cut two holes in the top of the trunk, so the bowls fit in and hang by their rims. (The stainless steel kind work best for this setup.) Use the space inside to store treats, food, or other supplies. *Note:* If the trunk you have isn't quite high enough, attach wooden feet or lockable wheels to the bottom.

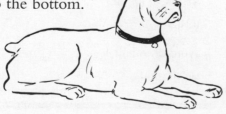

TIP The space under a child's bed seems tailor-made for storing toys, games, craft supplies, and even foldable clothes. But you don't have to go out and buy special storage containers. Just take a tip from Grandma, and recycle a cast-off plastic **WADING POOL.**

TIP A plastic **WADING POOL,** lined with a thick layer of newspapers, makes a fine nursery for newborn puppies or kittens. The sides are high enough to keep the babies in (at least for a while), but low enough so that Mom can come and go easily. And because the pool is watertight, you can put it anywhere without risking damage to wood floors or carpeting.

TIP If you come across a big old **WASHTUB** like the one Grandma Putt had, turn it into a rainy-day entertainment center for a small child. Fill it almost to the brim with dried beans, and toss in measuring cups, a funnel, and a few well-rinsed lids from detergent bottles or spray-paint cans. Then give it to anybody between the ages of about 3 and 6. (That's old enough not to swallow the beans, but young enough to enjoy tossing them around.)

The great
OUTDOORS

TIP You've just found a box of old, scratchy (or even broken) **AUDIOTAPES.** Who on earth would want to keep those? Well, if you want to chase birds out of newly planted seedbeds, the answer is *you!* To launch your scare campaign, break the cassettes open, or simply unroll the tape if you've got the old-time reel type. Then push a stake into the ground at either end of each planting bed, roughly in the center, and string the tape between them, about 1 foot off the ground. Stretch it good and tight, so that it hums as it vibrates in the wind. Birds don't like that sound one little bit, and when they hear it, they'll get outta there fast!

TIP Do you have a **BABY BATH-TUB** that's outlived its original purpose? Then do what Grandma Putt did when all the wee folks in her family had graduated to bigger bathing quarters: Use that tiny tub to baby your fresh-picked produce. When you go out to the garden to harvest your vegetables, take the bathtub with you, and fill it with cold water from the hose. As you

ONE MORE TIME

Are winged diners beating you to your fruit harvest? Well, don't give up without a fight. And remember: Victory could be as close as your (or your grandma's) attic. Just look for any of this **BRIGHT, SHINY STUFF.** Then, either set it on the ground among the birds' targets, or hang it from the branches of your fruit trees and bushes:

▷ **Aluminum pie and cake pans**

▷ **Bells**

▷ **Christmas tree tinsel or shiny silver garlands**

▷ **Life-size statues of cats, owls, foxes, or dogs**

▷ **Pinwheels**

▷ **School pennants**

▷ **Small flags**

▷ **Small mirrors**

▷ **Strips of Mylar®**

▷ **Whirligigs**

▷ **Wind chimes**

▷ **Wind socks**

pick your peas, beans, or what-have-you, drop them into the drink. They'll stay crisp longer, and they'll get a good prewashing before you take them indoors.

TIP If you've got an old **BAD-MINTON NET** tucked away in the attic, you've got a dandy instant trellis for annual flower vines or up-and-coming vegetables like cucumbers, small melons, and peas. Just sink a couple of posts in the ground, attach the net, and bingo! Your garden just got sporty! (If you'd prefer a more decorative trellis, check out the suggestions in the One More Time box on page 350.)

TIP You probably don't think of **BADMINTON RACKETS** as pest-control tools, but if you're facing an invasion of flea beetles, a pair of these birdie-whackers can rush to your rescue. Just cover the face of each racket with a plastic bag, pull it tight, and fasten it with tape or a twist tie. Coat the plastic with petroleum jelly, or spray it with a commercial stickum like Tanglefoot®, so it's ultra-gooey. Then hold a racket on each side of a beetle-ridden plant, and gently jiggle the foliage with your knee. The beetles will leap off

the leaves and onto your traps. Then all you have to do is pull off the bags and drop them into the trash.

TIP Despite their names, plum curculios and fruit-tree leaf rollers don't confine their destruction to plums or fruit trees. Besides their namesake crop, the plum pests target almost every tree fruit under the sun, as well as blueberries. The leaf rollers go after bramble fruits, and just about any deciduous tree and shrub you can name, including roses. If these villains are making a mess of your landscape, go after 'em with Grandma Putt's weapon of choice: a **BASE-BALL BAT.** Here's your game plan: When the first blossoms appear on your tree, spread old sheets on the ground under the branches. Then wrap your bat in a big, thick towel or similar padding, and whack the branches. Depending on the pests in question, they'll come tumbling down (in the case of the curculios) or drop to the ground on silken strands (the leaf rollers). Your mission is to gather up the sheets and shake the hooligans into a bucket of vinegar. One word of caution: If you use this trick on shrubs or fruit bushes, just jostle the stems and branches gently; don't try to hit one over the left-field wall!

The best trellises don't simply support vining plants; they also add visual pizzazz to a garden. If you'd like an out-of-the-ordinary touch for your landscape, whether you're growing flowers or ornamental edibles, you just might find the perfect **DECORATIVE RELIC** in your (or someone else's) attic. Consider these possibilities:

▷ **Iron garden gates**

▷ **Iron window bars**

▷ **Multipaned window frames (minus the glass, of course!)**

▷ **Old doors**

▷ **Old wooden ladders**

▷ **Orphaned brass or iron headboards or footboards**

▷ **Shutters**

Turning Your Treasure into a Trellis

All vines grow in one of four ways, and depending on which type you have and the structure you've found to support them, you may need to make a few adaptations. Here's the lowdown on that score:

▷ **Clinging vines.** These hangers-on, such as Boston ivy, climbing hydrangea, and trumpet creeper, send out rootlets or "holdfasts" that latch on to any surface they encounter. Just plant them at the base of your chosen support, and stand back—they'll be off and scrambling before you can say "Cover that door!"

▷ **Procumbent, a.k.a. scrambling, vines.** This category, which includes asarina, indeterminate tomatoes, and some varieties of honeysuckle and jasmine, lacks any support mechanism. That means you'll need to attach them to your trellis. (Climbing roses, which technically speaking are not vines, need to be treated the same way.) Fortunately, it's a simple job. If you're using an open-work structure, like a lacy iron gate or window frame, use twine or twist ties to fasten the growing stems to various uprights and cross pieces. In the case of a flat surface, like a door, insert screws or nails, and tie the stems to them.

▷ **Tendril vines.** Cup-and-saucer vine, sweet peas (garden peas, too), and scarlet runner beans fall into this category. They grab on to their supports using little shoots that grow out from the main stem. If your trellis has plenty of openings, surrounded by slender pieces—either vertical, horizontal, or diagonal, vines of this type should perform well without any special help on your part. To customize shutters, doors, or other flat surfaces, attach a piece of nylon netting or lengths of twine for the plants to climb on.

▷ **Twining vines.** These include morning glory, moonflower, and climbing nasturtiums, and they do exactly what their name implies: They wind themselves around their supports as they grow. For these guys, your action plan is exactly the same as the one described for tendril vines, above.

TIP You almost never see a blackboard anymore. They've nearly all been replaced by smooth, white boards and felt-tip markers. And those of us who still remember the ear-numbing sound of chalk shrieking across that matte surface say "Good riddance!" But that's *not* what you want to say about a **BLACKBOARD ERASER.** If you still have one of those babies lying around (the old felt kind), tuck it into your car's glove compartment. Then, whenever the windows steam up, pull out the eraser, and wipe away the condensation. (I learned this terrific tip from a retired school teacher who was a friend of Grandma Putt's.)

TIP Once raccoons have staked their claim on your territory, they can be all but impossible to get rid of. But here's one trick that worked like a charm for Grandma— that is, when their target was her garbage cans, the bird feeder on her porch, or anything else that was close to an electrical outlet. Just find some **BLINKING CHRISTMAS TREE LIGHTS,** and string them up on the feeder pole, or on the wall next to the cans. The on-again, off-again lights will make the vexing varmints vamoose—vigorously!

In Grandma's Day

At all of our family barbecues, there was always one thing you could count on: A nonstop round of **BADMINTON** matches. In fact, it was such a normal part of our summer routine that, as a small child, I thought Grandma and Grandpa had invented the game just for us! When I got a little older, Grandma told me the real story of this perennial Putt pastime (or at least one version it). She said it started thousands of years ago in ancient Babylonia, as a fortune-telling ritual. Two people would hit a lightweight, feather-tipped ball back and forth, and the length of time they kept it in the air foretold how long the players would live. Over the centuries, the ceremony evolved into a game, and spread far and wide, including to India, where it was called *poona*. When British Army officers arrived in India in the 1860s, they went gaga for the game, and took it back to England. There, in 1873, it made a big hit at a party given by the Duke of Beaufort at his estate, called (you guessed it) Badminton. A few years later, the sport made its way to the Big Apple, where the Badminton Club of New York was formed in 1878.

TIP Got a couple of old **BOWLING BALLS** around? Take them outside, and tuck them into your flower beds. (In case you haven't been keeping up with the glossy magazines lately, colorful tenpin and duckpin balls are all the rage in garden-design circles!)

TIP Your old croquet set seems to have vanished—except for those beautiful wooden **CROQUET BALLS.** Don't let 'em go to waste. Drill holes in them and use them as colorful finials on a garden fence.

TIP You bought a new canvas **HAMMOCK** and sent the old one to the attic, because you figured it might come in handy someday. Well, if you're having a brutal heat wave, and your tender plants are withering in the sun, that someday is now! Just get some stakes of the length you need, pound them into the soil around your planting bed, and lay the hammock on top. Presto—instant relief!

TIP An old canvas **HAMMOCK** makes a perfect cover for a load on your car's roof rack or in the back of a pickup truck.

TIP When autumn leaves start to fall, use Grandma Putt's favorite removal technique: Rake them up, toss them in an old canvas **HAMMOCK,** and haul them off to the compost pile.

TIP When electric heating pads came into widespread use in the 1950s, a whole lot of **HOT-WATER BOTTLES** (including Grandma's) got tucked away in attics, and on the top shelves of linen closets, all across the country. Well, how about bringing your handy heater out of retirement and turning it into a kneeling pad for hands-and-knees gardening chores? Just open up the end, and fill the rubber pouch with soft cloths, old pantyhose, or small chunks of foam. Use a knitting needle or chopstick to shove the material all the way to the end. Don't overdo it, though. You want enough stuffing to create a comfortable cushion, but not so much that the bottle becomes rigid.

TIP Nothing puts a damper on a backyard barbecue like a bunch of bugs flitting around and landing on your food—leaving all kinds of nasty germs behind. You could protect your vittles with some of those fancy mesh food tents they sell in catalogs. Or you could foil the rascals the way Grandma did: Clean up some old **LAMPSHADES,** drape a piece of muslin over each one (so the opening on top is covered), and set them over your serving dishes.

ONE MORE TIME

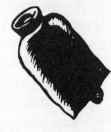

Calling all weekend warriors! The next time you need sturdy plant stakes, check out your stash of over-the-hill **SPORTS EQUIPMENT.** Any of these winners will keep your floppy flowers or vegetables on the up-and-up:

▷ **Golf clubs**

▷ **Hockey sticks (sink the blade end into the soil)**

▷ **Pool cues**

▷ **Posts from badminton or volleyball nets**

▷ **Ski poles**

▷ **Stakes from a croquet set (for smaller plants)**

▷ **Walking sticks**

TIP When you no longer need a **MESH PLAYPEN** to corral toddlin' tykes, move the enclosure to the garden shed, and tote it around the yard as you rake leaves in the fall. It's the perfect holder: roomy, lightweight, and (thanks to the open-weave panels) all but windproof.

TIP A wheelbarrow is one of the most useful pieces of equipment a gardener could ask for—except on days when the ground is mucky, and you've got the barrow loaded with compost, transplants, or yard debris. Then the wheel sinks in so far you can barely budge the thing. Well, I've found the solution to that frustrating problem: On wet days, I leave my wheelbarrow in the shed and use an old **PLASTIC SNOW SAUCER.** No matter how heavy the load is, that round-bottomed sled glides along smoothly over the mud, and wet grass, too.

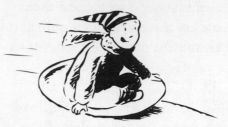

TIP One of my favorite garden "tools" is an old **ROLLING GOLF BAG** that came straight from the attic. I slide hoes, rakes, and shovels into the plastic tubes, and the zippered pockets hold hand tools, seed packets, and all kinds of odds and ends. Best of all, the big wheels make it a cinch to pull the bag right along behind me.

TIP When I gave Grandma Putt a new marble **ROLLING PIN** for Mother's Day one year, she took her old, wooden one out to the garden shed and gave it new life as a dibble for setting out transplants. All she had to do was push one of the handles into the prepared soil, and—voilà—a perfect planting hole!

TIP If you're a snake-o-phobe like me, even a **RUBBER SNAKE** can make you jump when you come upon it suddenly. Well, it does more than that to squirrels, mice, and other garden-variety pests—it

---

ONE MORE TIME

When an all-cotton canvas **HAMMOCK** gets too ratty even for lawn and garden chores, cut it into thin strips, and toss 'em on the compost pile, or bury them in your garden. That fabric will break down into fine, soil-building humus.

---

scares the livin' daylights out of them! So if you've got a few fake serpents stashed away, turn them loose on the lawn to keep small varmints on the run.

TIP Got an old **SCREEN DOOR** with a frame that's, shall we say, seen better days? Then you've got an extra-large garden sifter. When you need big supplies of fine compost or topsoil for a new bed, prop up the door, right on site, on plastic milk crates, 5-gallon buckets, or even sturdy cardboard boxes. Then sift your stuff right through the screening.

TIP Whatever you do, hang on to all the **SHEER WHITE WINDOW CURTAINS** you come by. Then use them, as Grandma Putt did, to protect your plants from light frosts and bad bugs. They work just as well as the most expensive row covers. What's more, they hold up even better. When they've done their job—either at the beginning or the end of the growing season—just toss 'em in the washing machine, and stash them in the garden shed until you need them again. (But be careful not to snag the fabric on rose canes or bramble-fruit bushes.)

Put 'Em Here

Garden centers and catalogs sell a zillion kinds of planting pots. But when it comes to adding real pizzazz to a garden, nothing beats a few plants that are nestled into (shall we say) unconventional containers—such as these **SOIL-WORTHY TREASURES** of all sizes that you might have in your attic. Depending on the composition, and value, of your container, you may want to use it as an outer liner, and set a potted plant (or several) inside.

Small	Medium	Large and Extra-Large
Canister sets	Birdbaths	Bathtubs
Ceramic bowls	Bushel baskets	Battered rowboats or canoes
Children's sand pails	Dresser drawers	Sandboxes and wading pools
Chimney pots	Galvanized buckets	Washtubs
Coal scuttles	Iron kettles	Watering troughs
Decorative tins	Sinks	Wooden barrels
Rubber boots	Tool caddies	Wooden farm wagons
Watering cans	Wooden wine crates	

It's a Frame-Up!

If you've looked at **TOPIARY FRAMES** in a garden center lately, you know that some of these fancy plant supports can cost a bundle. But there may be an over-the-hill something lurking in your attic that could form the base for a three-dimensional green "sculpture." Here are some likely finds and the ways to turn them into upscale garden art. As for what the living cover should be, to get all-but-instant gratification, plant seeds or transplants of an annual vine at the base of your frame. They'll scramble up and over the framework in a flash. Good candidates include morning glories, gourds, sweet potato vine, or hyacinth beans. For a more permanent show, go with a perennial such as silver lace vine, honeysuckle, Dutchman's pipe, or English ivy.

Fabulous Find	The Conversion Process
Artificial Christmas tree	Strip off the fake needles and bury the base in a prepared planting bed or a large pot.
Child-size tepee frame	Set up the poles, cover the framework with nylon netting, and secure it to the ground with U-shaped metal pins.
Decrepit lawn chair	Remove any fabric or webbing (but leave any metal springs or seat supports). Then, either sink the legs 2 or 3 inches into your prepared planting bed, or anchor the bottom bars to the soil with U-shaped metal pins.
Lampshade	Pull off any remaining parchment or fabric, and set the wire framework on top of the soil in a pot.
Old patio umbrella	Take off whatever's left of the cover. Sink a 6- to 8-inch length of PVC pipe into your prepared soil, and insert the umbrella shank. If it wobbles inside the pipe, firm it up with pebbles or wooden shims.
Rusty iron bed frame	Haul it out, set it up in a large planting bed, and push the edges a few inches into the soil. Spread a sheet of hardware cloth or chicken wire between the bed rails to form the "mattress," and secure it with loops of wire.
Screen door frame with ornamental insert	Attach it to posts set into the ground.
Wire reindeer from an old Christmas display	Using U-shaped metal pins, attach the feet to the soil in either a prepared planting bed or a large container (depending on the size of the critter).

TIP You've been hankering for a potting bench, but you don't want to pay the prices they charge for the things in fancy garden shops and catalogs. How about that **SIDE-BOARD** that's taking up space in your attic? The top will give you a nice, big work surface. The inside shelves can hold containers, potting mix, and fertilizer. You can screw hooks into the ends of the cabinet and hang up hand tools. And you can't beat the price! No sideboard available? A desk, vanity table, or low dresser will work just as well.

TIP Grandma Putt saved seeds from nearly all of her annual flowers, herbs, and vegetables. That added up to a *lot* of seeds to keep track of, but she had the system down pat. In the fall, after she dried the seeds, she put each kind in a small, clean glass bottle that once held spices, pills, or gift-basket condiments. She wrote the vital stats, like the plant name and the seed-collection date, on masking tape, and stuck it to the bottle. Then she stored the containers in old wooden **SPICE RACKS** hanging on the wall of her garden shed, where the air stayed cool, but not freezing, and no direct sunlight reached the seeds. When spring planting time rolled around, those seeds were rarin' to grow!

TIP Are slugs munching their way through your garden? Well, you don't have to put up with their shenanigans. Just patrol the premises with your trusty sidearm—a **SQUIRT GUN** filled with vinegar—and when you see one of the slimy villains, let him have it right in the back! (After all, when it comes to pest warfare, no law says you have to honor the Code of the West.)

TIP Grandma was always looking for clever ways to display her container plants. On one corner of her porch, she used an old wooden **STEPLADDER** that she'd painted to match the trim on her house.

TIP Do you still have the **SWING SET** that your children stopped using 20 years ago? Well, haul that thing out of the attic and use it to support a hammock. Take off all the hardware that held the sliding board, swings, and so forth. Paint the metal framework in a color that blends with your outdoor decor. Then hang your hammock between the A-shaped ends.

ONE MORE TIME

Even when old **TEA AND COFFEE CUPS** have lost their handles, they're still fine to drink from—especially when the imbibers are beneficial insects who are fighting off bad-guy bugs in your garden. Just sink each cup into the soil, to within ¼ inch or so of its rim, and fill it with water. Your pint-size, multilegged posse will thank you!

TIP As Grandma Putt was starting to get on in years, she found a new gardening interest: collecting different kinds of mint. She had dozens of yummy-smelling varieties, including chocolate, apple, and pineapple. She grew them in pots and displayed them on old wheeled **TEA CARTS** that she pulled from her (and her friends') attics. The containers kept the mint from sending its rampaging roots all through the garden, and the rolling carts performed a quartet of good deeds: They added a decorative touch to the landscape, kept soilborne pests and diseases at bay, and made it easy for Grandma to wheel her green pals indoors when cold weather arrived. Best of all, the carts put the plants at a height that made them easy for Grandma to tend—even on days when her back was a little on the stiff side.

TIP Some of the best plant labels I've ever had came right out of Grandma Putt's attic. No, they weren't old labels that she had used—they were **VENETIAN BLINDS.** I just cut the cords that held all the slats together, then cut each of those slats into pieces about 8 inches long. The wide strips gave me plenty of room to write my plants' names and anything else I needed to know, like the planting date, expected sprouting time, and probable harvest date. (I used an indelible marker, of course.) I stuck the labels into the soil, and they stayed right on the job through rain, wind, sleet, and even an early snow or two!

TIP Your kids long ago outgrew their **WADING POOL.** Furthermore, you've just installed a backyard swimming pool, so you might as well toss that shallow plastic relic, right? Wrong! Set it next to the big pool, and encourage folks (grown-ups and kids alike) to dunk their feet in it, thereby leaving dirt and grass behind, before diving into the deeper water.

TIP Believe it or not, my childhood **WAGON** has never seen the inside of anybody's attic. When I outgrew that little red vehicle, Grandma adopted it, and it became one of her favorite garden helpers. Every spring, she used it to harden off the new seedlings that she'd started indoors. Now it "lives" at my place, where I use it for exactly the same purpose. (If you don't speak gardening lingo, *hardening off* means taking baby plants into the fresh air and sunshine for brief, ever-increasing, periods of time each day, to get them used to outdoor life.)

TIP Later on in the season, Grandma turned my **WAGON** into a movable display stand for tender container plants. Besides adding visual pizzazz to her garden, it gave her a fast, easy way to whisk the pots to shelter when a storm came up, or an early (or late) frost threatened.

TIP A **WAGON** can come in mighty handy for nongardening chores, too. For instance, it's the perfect vehicle for carting groceries from your car to your house, or lugging firewood from the wood pile to your hearth.

GRANDMA PUTT'S
Secret Formulas

A TABLE TO GROW

If your attic offers up a nifty old wagon, turn it into a portable, greenery-filled table for your deck, patio, or yard. Here's all there is to it.

Drill with ½-inch bit (optional)
Old metal wagon*
Clear, rust-resistant spray varnish
Potting mix
2–4 glass or ceramic tiles
Low-growing, spreading plants**

Drill six or eight drainage holes in the bottom of the wagon, if you'd like.*** Spray the bottom and sides with the varnish. When it's dry (check the label for timing), fill the wagon to within about 3 inches of the rim with potting mix. Place the tiles on the surface to hold drinks and snacks. Then set your plants into the soil, and water lightly.

* Or substitute a vintage wheelbarrow or a child's pedal-powered jeep or dump truck with a roomy rear cargo area.

** Good choices include pennyroyal, Irish moss, Corsican mint, or—for sweet scent and nighttime viewing pleasure—white sweet alyssum.

*** As long as you water often but lightly, this step isn't really necessary.

INDEX